T0250405

Supramolecular Design for Biological Applications

Supramolecular Design for Biological Applications

Edited by
Nobuhiko Yui

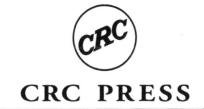

CRC PRESS

Boca Raton   London   New York   Washington, D.C.

Library of Congress Cataloging-in-Publication Data

Supramolecular design for biological applications / Nobuhiko Yui, editor.
    p. cm.
  Includes bibliographical references and index.
  ISBN 0-8493-0965-4 (alk. paper)
  1. Supramolecular chemistry. 2. Biochemistry I. Yui, Nobuhiko.

QP801.P64 2002
572.8—dc21
    2001043887

Visit the CRC Press Web site at www.crcpress.com

Foreword

The Sixth World Biomaterials Congress held in Kamuela, HI, in May 2000 featured 10 workshops. Dr. Nobuhiko Yui organized the workshop titled "Supramolecular Approach to Biological Function" that focused on modulation, alteration, and mimicking of biological functions by a new family of molecular assemblies. He urged presenters to use supramolecular approaches to provide innovative ideas for developing novel biomaterials. The success of the workshop led Dr. Yui to consider producing a comprehensive book detailing the applications of supramolecular science to biological functions. He intended the scope and focus of the book to go beyond contents presented at the workshop, and I believe he and his authors succeeded in producing a useful, high-quality book that covers all the important aspects of this very specialized field of life science.

Three factors have fueled the tremendous progress in supramolecular design for biological applications. The first is the invention of a number of precision polymerization techniques that allow us to design macromolecular compounds. We can prepare precisely designed polymers, controlling their molecular weight and its distribution. Techniques like size exclusion chromatography and mass spectroscopy greatly aided these efforts. Another factor is the explosion of novel diagnostic and therapeutic technologies. The scope of biomedical engineering has been widened, and now includes design of hybrid artificial organs using tissue engineering, artificial vectors for gene therapy, and novel and effective drug delivery and targeting systems. The final factor is advanced instrumentation. Techniques such as scanning probe microscopy and atomic force microscopy allow us to carry out real-time observations and perform molecular manipulations. We could only imagine these until quite recently.

The basic concepts of supramolecular architecture and mimicking biological functions are by no means new. Early researchers driven by the need to understand the structures and functions of living organisms built the foundations of modern natural science. Specialized research then accelerated progress, particularly in life science and information technology, in the past 20 years. Supramolecular design for biological applications is the next great frontier of life science. Yui's book discusses its history and basic concepts, provides a much-needed update of recent developments, and suggests future research directions that will allow this exciting branch of science to realize its full potential in the new century. I would like to offer Dr. Yui and his authors my congratulations on the production of a landmark book that will be of great value to researchers who will find new biomedical and other applications for supramolecular chemistry.

Teiji Tsuruta
Emeritus Professor
University of Toyko
Tokyo, Japan

The Editor

Nobuhiko Yui, Ph.D., is currently a professor in the School of Materials Science, Japan Advanced Institute of Science and Technology, Ishikawa, Japan. He earned his Ph.D. in applied chemistry from Sophia University, Japan, in 1985. Dr. Yui then joined the Institute of Biomedical Engineering of Tokyo Women's Medical College as an assistant research professor. While at Tokyo Women's Medical College, he spent a year as a doctoral research fellow at the University of Twente, The Netherlands. In 1993, Dr. Yui became an associate professor at the Japan Advanced Institute of Science and Technology; he became a full professor in 1998.

Dr. Yui is a member of the Controlled Release Society (CRS), the American Chemical Society, the New York Academy of Sciences, the Japanese Chemical Society, the Japan Society of Polymer Science, the Japan Society of DDS (Drug Delivery Systems), the Japanese Society for Biomaterials, and the Japanese Society of Artificial Organs. He served as a board member of the Japanese Society of Artificial Organs, the Japanese Society for Biomaterials, and the Japan Society of DDS. He is on the Board of Scientific Advisors of the Controlled Release Society (CRS) and the Editorial Board of the *Journal of Biomaterials Science, Polymer Edition*.

Dr. Yui served as the secretary for the first and second Asian International Symposiums on Polymeric Biomaterials Sciences that succeeded in strengthening Asian research interests in biomaterials and drug delivery systems (1996–2000). He recently helped organize the sixth World Biomaterials Congress Workshop entitled "Supramolecular Approach to Biological Functions." He received the Award for Outstanding Research from the Society for Biomaterials of the U.S. in 1985, the 49th Worthy Invention Award from the Science and Technology Agency of Japan in 1990, the Young Investigator Award from the Japanese Society for Biomaterials in 1993, the CRS–Cygnus Recognition Award for Excellence in Guiding Student Research from the CRS in 1997, and the Best Paper Award from the Japanese Society of Artificial Organs in 1997.

Dr. Yui is the author of more than 180 scientific papers. His current major research interests include the molecular design of biodegradable and/or smart polymers with unique supramolecular structures such as polyrotaxanes, molecular tubes, and interpenetrating polymer networks.

Contributors

Kazunari Akiyoshi, Ph.D.
Graduate School of Engineering
Kyoto University
Kyoto, Japan

Katsuhiko Ariga, Ph.D.
ERATO Nanospace Project
Japan Science and Technology
 Corporation
Tokyo, Japan

Keiji Fujimoto, Ph.D.
Faculty of Science and Technology
Keio University
Tokyo, Japan

Taichi Ikeda, Ph.D.
School of Materials Science
Japan Advanced Institute of Science
 and Technology
Ishikawa, Japan

Kazuhiko Ishihara, Ph.D.
Graduate School of Engineering
University of Tokyo
Tokyo, Japan

Nobuo Kimizuka, Ph.D.
Graduate School of Engineering
Kyushu University
Fukuoka, Japan

Akio Kishida, Ph.D.
Department of Biomedical Engineering
National Cardiovascular Center
 Research Institute
Osaka, Japan

Mizuo Maeda, Ph.D.
Graduate School of Engineering
Kyushu University
Fukuoka, Japan

Atsushi Maruyama, Ph.D.
Department of Biomolecular
 Engineering
Tokyo Institute of Technology
Tokyo, Japan

Takashi Miyata, Ph.D.
Faculty of Engineering
Kansai University
Osaka, Japan

Yuichi Ohya, Ph.D.
Faculty of Engineering
Kansai University
Osaka, Japan

Tooru Ooya, Ph.D.
School of Materials Science
Japan Advanced Institute of Science
 and Technology
Ishikawa, Japan

Kinam Park, Ph.D.
School of Pharmacy
Purdue University
West Lafayette, Indiana

Yong Qiu, Ph.D.
School of Pharmacy
Purdue University
West Lafayette, Indiana

Takeshi Serizawa, Ph.D.
Faculty of Engineering
Kagoshima University
Kagoshima, Japan

Tetsuji Yamaoka, Ph.D.
Department of Polymer Science and
 Engineering
Kyoto Institute of Technology
Kyoto, Japan

Masayuki Yokoyama, Ph.D.
Institute of Advanced Biomedical
  Engineering and Science
Tokyo Women's Medical University
Tokyo, Japan

Nobuhiko Yui, Ph.D.
School of Materials Science
Japan Advanced Institute of Science
  and Technology
Ishikawa, Japan

Acknowledgments

I am very pleased to acknowledge Dr. Teiji Tsuruta, Emeritus Professor at the University of Tokyo, for encouraging this work and contributing valuable comments to each of the chapters included in this book. Dr. Tsuruta is one of the pioneers of polymeric biomaterials and has promoted research in the field since 1970. I found his sincere attitude toward young contributors very helpful. Dr. Tsuruta possesses a rare combination of scholarship and humanity. His unique ability to guide, assist, and inspire continues to motivate the contributors.

I thank all the contributors for their willingness to work with me on this book. I also wish to thank Drs. Akio Kishida, Tetsuji Yamaoka, and Yuichi Ohya for planning the content of this book.

Table of Contents

SECTION III Future Aspects of Supramolecular Architectures

1 General Introduction

Nobuhiko Yui, Akio Kishida, Tetsuji Yamaoka,
and Yuichi Ohya

CONTENTS

1.1 PERSPECTIVES

Science is knowledge we use to understand nature. People are always inspired by nature, and have tried to understand and utilize the laws of nature through scientific approaches. In the 20th century, technological innovation progressed at an accelerated pace and permeates almost every facet of our daily lives. The acceleration of both science and technology has led to remarkable advances, and this is especially true in the area of medicine. For example, surgery was used rarely as a therapeutic measure until the 19th century. A huge number of new therapeutic methodologies have been developed, and improvement and enhancement of the human body by artificial materials is one of the most successful innovations in the last century. These successes are largely due to fundamental scientific research into the interactions of artificial materials and living organisms. Technological effort has revolutionized our health care systems, surgery plays a prominent role in curing diseases, and further scientific exploration into these fields continues to bring about unique advances in medical treatment.

One example of this technological innovation is the artificial organ, a product that was an early result of modern scientific advances. The first artificial kidney attracted widespread attention and ignited an outbreak of biomedical engineering. Researchers in the areas of materials, mechanical engineering, electronics, and information technology devoted their efforts to developing artificial organs and other medical devices. Their efforts yielded remarkable achievements such as the artificial heart, artificial kidney, artificial blood vessel, artificial lung, and pacemaker. The concept of biomaterials was proposed and quickly became an indispensable factor in medical engineering. The editorial preface of the first issue of the *Journal of*

Biomaterials Science, Polymer Edition in 1989 defined *biomaterials* as materials that are used in contact with tissue, blood, cells, proteins, and any other living substance.[1] Fundamental research on biomaterials also contributed practical pharmaceutical biomaterials applications such as the controlled release of biologically active agents and drug targeting.

The majority of biomaterials research efforts centered on utilizing well-known polymeric materials for certain purposes. Since the early 1960s, polymeric materials were thought to have much potential in medical and pharmaceutical applications such as artificial blood vessels, artificial hearts, cardiovascular devices, implantable drug carriers, and surgical repair materials.[2] However, it is obvious from the literature that conventional approaches using common polymeric materials have met with limited success for biomedical use.

For instance, the use of polymeric materials has been well recognized to produce undesirable foreign body reactions resulting in the failures of biomedical devices implanted in living bodies. Thus, biocompatible, especially blood-compatible, polymeric surfaces have been the focus of U.S. projects in the 1970s, particularly for the design of totally replaceable artificial hearts. The majority of research on biomaterials has been based on conventional and classical polymer sciences. The physical properties of polymeric materials were first predicted by P. J. Flory in the early 1950s.[3] He established the basic concepts of polymeric materials including block copolymers, graft copolymers, and cross-linked polymeric networks.

Biomaterials studies attempted to prevent foreign body reactions, but met with limited success based on classical polymer science in the 1970s and 1980s. Polymeric surfaces that reduce physicochemical interaction with blood components were proposed. The minimizing interfacial free energy hypothesis was a famous example that used hydrogels as blood-compatible surfaces. However, further difficulties in establishing ideal blood-compatible surfaces have arisen.

Further research into blood–materials interaction revealed that blood clotting reactions influenced by the surfaces were found to occur systemically throughout the blood circulation, not only on the surfaces. This is known as microembolization and is often observed in the capillaries and kidneys. Another issue that arises in chronic blood–material interactions when the hydrophilic surfaces are exposed to blood for a long period is calcification. Further, protein adsorption prior to platelet adhesion has been significant and temporal, which presents difficulties when the process is performed on non-fouling surfaces.

Hydrophilic–hydrophobic microdomain-structured surfaces seen in some block and graft copolymers have been studied in attempts to prevent platelet activation, but the mechanistic aspects of these microstructures have not yet been fully revealed. As an alternative, the development of novel biomaterials surfaces using biologically active molecules was proposed in the 1980s. Immobilization of an anticoagulant on polymeric surfaces is a typical example of such a blood-compatible surface. In the 1990s the interests of many researchers shifted toward other aspects of biomedical applications, leaving these problems unresolved. One persistent problem is the reconstruction of damaged tissues using cell culture techniques on polymeric surfaces or three-dimensional scaffolds. The introduction of biologically active molecules and/or biospecific ligands into biodegradable polymers has been a general strategy that has succeeded to a certain extent in the form of implantable tissue devices. This success is mainly attributed to help from molecular cell biology. This is only one example of how biomaterials have been designed and used to achieve a certain goal but failed to meet it. Other biomaterials including biodegradable polymers, polymer–drug conjugates, and biomimetic polymers have similar prospects for application as biomedical devices.

The ultimate goal of using biomaterials is to restore the functions of natural living tissues and organs. In many cases in biomaterials research, the original idea has not been fully realized, and unexpected issues such as the complicated reactions of the body including systemic foreign body reaction caused by incomplete design of biomaterials based on conventional polymer sciences presented much more difficult problems.

In order to solve these issues and design tailor-made biomaterials, the cooperation of biomaterials science and other interdisciplinary sciences is necessary. New ideas about the relation between the primary structures and physical properties of polymers may disturb our thinking about biomaterials design. Indeed, looking at biological systems in nature, molecular association via noncovalent bonding is a well organized component of biological hierarchy. The examination of structures and functions of several biological devices revealed the importance of utilizing molecular interaction in biomaterials design. Thus, the focus of biomaterials design should shift toward the development of novel polymeric architectures based on new molecular science. Through careful observation of the living body, one finds that biological systems have supramolecular structures.

The characteristics of supramolecular structure in nature are as follows: (1) the system consists of various kinds of molecules, (2) the system has a self-assembled structure, sometimes accompanied by hierarchical order, (3) the system uses integrated and synergistic interaction that contains multiple reaction pathways reacting to one signal, (4) the system changes its reactivity dynamically, and (5) weak interaction such as hydrophobic interaction is important to maintain the system.

On the basis of this host–guest chemistry, a new field of science designated *supramolecular chemistry* was born and has become the next great frontier of modern science. During the 1990s, progress in supramolecular chemistry led to the fascinating new field of macromolecular architecture, which aims to mimic supramolecular systems in nature. Some research groups are now struggling to develop new areas of molecular assemblies for biological application. New synthetic methods based on supramolecular chemistry have created branched, cyclic, mechanically locked, cross-linked, star-shaped, and dendritic architectures. These new macromolecular architectures are mainly constructed by inter- and intramolecular interactions. Since many studies on supramolecular chemistry arose from sophisticated knowledge of biological systems, it is natural that researchers would devote themselves to supramolecular chemistry. Supramolecular chemistry is unique in that it is the chemistry of integration, not reduction. The main objectives of supramolecular chemistry are the controls of both molecular interaction and the three-dimensional arrangements of molecules. Further development and integration of these technologies will make it possible to build an organized system that will realize novel biological functions.

The purpose of this book is to advance the understanding of supramolecular-structured biomaterials and associated issues regarding the biological functions of these materials. The focus is on the modulation, alternation, and emulation of biological functions by a new family of molecular assemblies. The authors of each chapter provide innovative concepts for developing novel biomaterials for diagnosis, drug administration, and environmental protection via the supramolecular approach.

This chapter introduces perspectives of supramolecular chemistry that emphasize recent trends in materials design. Such approaches are seen as promising methods for the design of novel biomaterial functionality. Definitions and classifications of supramolecular architectures are also introduced, although these architectures are not always used as biomaterials. Finally the goals of this book are outlined in an attempt to give the reader a greater understanding of its purpose.

1.2   WHAT IS SUPRAMOLECULAR ARCHITECTURE?

Supramolecular chemistry may be defined as utilizing molecular interaction and complexation to produce specifically ordered structures. F. Vögtle defined it as chemistry "beyond the molecule" — the chemistry of customized intermolecular interaction.[4] J.-M. Lehn stated the goal of supramolecular chemistry was gaining control over intermolecular bonds beyond the molecular chemistry based on covalent bonds.[5] Supramolecular chemistry focuses on molecular association and complexation based on noncovalent molecular interactions. The basis of these molecular forces has been studied since the 1950s and is well understood as the thermodynamics of molecular interactions.

Supramolecular chemistry is not a simple correction of the term "host–guest chemistry." The progressive image of supramolecular chemistry should involve use of a wide range of molecular interactions to construct shape-specific architectures and determine their possible functionalities. A thorough understanding of the concept of chemistry "beyond the molecules" will be essential for examining this topic. For example, interlocked molecules such as rotaxanes may be prepared based on basic knowledge of host–guest chemistry. These materials have far-reaching potential for performing novel functions that are beyond the scope of host–guest chemistry.

The formations of several molecular assemblies are believed to be both enthalpy- and entropy-driven. Noncovalent interactions, which contribute to increases in negative enthalpy for constructing supramolecular structures, include van der Waals interaction, hydrogen bonding, electrostatic interaction, and coordination bonding. The role of entropy change in molecular complexation should be also considered. In particular, the freeing of structured water molecules from a certain molecular system, one of the major events in hydrophobic effect, is a well-known phenomenon that increases the entropy of the system.

The creation of molecular assemblies from each molecule through intermolecular forces will be one of the feasible approaches to constructing supramolecular architectures. Anisotropic structures of supramolecular architectures seen in one-, two-, and three-dimensional regions will also be of great interest. This cutting-edge technology has been used to find variations of host–guest complexations, sometimes related to stereo-specific recognition of certain molecules. This technique had been limited to low molecular weight compounds in the past.

Cyclodextrin (CD) chemistry is representative of this area of research, and CD has been widely used as a suitable model of artificial enzymes. Interfacial phenomena such as the formation of lipid bilayers and micelles observed in surface active molecules have been studied extensively. The dimensions and scales of molecular assemblies have been increased. Thus far, the materials studied have been limited to those with relatively low molecular weights. Supramolecular chemistry now involves a variety of materials and molecular weights and includes their potential applications in biomaterials.

Recent advances in supramolecular chemistry expanded the concept of supramolecular architecture to noncovalent molecular association and complexation. Though some molecules may be constructed through covalent bonds, one of the characteristics of supramolecular architecture is a well-organized structure sometimes accompanied by a hierarchical order measured in nanometers or on a larger scale. The concepts and structures of supramolecular architectures are summarized in Table 1.1.

TABLE 1.1 Summary of Supramolecular Architectures

Architecture	Description
Molecular assemblies by host-guest chemistry	Organized complexes to be formed by intermolecular interaction among the molecules having definite structure
Interlocked molecules	Physically locked or entrapped molecules such as rotaxanes, catenanes and knots
Langmuir Blodgett films—liposomes	Two- or three-dimensional architectures via hydrophobic (lipophilic) interaction among the surface-active compounds
Liquid crystals	Liquid-crystalline state achieved with mesogenic compounds or molecular associations
Self-organized assembly membrane (SAM)	Organized monolayers derived from the interaction of surface with terminal groups of molecules
Polymeric micelles	Closed association of polymers by inter- or intramolecular interactions in solution
Microphase separated structures	Phase separation derived from inter- or intramolecular immiscibility of copolymers of polymer blend to induce microstructures
Gel interpenetrated structures	Three-dimensionally cross-linked polymer networks containing solvents, and mutually penetrated networks
Alternative absorption membranes	Layer-by-layer structures produced with two (or more) components by repetition of different absorption
Dendrimers and fullerenes	Molecules having highly ordered shapes constructed by covalent bonding
Biological molecules	Proteins, nucleic acids, etc. that have ordered three-dimensional structures, and their assembly

Supramolecular architecture involves well-designed and long-range structures. This does not simply mean ordered (regular) structures; it also means spatially specific structures optimally designed for performing special functions. Consequently, even artificial enzymes such as catalytic antibodies and ribozymes are included in this category. Supramolecular chemistry has involved, absorbed, and unified facets of physical chemistry, organic chemistry, biochemistry, inorganic chemistry, and polymer chemistry, which were earlier considered separate scientific specialities.

We cannot ignore the great contributions of analytical instruments and technologies to the advancement of supramolecular chemistry. Advanced analysis technologies have contributed extensively to our ability to characterize the molecular interactions and structures of supramolecular architectures, and allowed us to understand the molecular dynamics, thermodynamics, and kinetics of complexation reactions. For example, isothermal titration calorimetry (ITC) provides precise information on the thermodynamic parameters of host–guest complexation. Surface plasmon resonance spectroscopy is used to analyze transient protein adsorption phenomena on biomaterials' surfaces. High-resolution nuclear magnetic resonance (NMR) apparatus can determine the precise distances of detailed dipole–dipole interactions in molecular assemblies. Cumulative spectral studies using UV-visible, fluorescent, and circular dichroism spectroscopy give us important information about structures and conformations of molecules and molecular assemblies. Table 1.2 summarizes the representative analytical instruments and technologies used in supramolecular chemistry. In later chapters, many of these advances in analytical instruments and methods are explained in detail.

1.3. SUPRAMOLECULAR ASSEMBLY IN BIOLOGICAL SYSTEMS

Nature utilizes the advantages of the supramolecular structures to their full potential. A DNA molecule bears all the one-dimensional information about the human body which has three-dimensional architecture. The information carried by DNA is inherited by RNA and translated further while still in its one-dimensional state. Ultimately, these one-dimensional molecules serve various functions by forming neat three-dimensional structures.

Ribozyme, also known as RNA, exerts enzymatic activity and assesses the three-dimensional structures based on hydrogen bonding of the nucleosides. The enzymes, which also possess one-dimensional primary molecular structures, form secondary structures, called α helices or β–sheets, tertiary structures in which parts of the secondary structures are assembled, and quaternary structures. These hierarchical structures are formed mainly by noncovalent interactions and disulfide bonds. It is important that various functional groups and/or residues are spatially arranged in appropriate positions in the three-dimensional structures of these ribozymes and enzymes. This is one of the key factors for the specific recognition of the chemical structure of the substances. To achieve such spatially controlled arrangements with

TABLE 1.2 Analytical Instruments and Technology Used in Supramolecular Chemistry

Analytical Goal	Instruments and Technologies
Molecular interaction and thermo-dynamics	NMR, ITC, DSC, QCM, surface plasmon resonance spectroscopy
Structural analysis	NMR, FT-IR, x-ray or neutron diffraction, ESI-MS, MALDI-TOF-MS
Information expressed in nanometer or mesoscopic scales	SEM, TEM, AFM, STM, SNOM, XPS, DLS, SLS
Purification and separation	HPLC, capillary electrophoresis

NMR: nuclear magnetic resonance, ITC: isothermal titration calorimetry, DSC: differential scanning calorimetry, QCM: quartz crystal microbalance, FT-IR: Fourier transform infrared spectroscopy, ESI-MS: electron spray ionization mass spectroscopy, MALDI-TOF-MS: matrix-assisted laser desorption ionization time-of-flight mass spectroscopy, SEM: scanning electron microscopy, TEM: transmittance electron microscopy, AFM: atomic force microscopy, STM: scanning tunneling microscopy, SNOM: scanning near-field optical microscopy, XPS: x-ray photoelectron microscopy, DLS: dynamic light scattering, SLS: static light scattering, HPLC: high-performance liquid chromatography.

only covalent bonding, it is necessary to design huge compounds with extremely complicated chemical structures.

Another important role of the supramolecular structure in nature is the achievement of dynamism. Since enzymes recognize the substrates through noncovalent interactions, the substrates can be dissociated after the reactions and the enzymes act against the other substrates again. Some proteins change their three-dimensional structures to express different activities by phosphorylation. Such activity changes are reversible in response to phosphorylation/dephosphorylation at specific sites of the proteins; this reversibility is the basic characteristic of biological actions. Cell division becomes possible because plasma membranes are formed through weak hydrophobic interactions of phospholipids. Even bone tissue, which seems to be static in the body, possesses a well-organized structure. Bone units made of collagen fibrils with hydroxyapatite crystals produce bone resorption and osteogenesis. These activities cannot be achieved by covalent bondings that are difficult to dissociate under physiological conditions. Thus, living organisms require supramolecular structures to perform sophisticated functions that cannot be achieved solely through covalent bonding. The supramolecular structure is indispensable for the formation of a three-dimensional structure using one-dimensional information.

1.4. CONSTRUCTION

The research on supramolecular structures advanced beyond understanding living tissues and now enables us to utilize these structures as biomaterials. The aim of this book is to apply recent advances in supramolecular approaches to biomedical and pharmaceutical functions. The selection of supramolecular architectures to be discussed was based upon our success in organizing the 6th World Biomaterials Congress Workshop entitled "Supramolecular Approach to Biological Functions" held in May of 2000.[6] Two Japanese government-supported scientific research programs, "New Polymers and Their Nano-organized Systems" (1996–1999)[7] and "Molecular Synchronization for Design of New Materials Systems" (1999–2003) were also instrumental in our selection of authors and topics for this book.

Incorporating supramolecular chemistry into the field of materials science is of great importance because of the great number of potential biological applications. In early 2000 U.S. President Clinton advocated strong political support for nanotechnology including development of supramolecular biomaterials. A report titled "National Nanotechnology Initiative: Leading to the Next Industrial Revolution," launched by the Interagency Working Group of the National Science and Technology Council's Committee on Technology, suggests the potential for nanotechnology's utilization in biorelated fields including medicine, health, environmental conservation, biotechnology, and agriculture.

The themes and contents of this book were carefully chosen and divided into three sections: basic strategy for supramolecular architectures, biological application of supramolecular architectures, and future aspects of supramolecular architectures. In Section I, hydrophobic, hydrogen bonding, electrostatic, and other intermolecular interaction are explained in order to illustrate the principal molecular forces involved in constructing supramolecular architectures. Physical adsorption, gel and interpenetrating polymer networks, and interlocked molecules are introduced as representatives of novel supramolecular architectures constructed through inter- and intramolecular interactions.

In Section II, biodegradable polymers, stimuli-responsive materials and surfaces, and soft and hard tissue substrates are introduced as examples of potential applications for biomaterials design. Finally, drug delivery, drug targeting, gene delivery, sensing and diagnosis, biomimetic functions, and cellular modulation using the supramolecular approach are discussed.

The chapters ahead will illuminate the principles of molecular forces, and variations of supramolecular architectures based on each molecular force will be explained. Illustrations of molecular forces and supramolecular architectures in every chapter are intended to enhance understanding of the sizes of the architectures and the distances between molecules.

The goal of this book is to introduce the potential uses of supramolecular architectures in biomaterials. We cannot cover all aspects of supramolecular approaches in this book. For instance, shape-specific molecular architectures such as dendrimers and fullerenes are not included because these molecules are constructed via covalent bonding, and have been covered in many reviews and monographs. Recent progress in other supramolecular chemistry-based polymeric architectures is summarized in the last chapter.

This book is recommended for graduate students, academic researchers, and industrial researchers working in biomaterials science and technology, especially those interested in supramolecular chemistry. In the decades to come, the new field of functional biomaterials will be explored further, yielding a greater understanding of supramolecular chemistry.

ACKNOWLEDGMENTS

The authors are grateful to Jonathan Fulkerson for his critical reading of the manuscript.

REFERENCES

1. Tsuruta, T. et al., Editorial, *J. Biomater. Sci. Polym. Ed.*, 1, 1, 1989.
2. Tsuruta, T. et al., Eds., *Biomedical Applications of Polymeric Materials*, CRC Press, Boca Raton, 1993.
3. Flory, P.J., *Principles of Polymer Chemistry*, Cornell University Press, Ithaca, NY, 1953.
4. Vögtle, F., *Supramolecular Chemistry*, John Wiley & Sons, Chichester, 1991.
5. Lehn, J.-M., *Supramolecular Chemistry: Concepts and Perspectives*, VCH, Weinheim, 1995.
6. Proceedings of the 6th World Biomaterials Congress Workshop, *Supramolecular Approach to Biological Functions*, Japanese Society for Biomaterials, May 14, 2000.
7. Kunitake, T. et al., Eds., *Precision Polymers and Nano-Organized Systems*, Kodansha, Tokyo, 2000.

SECTION I

*Basic Strategy for
Supramolecular Architectures*

2 Hydrophobic Effects

Kazunari Akiyoshi

CONTENTS

2.1 INTRODUCTION

Hydrophobic effect is one of the main factors of the self-organization of biomolecules. For example, hydrophobic interactions are the major determining factors for the folding of proteins and the construction of biomembranes. Such functional architectures in living systems are constructed from many amphiphilic molecules that contain both hydrophilic and hydrophobic groups. The amphiphilic molecules self-assemble in water. This section deals with the fundamentals of hydrophobic effect and the self-assemblies of amphiphilic substances.

2.2 HYDROPHOBIC HYDRATION

The hydrophobic effect can be explained in terms of hydrophobic hydration and hydrophobic interaction.[1] Abnormal thermodynamic properties are observed when hydrophobic molecules such as hydrocarbons are dissolved in water.[2] For example, the dissolution of hydrocarbon is an exothermic process. The solubility of methane in water increases at lower temperatures. Such behavior in water differs markedly from that in other polar solvents such as methanol. The free energy (ΔG) of the transfer of n-butane from bulk liquid to water at 25°C is about 24.5 kJ mol^{-1}, and ΔH and TΔS

0-8493-0965-4/02/$0.00+$1.50

are −4.3 and −28.7 kJ mol[-1], respectively. Significant decreases in entropy accompany the dissolution of hydrophobic molecules in water.

Frank and Evans proposed an iceberg concept, in which water molecules form a microiceberg around a hydrophobic molecule when it is dissolved in water at room temperature.[3] The structures of water molecules around hydrophobic molecules become more crystalline compared to those of bulk water. They named this phenomenon hydrophobic hydration. Due to the decrease in entropy caused by iceberg formation, evaporation entropy becomes significantly higher. Furthermore, when various alkanes composed of different numbers of hydrocarbons are transferred from bulk liquid to water, the decrease in entropy is roughly proportional to the sizes of the surface areas of the hydrocarbons. This can be explained in terms of an increase in the number of water molecules that surround the surfaces of hydrophobic molecules.

2.3 HYDROPHOBIC INTERACTION

What would happen in the case of many hydrophobic molecules? When the numbers of hydrophobic molecules increase in water, the total free energy increases due to hydrophobic hydration. Hydrophobic molecules tend to aggregate to avoid contact with water molecules. As a result, the overall hydration of hydrophobic molecules becomes low, and thus the free energy for the entire solution decreases. Hydrophobic attraction is the phenomenon by which nonpolar substances minimize contact with water molecules in water.

Kauzmann showed that interactions among hydrophobic amino acid residues in polypeptides play a decisive role in the formation of higher-order structures of proteins in an aqueous solution, and called this phenomenon hydrophobic bonding, to distinguish it from van der Waals interactions.[4] Since then, this issue has received much attention. The hydrophobic bonding phase is suggestive of chemical bonding. However, no real chemical bonds exist between hydrophobic molecules. Therefore, Nemethy-Scheraga and Ben-Naim called this self-assembly of *hydrophobic interaction* and proposed statistical mechanics theories describing this behavior.[5] The theoretical and experimental research on the unique properties of water molecules has continued since then.

Figure 2.1 is a schematic representation of the behavior of hydrophobic molecules in water. In the figure, (a) represents hydrophobic hydration, in which networks of water molecules surround a hydrophobic molecule; (b) represents a model for hydrophobic interactions, in which molecules like those seen in (a) tend to self-assemble to avoid contact with water as much as possible. As a result of this kind of aggregation, the amount of structured water surrounding the solute decreases. However, the results of recent structural and spectroscopic studies show that (b) is not necessarily valid in the hydrophobic interaction model. It is generally accepted that interactions among hydrophobic molecules are due to solvent-separated hydrophobic pair interaction (c), not direct contact.[6] One layer of the hydration remains.

Strong interactions between hydrophobic molecules in water cannot be explained in terms of van der Waals forces, by which the interactions between

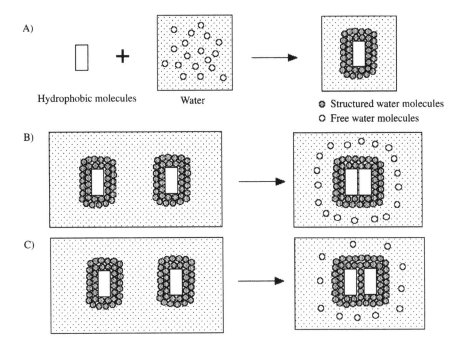

A)

Hydrophobic molecules   Water

⊕ Structured water molecules
○ Free water molecules

B)

C)

FIGURE 2.1 Schematic representations of hydrophobic hydration and hydrophobic interaction. (a) Model of hydrophobic hydration; hydrophobic molecule is surrounded by structured water molecules, (b) model of hydrophobic interaction; self-assembly of hydrophobic molecules to avoid contact with water as much as possible, (c) another model of hydrophobic interaction; solvent-separated hydrophobic pair interaction.

hydrophobic molecules in water are expected to be weakened. It is clear that bonding is not involved in interactions among hydrophobic molecules. The interaction between two hydrophobic molecules is primarily attributable to the rearrangement of hydrogen bond configurations in the overlapping solvation zones.[2] In any event, the fundamentals of hydrophobic interactions are still debated today.[7-10]

2.4   HYDROPHOBIC SURFACES: ATTRACTIVE HYDROPHOBIC FORCES

The hydrophobic interaction described above also occurs between two hydrophobic surfaces in water. In the past, it was difficult to determine the distance dependency for hydrophobic interactions experimentally. However, it is now possible to directly measure forces between two macroscopic surfaces using surface force apparatus.[2,11] This apparatus measures attractive and repulsive forces between two surfaces directly as a function of intersurface distances on the molecule level. It is also possible to measure separation force by determining the force required to pull apart two contacting surfaces.

The results of surface force measurements show that a hydrophobic surface exhibits strong long-range attractive forces in aqueous solution. The hydrophobic forces are significantly stronger than van der Waals forces. For example, in the interactions between uncharged mica surfaces modified with hydrophobic layers of a polymerized dialkyl ammonium amphiphile, attractive forces of up to 250 nm were seen in pure water. The surfaces jumped and came into contact at 76 nm.[12] The data for the attractive forces, however, are scattered in magnitude over a wide range (10 nm to 500 nm), depending on the methods used to prepare the hydrophobic surface. The reason for this type of long-range attraction is not yet known. Possible explanations include (1) the conformation of water molecules, in particular the hydrogen bond network,[13] (2) the electrostatic fluctuation between surfaces or the hydrodynamic fluctuation of water,[14] (3) spontaneous cavities,[15,16] (4) submicroscopic bubbles,[17] or nanobubbles bridging the two surfaces.[18]

Long-range attractive hydrophobic forces could explain numerous phenomena such as the rapid agglomeration of hydrophobic particles in water,[19] the fragility of water membranes on hydrophobic surfaces,[20] and the self-assembly of amphiphilic substances or biomolecules.

2.5 SELF-ASSEMBLY OF AMPHIPHILES

2.5.1 FORMATION OF MOLECULAR ASSEMBLY

Amphiphiles are compounds composed of both hydrophilic and hydrophobic groups. Sodium dodecyl sulfate (SDS) is a well-known amphiphile. The dodecane, which corresponds to the hydrophobic group of SDS, dissolves in water to some degree; however, above a certain concentration, it forms another phase via hydrophobic interaction-induced aggregation. The addition of further dodecane increases the concentration only in the separated phase, while the concentration in the aqueous phase remains unchanged. Consequently, water and oil phases are formed. SDS also forms a separate phase beyond the solubility limit for individual molecules (Figure 2.2). The resulting phase is an aggregate called a micelle that is dispersed in a solution.

Due to very favorable interactions between hydrophilic head groups and water, polar heads tend to retain contact with water, while hydrophobic groups aggregate to avoid contact with water. Due to these opposing behaviors, spherical aggregates are formed, each consisting of about 60 SDS molecules. The concentration of amphiphiles, of which 50% form micelles, is referred to as the critical micelle concentration (CMC). The CMC for SDS is -10^{-3} M. Micelles are thermodynamically stable aggregates. In general, molecules with a high degree of hydrophobicity can form aggregates at lower concentrations. For example, phospholipids in biological membranes usually have two long alkyl chains, and their CMCs are very low at -10^{-10} M. Hence, phospholipid molecules, in the equilibrium state form very stable aggregates. Amounts of free phospholipids in water are negligible. The use of organized polymerized systems based on amphiphilic monomers has been reported for improving the stability of the molecular assembly.[21]

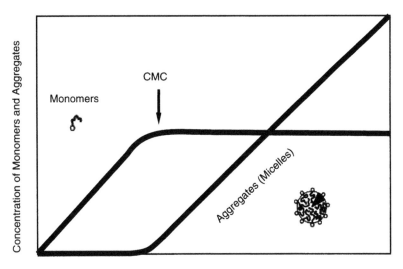

FIGURE 2.2 Monomer and aggregate concentrations as a function of total concentration of surfactant.

2.5.2 MORPHOLOGIES OF AGGREGATES

Amphiphilic molecules form various types of aggregates such as spherical micelles, nonspherical micelles, vesicles, bilayer membranes, and reverse-phase micelles. How are the structures of aggregates determined? Israelachvili and colleagues proposed that the geometric packing of amphiphiles determines the structures of aggregates.[2] They defined a packing parameter $v/a_0 l_c$, where a_0 represents the optimal surface area, v is the hydrocarbon volume, and l_c is the critical chain length. This value is an indicator of whether amphiphiles form spherical micelles, nonspherical micelles, vesicles, bilayer membranes, or reverse-phase micelles. For example, cone-shaped molecules such as SDS may form spherical micelles. However, this hypothesis may not be realistic because cone-shaped molecules do not actually exist.[22] Other proposed micelle structure models include a statistical lattice model,[23] a three-dimensional block model,[24] and a reef or rugged micelle model.[25] The last two models explain the *trans* structures of the CH_2 groups of hydrocarbon chains, and also imply that the majority of hydrophobic domains of amphiphiles come in contact with water.[26]

Kunitake and colleagues first reported that simple dialkyl ammonium salts form bilayer membranes.[27] They synthesized many amphiphiles and discussed structural factors of the formation of bilayer membranes. According to the geometric packing model, single-chain amphiphiles could form micelles. However, due to the improved molecular orientation, single-chain amphiphiles having aromatic rigid segments, such as azobenzene, sometimes form bilayer membranes. Depending on designs, amphiphiles with three or four alkyl chains could form bilayer membranes (Figure 2.3). Moreover, various aggregate morphologies, such as vesicles, globules, rods, tubes, and disks could be obtained by slightly changing the molecular structures of the amphiphiles. Consequently, amphiphiles with similar structures can also produce various aggregate morphologies. The assumption for the packing parameter is that the hydrocarbon chains of amphiphiles are completely in the liquid state. However, when hydrocarbon chains are in the gel state, the parameter becomes more complicated. The structures of molecular aggregates are determined by molecular shape, intermolecular stacking (i.e., the degree of binding and repulsion between molecules), and molecular alignment (i.e., the degree of bending within monomers).

Self-assemblies of amphiphilic molecules have been widely applied as biomaterials. In particular, liposomes, which are vesicles consisting of lipids such as phosphatidylcholine, are used in various fields such as pharmacology, medicine, cosmetics, and the food industry.[28]

2.6 SELF-ASSEMBLY OF AMPHIPHILIC POLYMERS

Amphiphilic polymers comprise a class of water-soluble polymers consisting of both hydrophobic and hydrophilic segments in a polymer chain. Various types of amphiphilic polymers have been reported.[29-32] Figure 2.4 shows the typical structures of amphiphilic polymers. Amphiphilic polymers have become the focus of interest for use as biomaterials. In this section, the general characteristics of the amphiphilic polymers are discussed.

2.6.1 AMPHIPHILIC BLOCK COPOLYMERS

AB- or ABA-type amphiphilic block copolymers, which exhibit an appropriate balance of hydrophobicity and hydrophilicity, thermodynamically form micelles (polymer micelles) similar to those of low molecular weight surfactants. The CMCs of

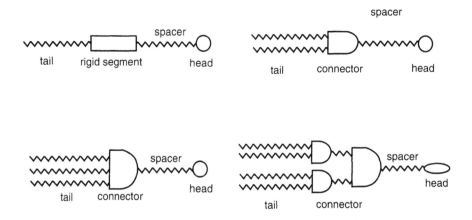

FIGURE 2.3 Schematic representations of bilayer-forming amphiphiles.

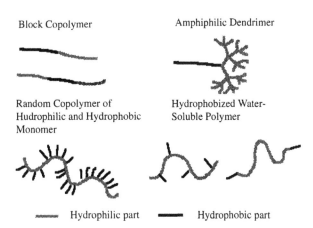

Block Copolymer   Amphiphilic Dendrimer

Random Copolymer of   Hydrophobized Water-
Hudrophilic and Hydrophobic   Soluble Polymer
Monomer

━━━ Hydrophilic part   ━━━ Hydrophobic part

FIGURE 2.4 Schematic representation of various amphiphilic polymers.

polymer micelles are quite low, and these micelles are stable compared to surfactant micelles. The block copolymers with higher hydrophobicities do not spontaneously dissolve in water. Such hydrophobic polymers first dissolve in appropriate solvents such as DMSO and ethanol, and then subsequently dialyze against water. In this process, polymer micelles with core-shell structures are formed. This type is called a kinetically frozen micelle,[33] and is much more stable than thermodynamically formed micelles. Polymers are not exchanged between micelles at near room temperature.[34] Hydrophobic polymer chains of the micelle exist in a glassy state and hydrophilic polymer chains that attract water maintain colloidal stability. Similar to low molecular weight amphiphiles, various aggregate morphologies, such as vesicles, globules, rods, and lamellar structures can be obtained by changing the molecular structures of polymer amphiphiles.[35]

It is relatively easy to trap a large number of hydrophobic drugs such as adriamycin into the hydrophobic cores of core-shell type polymer micelles.[36-38] The high colloidal stability (thermodynamic or kinetic) of polymer micelles gives them an advantage over low molecular weight surfactants as drug carriers. Biodegradable unimer micelles with dendritic structures have been designed as drug carriers.[39] ABC-type multiblock copolymers are of interest for possible application as a multifunctional polymer micelles, for example, as a stimuli-responsive polymer micelle.[40,41]

2.6.2 AMPHIPHILIC RANDOM COPOLYMERS

Amphiphilic polyelectrolytes such as poly(2-vinylpyridine), quaternized with n-dodecyl bromide, form compact conformations in water.[42] The long alkyl groups attached to the polyelectrolyte chain associate in water to form a micellar structure. Amphiphilic polyelectrolytes exhibit high surface activity and solubilize small hydrophobic molecules similar to surfactant micelles. These polymers have been called *polymer surfactant* or *polysoap*.[30,42] Usually, the balance between hydrophobicity and hydrophilicity in polymer surfactants is similar to that of low molecular weight surfactants. The CMCs of intramolecular micelles, however, are quite low because hydrophobic groups are attached to the polymer at high local concentrations. Polysulfonates modified with bulky hydrophobic groups having cyclic structures form unimolecular micelles in water through intramolecular self-association.[43,44] A polymer prodrug designed by Ringsdorf is based on this polysoap structure.[45] Several drugs and bioactive oligopeptides are hydrophobic. Such drug–polymer conjugates often form intramolecular micelles.[46-48]

2.6.3 HYDROPHOBICALLY MODIFIED WATER-SOLUBLE POLYMERS

Hydrophobically modified water-soluble polymers, also known as hydrophobized polymers, are water-soluble polymers which are modified only slightly by hydrophobic groups (less than 5 wt%).[32] The hydrophobicity of these polymers is quite low compared to polysoaps. Therefore, the association behavior of hydrophobized polymers is different from that of polysoap. The aggregation numbers of hydrophobic groups are relatively low due to steric hindrance by the hydrophilic polymer chain. Surface activity is lower due to the lower hydrophobicity compared to polymer surfactants. At relatively high polymer concentrations, intermacromolecular associations of polymers are induced through association of hydrophobic groups, resulting in a marked increase in the viscosity in solution. For this reason, hydrophobized polymers are often used as viscosity modifiers. At higher polymer concentrations phase separation or gelation is observed.

Unique nanoparticles with hydrogel structures formed by the self-assembly of hydrophobized polysaccharides have been reported.[49-51] Pullulan derivatives with highly hydrophobic groups such as cholesterol form monodispersive nanoparticles through intermacromolecular association in water.[49] The nanoparticles exhibit hydrogel structures in which the cross-linking points represent the hydrophobically associated domains of hydrophobic groups. This type of self-assembly is different from those of polymer micelles or polysoap, and is a new method for preparing monodispersed hydrogel nanoparticles.[52,53] The hydrogel structure is suitable for trapping various proteins under mild conditions.[54,55] Hydrogel nanoparticles of hydrophobized pullulans have been widely used as carriers for anticancer drugs,[56] insulin,[57] and vaccines,[58,59] and also as artificial molecular chaperones.[60]

2.7 HYDROPHOBICITY OF BIOMOLECULES

Lipids in biomembranes are typical examples of amphiphilic molecules. Nucleic acids such as DNA and RNA are amphiphilic polymers in which the amphiphilic nucleotides (relatively hydrophobic heterocyclic bases, hydrophilic sugars, and phosphate ions) are polymerized. Proteins are amphiphilic copolymers consisting of both hydrophilic and hydrophobic amino acids. Their hydrophobicity is relatively high even in water-soluble globular proteins. Most proteins are comprised of 50%

hydrophobic amino acids. The main driving force of folding for proteins is hydrophobic interaction, as suggested by Kauzmann. In the evolution process, such hydrophobic polypeptides were selected in order to realize compact intramolecular functional structures. Due to their high hydrophobicity, however, proteins tend to associate intermolecularly and eventually precipitate. For example, proteins easily aggregate and precipitate after heating. Nonnative proteins such as nascent proteins or heat-denatured proteins lose their compact conformations and expose their hydrophobic domains. Therefore, such proteins tend to aggregate spontaneously . To prevent the aggregation of proteins in the process of folding or heat stress, molecular chaperones exist in living systems. They are molecular machine systems consisting of a series of proteins that recognize and trap nonnative proteins mainly by hydrophobic interaction.[61,62] Through this entrapment, aggregation is inhibited and folding is assisted using the energy of ATP.

Saccharides may appear to be hydrophilic, but, some exhibit amphiphilic behavior. In fact, both hydrophilic –OH groups and hydrophobic –CH groups exist on the surface of a saccharide molecule. For example, cyclodextrins have hydrophobic cavities that trap hydrophobic molecules in water. Linear dextrin and amylose also exhibit hydrophobicity.[63,64] The importance of hydrophobic interactions in saccharide–saccharide interactions on the cell surface in cell–cell adhesion has been suggested.[65,66]

Hydrophobic interaction is a basic requirement for constructing supramolecular architectures in living systems and in artificial systems. This interaction is effective only in aqueous solution. Due to the hydrophobicity of biomolecules, hydrophobic interaction is very important in the design of various biomaterials. Recent results of the distance dependency for hydrophobic interactions and the long-range attractions between hydrophobic surfaces offered useful information about various biological phenomena and possible designs of novel dynamic molecular assembly systems.

REFERENCES

1. Tanford, C., *Hydrophobic Effect*, Wiley, New York, 1973.
2. Israelachvili, J., *Intermolecular Surfaces*, 2nd Ed., Academic Press, New York, 1992.
3. Frank, H.S. and Evans, M.W., Free volume and entropy in condensed systems III. Entropy in binary liquid mixtures; partial molal entropy in dilute solutions; structure and thermodynamics in aqueous electrolytes, *J. Chem. Phys.*, 13, 507, 1945.
4. Kauzmann, W., Some factors in the interpretation of protein denaturation, *Adv. Protein Chem.*, 14, 1, 1959.
5. Ben-Naim, A., *Hydrophobic Interaction*, Plenum Press, New York, 1980.
6. Franks, F., Hydrophobic interactions: a historical perspective, *Faraday Symp. Chem. Soc.*, 17, 7, 1982.
7. Suzuki, K., The current state of research on water structure and hydrophobic interaction: on the extension of research since professor Kauzmann, *Hyomen*, 34, 43, 1996.
8. Shinoda, K., "Iceberg" formation and solubility, *J. Phys. Chem.*, 81, 1300, 1977.
9. Murphy, K.P., Privalov, P.L., and Gill, S.J., Common features of protein unfolding and dissolution of hydrophobic compounds, *Science*, 247, 559, 1990.

10. Soda, K., Structural and thermodynamic aspects of the hydrophobic effect, *Adv. Biophys.*, 29, 1, 1993.

11. Israelachvili, J.N. and Pashley, R.M., The hydrophobic interaction is long range, decaying exponentially with distance, *Nature*, 300, 341, 1982.

12. Kurihara, K. and Kunitake, T., Submicron-range attraction between hydrophobic surfaces of monolayer-modified mica in water, *J. Am. Chem. Soc.*, 114, 10927, 1992.

13. Attard, P., Long-range attraction between hydrophobic surfaces, *J. Phys. Chem.* 93, 6441, 1989.

14. Yaminsky, V.V. and Ninham, B.W., Hydrophobic force: lateral enhancement of subcritical fluctuations, *Langmuir*, 9, 3618, 1993.

15. Claesson, P.M. et al., Interactions between water-stable hydrophobic Langmuir–Blodgett monolayers on mica, *J. Colloid Interface Sci.*, 114, 234, 1986.

16. Bunkin, N.F. et al., Effect of salts and dissolved gas on optical cavitation near hydrophobic and hydrophilic surfaces, *Langmuir*, 13, 3024, 1997.

17. Parker, J. L., Cleasson, P. M., and Attard, P., Bubbles, cavities, and the long-range attraction between hydrophobic surfaces, *J. Phys. Chem.*, 98, 8468, 1994.

18. Ishida, N. et al., Nano bubbles on a hydrophobic surface in water observed by tapping-mode atomic force microscopy, *Langmuir*, 16, 6377, 2000.

19. Xu, Z. and Yoon, R. H., A study of hydrophobic coagulation, *J. Colloid Interface Sci.*, 134, 427, 1990.

20. Tchaliovska, S. et al., Studies of the contact interaction between an air bubble and a mica surface submerged in dodecylammonium chloride solution, *Langmuir*, 6, 1535, 1990.

21. Ringsdorf, H., Schlarb, B., and Venzmer, J., Molecular architecture and function of polymeric oriented systems: models for the study of organization, surface recognition, and dynamics of biomembranes, *Angew. Chem. Int. Ed. Engl.*, 27, 113, 1988.

22. Fuhrhop, J.-H. and Koning, J., Membranes and molecular assemblies: The synkinetic approach, in *Monographs in Supramolecular Chemistry,* Royal Society of Chemistry, London, 1994.

23. Dill, K.A. and Flory, P.J., Molecular organization in micelles and vesicles, *Proc. Natl. Acad. Sci. U.S.A.,* 78, 676, 1981.

24. Fromherz, P., Micelle structure: a surfactant block model, *Chem. Phys. Lett.*, 77, 460, 1981.

25. Menger, F.M., The structure of micelles, *Acc. Chem. Res.*, 12, 111, 1979.

26. Menger, F.M. and Mounier, C.E., A micelle that is insensitive to its ionization state: relevance to the micelle wetness problem, *J. Am. Chem. Soc.*, 115, 12222, 1993.

27. Kunitake, T., Synthetic bilayer membranes: molecular design, self-organization, and application, *Angew. Chem. Int. Ed. Engl.*, 31, 709, 1992.

28. Lasic, D.D., *Liposomes: From Physics To Applications*, Elsevier, Amsterdam, 1993.

29. Glass, J.E., Ed., *Polymers in Aqueous Media: Performance through Association*, American Chemical Society, Washington, 223, 1989.

30. Shalaby, S.W., McCormick, C.L., and Butler, G.B., Eds., *Water-Soluble Polymers: Synthesis, Solution Properties, and Applications*, 467, American Chemical Society, Washington, 1991.

31. Morishima, Y., Unimolecular micelles of hydrophobically modified polysulfonates: potential utility for novel photo chemical systems, *Trends Polym. Sci.*, 2, 31,1994.

32. Dubin, P. et al., Eds., *Macromolecular Complexes in Chemistry and Biology*, Springer-Verlag, Berlin, 1994.

33. Xu. R. et al., Micellization of polystyrene–poly(ethylene oxide) block copolymers in water 5. A test of the star and mean-field models, *Macromolecules*, 25, 644, 1992.

34. Wang, Y. et al., Detection of the rate of exchange of chains between micelles formed by diblock copolymers in aqueous solution, *Polym. Bull.*, 28, 333, 1992.

35. Zhang, L. and Eisenberg. A., Ion-induced morphological changes in "crew-cut" aggregates of amphiphilic block copolymers, *Science*, 268, 1728, 1995.

36. Kabanov, A. et al., A new class of drug carriers: micelles of poly(ethylene)–poly(propylene) block copolymers as microcontainers for targeting drugs from blood to brain, *J. Control. Rel.*, 22, 141, 1992.

37. Kwon, G.S. and Kataoka, K., Block copolymer micelles as long circulating drug vehicles, *Adv. Drug Deliv. Rev.*, 16, 295, 1995.

38. Kataoka, K. et al., Doxorubicin-loaded poly(ethylene glycol)–poly(β-benzyl-L-aspartate) copolymer micelles: their pharmaceutical characteristics and biological significance, *J. Control. Rel.*, 64, 143, 2000.

39. Liu, H., Farrell, S., and Ulbrich, K., Drug release characteristics of unimolecular polymeric micelles, *J. Control. Rel.*, 68, 167, 2000.

40. Bae, T.H. et al., Biodegradable amphiphilic multiblock copolymers and their implications for biomedical applications, *J. Control. Rel.*, 64, 3, 2000.

41. Kurisawa, M., Yokoyama, M., and Okano, T., Gene expression control by temperature with thermo-responsive polymeric gene carriers, *J. Control. Rel.*, 69, 127, 2000.

42. Strauss, U.P., Gershfeld, N.L., and Crook, E.H., The transition from typical polyelectrolyte to polysoap. II. Viscosity studies of poly-4-vinylpyridine derivatives in aqueous potassium bromide solutions, *J. Phys. Chem.*, 60, 577, 1956.

43. Morishima, Y., Spectroscopic characterization of unimer micelles of hydrophobically modified polysulfonates, in *Multidimensional Spectroscopy of Polymers, Self-organization of Amphiphilic Polymers and Their Solution Properties,* American Chemical Society, Symposium Series 598, ACS, Washington, 490, 1995.

44. Morishima, Y. et al., Characterization of unimolecular micelles of random copolymers of sodium 2-(acrylamido)-2-methylpropanesulfonate and methacrylamides bearing bulky hydrophobic substituents, *Macromolecules*, 28, 2874, 1995.

45. Ringsdorf, H., Structure and properties of pharmacologically active polymers, *J. Polym. Sci. Symp.*, 51, 135, 1975.

46. Ulbrich, K. et al., Solution properties of drug carriers based on poly[N-(2-hydroxypropyl)methacrylamide] containing biodegardable bond, *Macromol. Chem.*, 188, 1261, 1987.

47. Patnum, D. and Kopecek, J., Polymer conjugates with anticancer activity, *Adv. Polym. Sci.*, 122, 55, 1995.

48. Duncan, R., Dimitrijevic, S., and Evagorou, E.G., The role of polymer conjugates in the diagnosis and treatment of cancer, *STP Pharm. Sci.*, 6, 237, 1996.

49. Akiyoshi, K. et al., Self-aggregates of hydrophobized polysaccharides in water. Formation and characteristics of nanoparticles, *Macromolecules*, 26, 3062, 1993.

50. Akiyoshi, K. et al., Microscopic structure and thermoresponsiveness of a hydrogel nanoparticle by self-assembly of a hydrophobized polysaccharide, Macromolecules, 30, 857, 1997.

51. Lee, K.Y. et al., Structural determination and interior polarity of self-aggregates prepared from deoxycholic acid-modified chitosan in water, *Macromolecules*, 31, 378, 1998.

52. Akiyoshi, K. et al., Controlled association of amphiphilic polymers in water: thermosensitive nanoparticles formed by self-assembly of hydrophobically modified pullulan and poly(N-isopropylacrylamides), *Macromolecules*, 33, 3244, 2000.

53. Akiyoshi, K. et al., Self-association of cholesterol-bearing poly(L-lysine) in water and control of its secondary structure by host–guest interaction with cyclodextrin, *Macromolecules*, 33, 6752, 2000.

54. Nishikawa, T., Akiyoshi, K., and Sunamoto, J., Macromolecular complexation between bovine serum albumin and self-assembled hydrogel nanoparticle of hydrophobized polysaccharides, *J. Am. Chem. Soc.*, 118, 6110, 1996.

55. Akiyoshi, K. and Sunamoto, J., Supramolecular assembly of hydrophobized polysaccharide., *Supramolecular Sci.*, 3, 157, 1996.

56. Taniguchi, I. et al., Cell specificity of macromolecular assembly of cholesteryl and galactoside groups-conjugated pullulan, *J. Bioactive Compatible Polymers*, 14, 195, 1999.

57. Akiyoshi, K. et al., Self-assembled hydrogel nanoparticle of cholesterol-bearing pullulan as a carrier of protein drugs: complexation and stabilization of insulin, *J. Control. Rel.*, 54, 313, 1998.

58. Gu, X-G. et al., A novel hydrophobized polysaccharide/oncoprotein complex vaccine induces *in vitro* and *in vivo* cellular and humoral immune responses against HER2 expressing murine sarcoma, *Cancer Res.*, 58, 3385, 1998.

59. Shiku, H. et al., Development of a cancer vaccine: peptides, proteins, and DNA, *Cancer Chemotherapy Pharmacol.*, 46, S77, 2000.

60. Akiyoshi, K., Sasaki, Y., and Sunamoto, J., Molecular chaperone-like activity of hydrogel nanoparticles of hydrophobized polysaccharide: thermal stabiliazation with refolding of carbonic anhydrase *B, Bioconjugate Chem.*, 10, 321, 1999.

61. Fink, A.L., Chaperone-mediated protein folding, *Physiolog. Rev.*, 79, 425, 1999.

62. Bukau, B. and Horwich, A.L., The Hsp70 and Hsp60 chaperone machines, *Cell*, 92, 351, 1998.

63. Balasubramanian, D., Raman, B., and Sivakama S., Polysaccharides as amphiphiles, *J. Am. Chem. Soc.*, 115, 74, 1993.

64. Wulff, G., Steinert, A., and Holler, O., Modification of amylose and investigation of its inclusion behavior, *Carbohydrate Res.*, 307, 19, 1998.

65. Kojima, N. and Hakomori, S., Specific interaction between gangliotriaosylceramide (Gg3) and sialosyllactosylceramide (GM3) as a basis for specific cellular recognition between lymphoma and melanoma cells, *J. Biol. Chem.*, 264, 20159, 1989.

66. Kojima, N. and Hakomori, S., Cell adhesion, spreading, and motility of GM3-expressing cells based on glycolipid-glycolipid interaction, *J. Biol. Chem.*, 266, 17552, 1992.

3   Hydrogen Bonds

Yuichi Ohya

CONTENTS

3.1   INTRODUCTION

Hydrogen bonding is probably the most important noncovalent interaction to think about in the development of biological or biomimetic supramolecular architectures. Water, the most ubiquitous medium in nature, forms strong intermolecular hydrogen bonds. However, hydrogen bonding is the major factor in three-dimensional structures of proteins and polynucleotides, the most typical biological macromolecules. The highly selective and directional nature of the hydrogen bonding system is ideal for the construction and stabilization of supramolecular architectures.

Hydrogen bonding is a weaker interaction compared with covalent or ionic bonding, and can therefore be switched on or off with energies that are within the range of thermal fluctuations at life temperatures. This means that the hydrogen-bonded molecules have dynamic characters around the thermodynamic equilibrium state. The weakness of the individual hydrogen bond is such that the bond is often not sufficient to provide the strength and specificity necessary for biological processes; however, this can be overcome by cooperation among and geometrical arrangement of a number of hydrogen bonds. The assembly systems of cooperative multiple hydrogen bonds may be stable and specific enough, but small energy supplies can make them dissociate as seen in the process of replication of DNA. Such dynamism and flexibility are the most essential characteristics for sustaining life.

The basic principles of the nature of hydrogen bonds are well described in the literature.[1-6] This chapter describes the basic and essential concepts of hydrogen bonding. Typical examples of natural and nonnatural hydrogen-bonded supramolecular architectures are introduced along with the methodologies to construct biomimetic and biologically functional supramolecular architectures using hydrogen bonding. For more examples, see References 7 through 16.

3.2 BASIC CONCEPT OF HYDROGEN BONDING

3.2.1 DEFINITION

Hydrogen bonds are formed when a donor (D) with an available acidic hydrogen atom is brought into intimate contact with an acceptor (A) carrying an available nonbonding lone pair (Figure 3.1). In the broadest sense, the definition proposed by Pimentel and McClellan[2] is that a hydrogen bond exists when there is evidence of a bond, and evidence that this bond specifically involves a hydrogen atom already bonded to another atom.

This definition does not specify the natures of the donor and acceptor atoms. Generally both D and A are highly electronegative atoms (O, N, F, Cl, Br, S) to form normal hydrogen bonding. However, the C of the hydrocarbon and the π-system may serve as a donor and an acceptor, respectively, to form weak hydrogen bonding. The idea that hydrogen bond is said to exist if the D$\cdots$A distance is closer than a van der Waals contact[17] was accepted as "the van der Waals radii cut-off criterion," and often taken as evidence for the presence of hydrogen bonding in x-ray diffraction crystallography analysis. However, this criterion was proposed in the period when hydrogen atoms could not seen in x-ray crystal diffraction studies. It is doubtful because

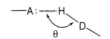

FIGURE 3.1 Hydrogen bond (linear type).

A = O, N, F, Cl, Br, S, π-system
D = O, N, F, Cl, Br, S, C

the D···A distance is also a function of the D-H-A angle and there are other objections.[4,5] Pauling's van der Waals radii and experimentally observed H···A distances in the solid state where oxygen was an acceptor are shown in Table 3.1. The distance between the hydrogen and acceptor atoms in normal hydrogen bonding is normally less than the sum of the van der Waals radii.

TABLE 3.1
Experimentally Observed D-H···A Hydrogen Bond Distances versus van der Waals Radii[a]

Type of bond DH A	Observed range of H A Distance (Å)	van der Waals radii[b] (Å)		
		W_H	W_O	Sum
OH---O<	1.44–2.10			
NH---O=C	1.58–2.05	1.2	1.4	2.6
NH---O<	1.60–2.40			

[a] Jeffrey, G.A. and Saenger, W., *Hydrogen Bonding in Biological Structures*, Springer-Verlag, Berlin, 1994.
[b] Pauling, L.C., *The Nature of the Chemical Bond*, Cornell University Press, Ithaca, 1939.

3.2.2 ENERGETICS

The enthalpy (ΔH) of hydrogen bonding is generally in the range of 10 to 40 kJ/mol for NH···O(N) or OH···O(N). Higher stabilization (>40 kJ/mol) may be observed when charged molecules are involved. In the cases of CH in hydrocarbons or π system, the strength should be much weaker (<10 kJ/mol). As formation of a hydrogen bond normally exhibits negative entropy change ($\Delta S<0$), the strength of hydrogen bonding has negative temperature dependence. Hydrogen bonding is essentially an electrostatic interaction; its strength strongly depends on the dielectric constant of the medium and becomes weaker in polar solvent. It is surprising that hydrogen bonding is a major interaction in biological supramolecular systems, although water, a polar solvent, is dominant. A number of techniques can enhance or support hydrogen bonding in nature, such as π–π stacking of nucleotide base pairs, hydrophobic pockets in proteins, and hydrophobic environments in lipid membranes.

3.2.3 DIRECTIONAL NATURE

The most important characteristic of the hydrogen bond is its directional nature. Optimal interaction can be predicted for a linear D-H-A arrangement with an angle (θ in Figure 3.1) around 180°. However, that is rarely found in solid-state structures that offer rich sources of corresponding geometries. The most probable angle observed for various samples of hydrogen bonds in the solid state is around 165°.[4]

This is consistent with the theoretical calculation for OH···O bonds using *ab initio* quantum mechanics on a model system.[18] However, this does not imply that linearity is not the most stable configuration for a hydrogen bond between isolated donor and acceptor molecules or between hydrogen-bonded dimers in the gas phase. Linear hydrogen bonding between one donor and one acceptor is energetically optimal, but is not common. Bent hydrogen bonds are often found in bifurcated configurations (Figure 3.2); in configuration 1, one hydrogen atom is located between three electronegative atoms, covalently bound to one and hydrogen bonded to the other two. The bifurcated hydrogen bond was first found in the crystal structure of glycin.[19] The bifurcation in configuration 2[2] is rarely observed in the crystalline state. To avoid confusion, the "three-centered" description was proposed for configuration 1 by Jeffery and Saenger.[4] Configuration 2 is observed in nucleosides only in conjunction with configuration 3. Nevertheless, the strong angular dependence of hydrogen bonding exists and it is useful for constructing artificial molecular organizations having well-defined structures.

3.2.4 POLARIZATION

Another characteristic of hydrogen bonding is polarization. The bonding between a partially positive hydrogen and a partially negative acceptor induces a dipole moment. Typically, the strength of the dipole moment of a hydrogen bond is calculated to be 3.5 D for peptide bonds in polypeptides. The dipole moment is often cancelled by neighboring hydrogen bonds in a reverse direction and such dipole–dipole interaction may stabilize the hydrogen bonding. However, when some hydrogen bonds are arranged in the same direction as found in the α-helices of polypeptides, a macro-dipole moment that may have an important role in biological system is formed.

Mainly based on an x-ray diffraction analysis, certain rules have been proposed for supramolecular assembly arising from the formation of hydrogen bonds within the system;[20-24] however, many factors influence the formation process that leads to the final supramolecular structure.

3.3 HYDROGEN BONDING IN BIOLOGICAL SYSTEMS

3.3.1 PROTEINS AND POLYPEPTIDES

Recognition and binding with small molecules or macromolecules via multiple weak interactions including hydrogen bonding are the primary events for protein's

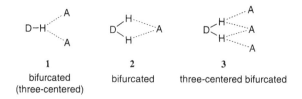

FIGURE 3.2 Bifurcated or three-centered hydrogen bond configurations.

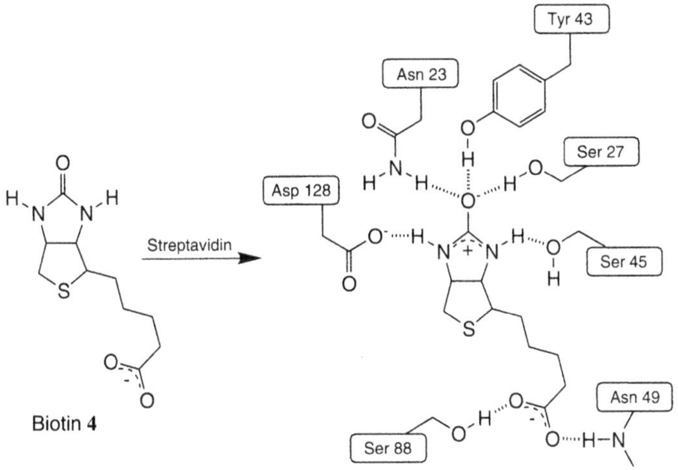

FIGURE 3.3 Binding of biotin (4) to streptavidin.[25]

bioactivities. An example of extremely efficient multiple binding ($K = 2.5 \times 10^{13}$ M^{-1}) of a small guest molecule (biotin) by a protein host (streptavidin) is shown in Figure 3.3.[25] Simultaneous actions of more than 10 weak hydrogen bonding, van der Waals, electrostatic, and lipophilic interactions produce a large binding free energy of −76 kJ/mol. Such specific and strong recognition and binding activities are derived from the geometrical arrangements of functional groups in the three-dimensional structures of proteins. For deeper understanding of protein structures, see References 26 and 27.

Since a peptide bond has both a donor (NH) and an acceptor (C=O) for hydrogen bonding, the hydrogen bonding plays a crucial role in the construction of three-dimensional structure of proteins. Electrostatic, van der Waals, hydrophobic (lipophilic), and π–π stacking interactions and coordination bonds are also important for forming final three-dimensional structures of proteins. However, secondary structures (α-helix, β-sheet, and turns) of proteins and polypeptides are formed mainly through hydrogen bonding of the amide bonds.

The α-helix (Figure 3.4) is a right-handed spiral secondary structure having favorable dihedral angles around α carbon (C_α). All the peptide bonds in the helix form hydrogen bonds that confer maximum stability. The relevant parameters of the α-helix are 3.6 residues per turn and 0.54 nm of pitch. The carbonyl oxygen of the (n)th residue forms a hydrogen bond with the NH group of the ($n + 4$)th residue (1←5 hydrogen bond). The side chain groups are directed outward from the helix axis. Each hydrogen bond in the polypeptide has 3.5 D of dipole moments. The hydrogen bonds in the α-helix are arranged in the same direction (helix axis). Therefore, the α-helix containing n hydrogen bonds has about 3.5n D of macro-dipole moment where the N terminal and the C terminal are the positive and negative poles,

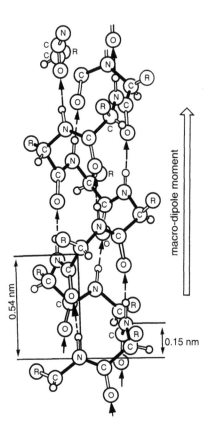

FIGURE 3.4 The structure of the α-helix and its macro-dipole moment. Hydrogen bonds are indicated by dotted lines with arrows.

respectively[27,28] (Figure 3.5). Positively charged amino acids (Glu, Asp) near *N* terminal and negatively charged amino acids (Lys, Arg) near *C* terminal stabilize the α-helix by canceling the macro-dipole moment.[29-31] Indeed, such locations are often found in naturally occurring proteins.[32] The dipole–dipole interactions among macro-dipoles or among macro-dipoles and charged groups (or ions) may also have supporting effects on the stabilization of three-dimensional structures of proteins and synthetic polypeptide assemblies and control the pKa of functional groups, stabilization of the transition state, and charge transfer behavior on enzymes.[33,34]

Another regular secondary structure is the β-pleated sheet (β-sheet) (Figure 3.5). The structures of β-sheets are parallel or antiparallel. Like α-helices, β-sheets have repeating dihedral angles and are stabilized by the maximum possible number of interchain hydrogen bonds. One stereochemical feature of the β-sheets is that amino acid side chains point alternately up and down, and adjacent side chains interact sterically to produce a right-handed twist.[35-37] Turns and random coils can be also involved in the secondary structures; β-turns are frequently used to give rise to a chain reversal. They are stabilized by main chain 1←4 hydrogen bonding. At least three types of β-turns, types I, II, and III, have been identified. The disordered secondary structures are called random coils.

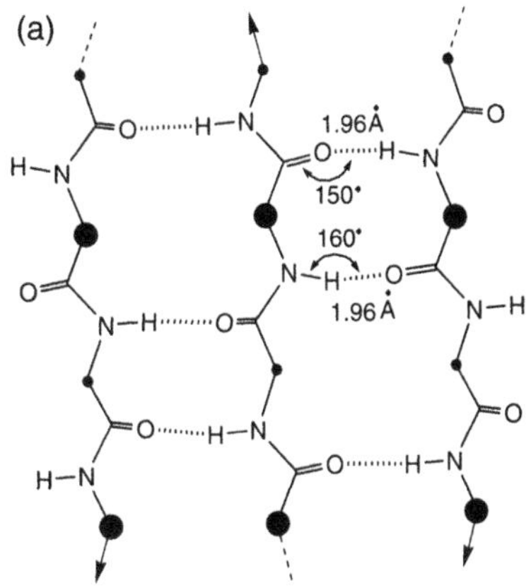

FIGURE 3.5 Geometry of (a) antiparallel and (b) parallel β-sheets, with average hydrogen bond distances and angles shown. C_α atoms are indicated by dots. If side chains point up (toward viewer), the dots are large, otherwise the side chains point down.[4,35,36]

Secondary structures can be combined to form super-secondary motifs. Figure 3.6 illustrates typical examples of super-secondary motifs, ββ′ (β hairpin), αα′ (α hairpin), and βαβ′ (Rossmann fold, two strands of β-sheet connected by an α-helix). The tertiary structure, which relates to the spatial relationship between secondary structural elements, is mainly constructed by combinations of such super-secondary motifs.

Based on these super-secondary motifs, the syntheses of artificial proteins having totally different primary structures have been extensively studied.[38-48] An artificial αβ barrel protein that is structurally similar to naturally occurring triose phosphate isomerase, was genetically synthesized using four repetitions of αβα′β′ super-secondary motifs.[40] DeGrado and coworkers developed the methodology using assembled α-helices (helix bundle) to produce novel artificial proteins[41,42] (Figure 3.7). Mutter and coworkers proposed a template-assembled synthetic protein (TASP) by attaching several α and/or β structures on oligopeptides (or other

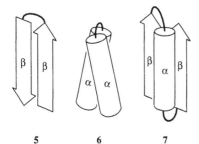

FIGURE 3.6 Representative super-secondary motifs: (5) ββ′ (β hairpin), (6) αα′ (α hairpin) and (7) βαβ′ (Rossmann fold). Cylinders represent α-helices while arrows represent β-strands.

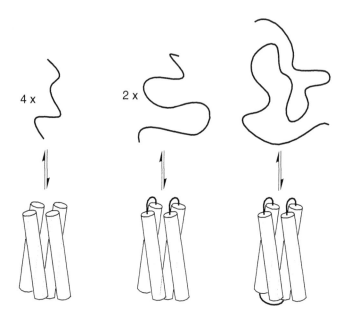

FIGURE 3.7 The incremental approach to the design of a four-helix bundle protein.[42]

suitable molecules) as templates[43-45] (Figure 3.8). These approaches to synthesizing artificial proteins exhibiting tailor-made structural and functional properties are called *de novo* designs. Synthesis of helichrome by Sasaki and Kaiser[46,47] and chymohelizyme by Stewart et al.[48] can be regarded as pioneer works for synthesis of artificial enzymes using such methodology.

3.3.2 NUCLEIC ACIDS

The macromolecular nucleic acids, deoxyribonucleic acid (DNA) and ribonucleic acid (RNA), are of prime importance in biology because they are responsible for the storage and expression of genetic information. The basic three-dimensional structure, right-handed double helix, of DNA was discovered by Watson and Crick in 1953.[49] The hydrophobic purine and pyrimidine bases are stacked in the center of the helix and the hydrophilic sugar–phosphate backbones are at the periphery. Bases are linked by hydrogen bonding in the base pairs such that adenine (A) in one strand opposes thymine (T) in the other strand, and guanine (G) opposes cytosine (C), so that one strand of DNA is said to be complementary to the other. Figure 3.9 illustrates Watson–Crick type hydrogen bonding between purine residues and pyrimidine residues. The π–π stacking and the hydrophobic interaction that allow the base pairs to avoid contact with water confer great stability to the double helix.

Double-stranded DNA exists in at least six forms (A through E and Z). More detailed information about the variation of double-stranded DNAs and RNAs are described in Saenger's book.[50] The B-form (Figure 3.10) is usually found under

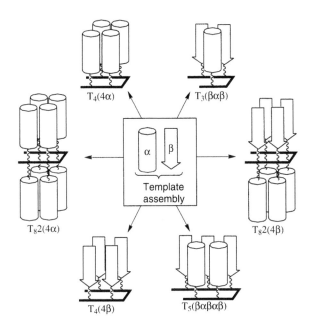

FIGURE 3.8 Variations of template-assembled synthetic protein (TASP) molecules.[43] Cylinders represent helices; arrows represent β-strands.

physiological conditions (low salt, high level of hydration). As for B-form double-stranded DNA, a single turn along the axis is 3.4 nm and contains ten base pairs, and the width of the double helix is about 2 nm. A major groove and a minor groove wind along the molecule parallel to the phosphodiester backbone. Some proteins and other molecules in these grooves can interact specifically with exposed atoms of the nucleotides, mainly by hydrogen bonding, and thereby recognize and bind to specific nucleotide sequences without disrupting the base pairing of the double helical DNA. Regulatory proteins can control the expression of specific genes via such

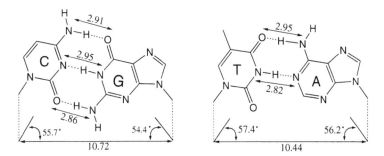

FIGURE 3.9 Watson–Crick type hydrogen bonding of purine residues and pyrimidine residues. Distances are shown in angstroms.

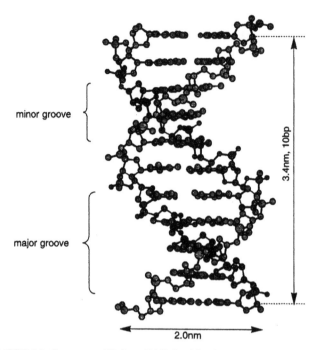

minor groove

major groove

3.4nm, 10bp

2.0nm

FIGURE 3.10 Structure of B-form DNA in side view.

interactions.[50] Many natural and synthetic DNA binding molecules via electrostatic interaction, groove binding (hydrogen bonding), or intercalation have been found.[50,51]

Besides Watson–Crick type hydrogen bonding, other kinds of hydrogen bonding patterns are possible among the bases.[4,50] Hoogsteen type hydrogen bonding is well known to form a triple helix (triplex) of DNA[52] (Figure 3.11). Pyrimidine oligonucleotides bind in the major grooves of Watson–Crick double-stranded DNA, with polypurine stretches resulting in triple-stranded structures.[53] The specificity in triplex formation is derived from Hoogsteen type hydrogen bonding in which thymine recognizes the AT base pair (T•AT triplet) and protonated cytosine recognizes the GC base pair (C⁺•GC triplet). In this motif, called the "pyrimidine motif" (Y•RY), the third strand is parallel to the central purine strand. There is another type of triplex. In the "purine motif" (R•RY)[54,55] consisting of A•AT (T•AT is also possible) and G•GC triplets (Figure 3.11), the third strand is antiparallel to the central purine strand and no protonation of pyrimidines is required. These triple-helical motifs are useful to recognize DNA specifically, and can regulate or modify their structures and functions.[53-56]

Quadruplex of DNA is well known for oligo-deoxyguanosine forming G-quartet (Figure 3.12a). Such structure is often found in teromere, which exists at the gene terminal and concerns aging of cells (Figure 3.12b).[57] Similarly the quadruplex structure, deoxyguanine, and isoguanine derivative form hydrogen-bonded cyclic tetramers, and "catch" Na⁺ or K⁺ ions between the central cavities of two sets of the

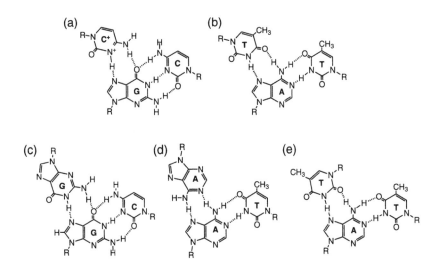

FIGURE 3.11 Nucleic acid base triplet by Watson–Crick and Hoogsteen type hydrogen bonding. (a) and (b) Pyrimidine motif (Y•RY), (c), (d), and (e) Purine motif (R•RY).

cyclic tetramers in organic solvents[58,59] (Figure 3.12c). The formation of the cyclic tetramer is strongly accelerated in the presence of high concentrations of metal ions. This is a typical example of host–guest cooperation; the guest (ion) accelerates the formation of the host. Columnar mesophase formation by stacking of quartets of guanine-related molecules was also reported.[60]

The structures of RNAs are also curious. Two strands of RNA having complementarity tend to form the A-form or A'-form of double helix.[50] Some RNAs, such as clover-leaf tRNAs[50] and hummer-head type ribozymes,[61] are known to form complicated three-dimensional structures via intramolecular hydrogen bonding. These three-dimensional structures are essential for the activity of tRNAs and ribozymes.

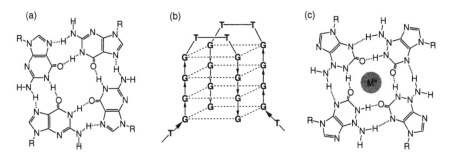

FIGURE 3.12 Structures of (a) G quartet, (b) the hairpin dimer of the telomeric end, and (c) isoguanine quartet metal ion complex.[58-60]

Although nucleic acids have supramolecular structures,[62] their elements, nucleotide bases, and analogues are quite useful for constructing supramolecular architectures because multiple hydrogen bonding can be easily prepared by combinations of them. Many supramolecular assemblies using oligonucleotides, nucleotide bases, and related compounds have been reported (see Sections 3.4. and 3.5).

3.3.3 Other Biological Molecules and Water

Other biological molecules, such as carbohydrates (saccharides and polysaccharides), are also biologically important and can form intra- or intermolecular hydrogen bonding with water and other molecules. For example, cellulose, a structural polysaccharide, has an intermolecular hydrogen-bonded crystal structure.[4,63]

Water molecules are essential components of biological processes. The structure of water has been the subject of intense research since the 19th century.[64] Water is said to form clusters of three- or four-coordinated water molecules (Figure 3.13) with mean lifetimes of about a nanosecond in the liquid state.[65] Most biological molecules are hydrated when they work.[66] It is important to consider the presence of water molecules to understand the three-dimensional structures of biological macromolecules and design biologically functional materials. To produce intra- or intermolecular hydrogen bonding in aqueous solution, negative free energy changes are required for the transition from the hydrated state to the hydrogen-bonded state.

To design polymeric biomaterials that interact with living bodies, it is important to understand the interactions of polymeric material surfaces with biological molecules such as proteins. It is necessary to consider the hydrated states and displacement of bound water molecules on the materials and proteins of the interaction processes.[67]

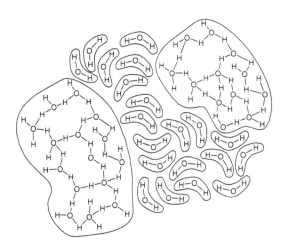

FIGURE 3.13 The Frank model of water clusters in liquid water. The water oxygens are three- and four-coordinated; those outside the cluster are nonbonded monomers.[65]

3.4 CONSTRUCTION OF SUPRAMOLECULAR ARCHITEC-TURE BY HYDROGEN BONDING

3.4.1 ASSOCIATION MODES

All modes of supramolecular assemblies can roughly be divided into two patterns: a closed association and an open association (Figure 3.14). A closed association is a mode by which a limited number of molecules associate noncovalently to form a definite size (or distribution) of association. An open association is a mode by which unlimited numbers of molecules associate noncovalently to form larger or infinite associations. The scale and the distribution of the size of an open-associated assembly generally depend on the concentration, temperature, and other extrinsic factors. We can find many examples of both patterns in biological systems. Hemoglobin is a tetrameric closed association consisting of two α-subunits and two β-subunits. Coat proteins of the tobacco mosaic virus form a type of open association. A biomembrane composed of lipid bilayers can be regarded as an open association with unlimited numbers of lipid molecules and membrane proteins; however, macroscopically, it is a closed association.

Closed and open associations are both important in biological systems. To construct functioning supramolecular architectures, it is the most important to control the association mode. Whether the association mode is open or closed, is regulated thermodynamically; it is enthalpy- and entropy-driven. Noncovalent interaction (not only hydrogen bonding) contributes to an increase in negative enthalpy; however, regular molecular association may lead to a decrease in positive entropy change. Consequently, the free energy change that determines the association mode depends on such factors. The steric (shape) factor that often results in van der Waals interaction and steric hindrance is also important for determining the mode of association. Many examples of closed and open associations are described in books and reviews.[7-16] Energetics and analytical methods for supramolecular assemblies are well described in Schneider's book.[15]

3.4.2 HYDROGEN-BONDED OPEN ASSOCIATION SYSTEMS

Open association is important for nanometer and larger scale architectures. Many stable open association systems have been found in crystals. See Figure 3.15. Carboxylic acids, such as benzoic acid (structure 8), are known to form dimers

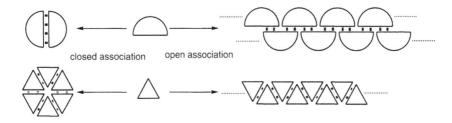

closed association   open association

FIGURE 3.14 Closed and open associations.

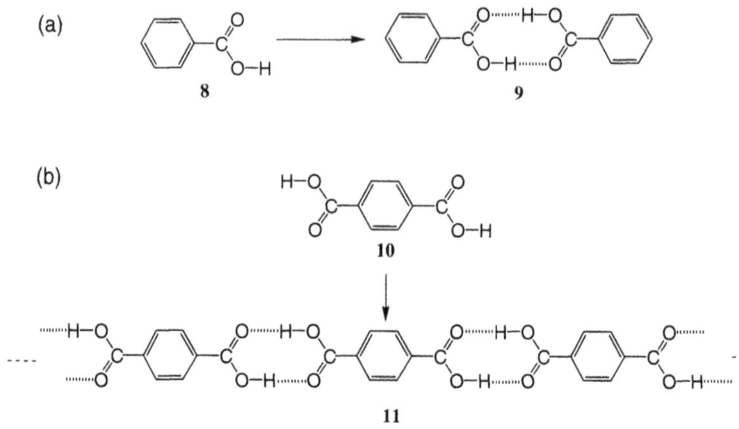

FIGURE 3.15 Associations of (a) benzoic acid (8) and (b) terephthalic acid (10).

(structure 9) by complementary hydrogen bonding in nonpolar solvents or in the solid state where O–H is a donor and C=O is an acceptor (Figure 3.15a).[68] The association mode of benzoic acid is a closed one. Terephthalic acid (structure 10) has two carboxylic acid groups at *para* positions. This *Janus** (two-faced) molecule is expected to form a linear open association (structure 11, Figure 3.15b). Two crystal structures are known for terephthalic acid, and linear infinite repetition of hydrogen bonding (structure 11) exists in both crystal systems.[69] On the *meta* isomer, isophthalic acid, the results are more complicated.

One can expect tape-type open association (structure 13) and cyclic closed hexagonal association (structure 14) for the isophthalic acid derivative (structure 12, Figure 3.16). Real crystal structure is the former.[70] Cyclic closed hexagonal association can be produced by introduction of a bulky group at the 5-position of isophthalic acid. The isophthalic acid derivative having a –OC$_{10}$H$_{21}$ group at the 5-position forms a crystal consisting of cyclic hexagonal associations (structure 14).[71] This example shows how the steric (shape) factor determines the association mode. As expected, the crystal structure of 1,3,5-benzenetricarboxylic acid (structure 15, Figure 3.17) is a two-dimensional honeycomb-type network (structure 16).[72,73] The void space, i.e., hole of a honeycomb network, is filled by another honeycomb network of structure 16.

These crystal structures can be regarded as superstructures of one- or two-dimensional hydrogen-bonded open associations through van der Waals and π–π stacking interactions. See Figure 3.18. There are some examples for hydrogen-bonded three-dimensional open associations.[74-78] 1,3,5,7-Adamantanetetracarboxylc acid (structure 17) forms a three-dimensional diamondoid network (structure 19).[76] The voids of the network are filled by another diamondoid network to form an

---

* Janus was an ancient Roman god, usually portrayed as a single figure with two faces looking in opposite directions.

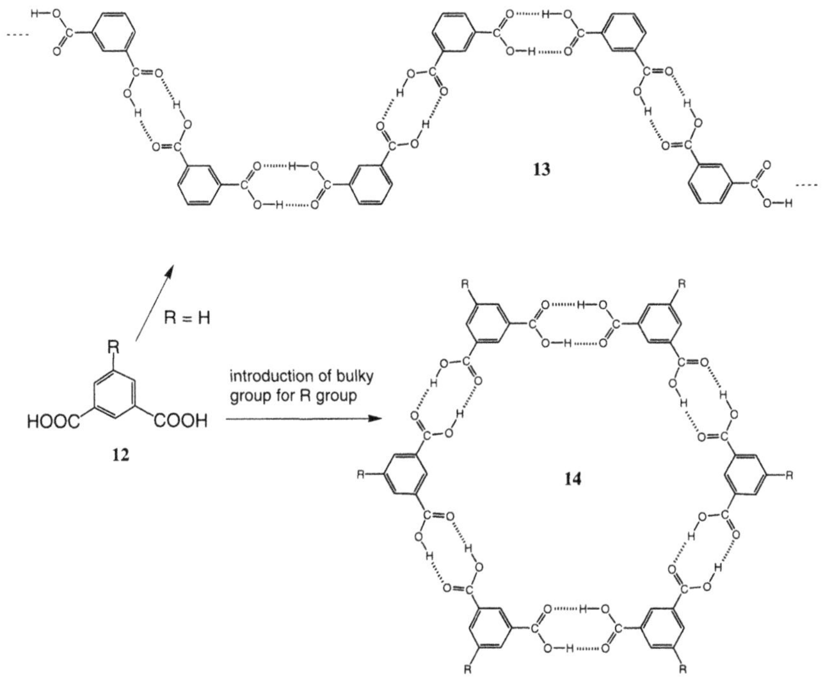

FIGURE 3.16 Two patterns of association of isophthalic acid derivatives (12): (a) crinkled tape (13) observed for (12) when R = H, and (b) cyclic hexagonal structure (14) observed for (12) when R = -C$_{10}$H$_{21}$.[70,71]

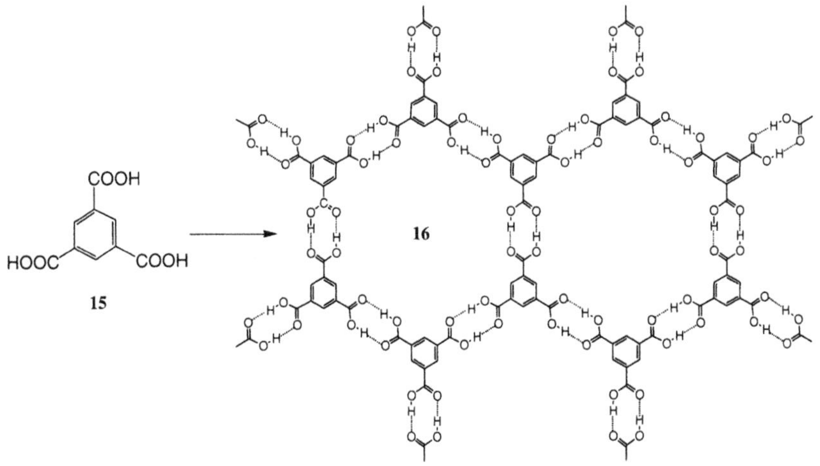

FIGURE 3.17 Honeycomb network (16) of 1,3,5-benzenetricarboxylic acid (15).[71,72]

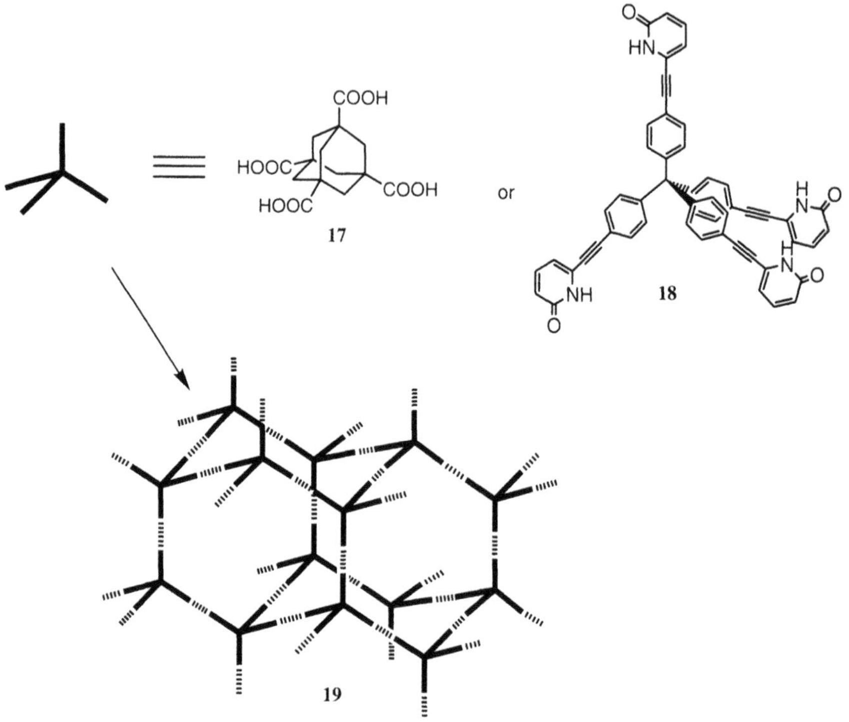

FIGURE 3.18 Interpenetrated diamondoid networks (19) arising from hydrogen-bonded 1,3,5,7-adamantanetetracarboxylic acid (17) and tetraarylmethane having pyridone units (18).[76,77]

interpenetrating structure. A similar diamondoid network by hydrogen bonding was reported for structure 18, which contains a rigid tetraarylmethane core with pyridone units held rigidly at a fixed distance from the core.[77,78] The larger voids of the network are also filled with interpenetrating networks and small guest molecules.

The diaminopyrimidinone derivative (structure 20, Figure 3.19) possesses three pairs of hydrogen bonding sites in self-complementary arrangement and can yield only a linear tape-type open association (structure 21), shown by the crystal structure of the octyl derivative.[79] Lehn pointed out the possibility that such linear arrays of protonatable or hydrogen-bonded sites may allow the directed long-range transfer of protons, thus functioning as a proton-conducting channel, i.e., as a proton wire.[7]

Figure 3.20 shows chemical structures reported by Ghadiri and coworkers.[39,80,81] A cyclic octapeptide, cyclo[–(D–Ala–Glu–D–Ala–Gln)$_2$–] (structure 22), forms a hydrogen-bonded nanotube (structure 23) having an internal diamer of 7 to 8 Å. Ghadiri also reported that another cyclic octapeptide with different side chains and the same chirality as structure 22 formed a trans-membrane ion channel in a lipid bilayer membrane.[39,82] Rod-like hydrogen-bonded open assocations by

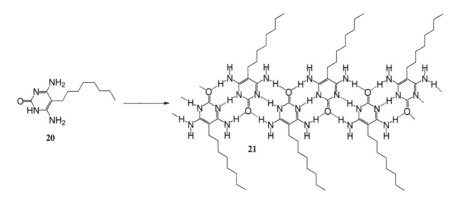

FIGURE 3.19 Hydrogen-bonded tape-like species (21) formed by self-assembly of self-complementary 4,6-diamino-5-octylpyrimidine-2(1*H*)-one (20).[79]

self-complementary molecules were also reported for structure 24 (Figure 3.21) in the solid state.[83]

Figure 3.22 shows the structure of the hydrogen-bonded cyanuric acid/melamine lattice. Cyanuric acid (structure 26) and melamine (structure 27) are simple compounds, but they possess 3/6 and 6/3 of possible donor/acceptor sites for hydrogen bonding, respectively, and are complementary to each other. Whitesides and coworkers reported the formation of a stable two-dimensional hexagonal lattice for a 1:1 complex of cyanuric acid and melamine in the solid state.[84] They also succeeded

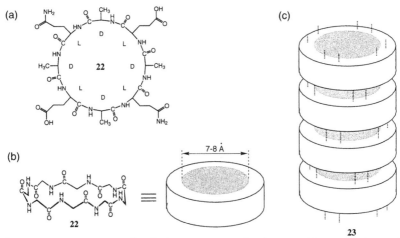

FIGURE 3.20 (a) Chemical structure of the peptide subunit cyclo [–(D–Ala–Glu–D–Ala–Gln)₂–] (22). **D** or **L** indicates amino acid chirality. (b) Side view of 22. For clarity, only backbone structure is represented. (c) Self-assembled tubular configuration (23) by intermolecular hydrogen bonding of 22.[80,81]

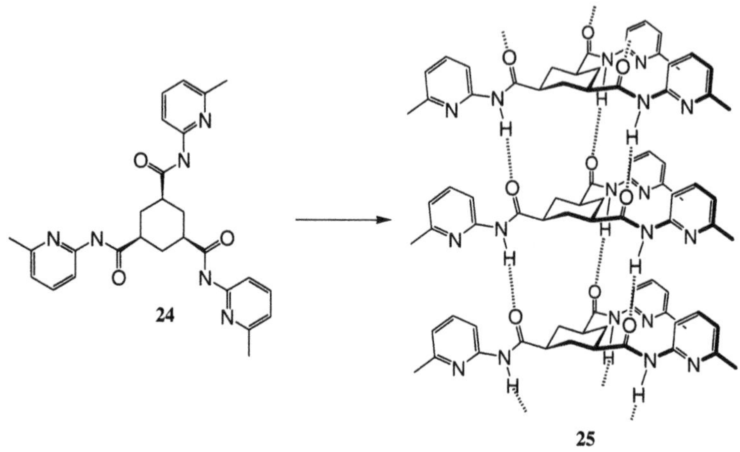

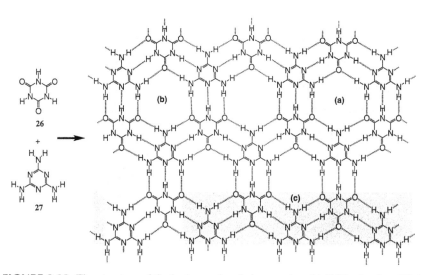

FIGURE 3.21 The structure of *cis,cis*-cyclohexane-1,3,5-tricarboxamide derivative (24) and its rod-like hydrogen-bonded self-assembly (25).[83]

in converting the insoluble open association to a soluble closed association.[85-92] We can find three types of basic assembly motifs in Figure 3.22: (a) the rosette (cyclic closed), (b) crinkled tape and (c) linear tape motifs. Some of such associations (Figure 3.23) — tape-type open (structure 30) or cyclic closed (structure 31) — were

FIGURE 3.22 The structure of the hydrogen-bonded cyanuric acid (26)/melamine (27) lattice.[84] Three types of assemblies found in solution and the solid state are observed: (a) the rosette, (b) crinkled tape, and (c) linear tape motifs.

reported for complementary 1:1 complexes of barbituric acid derivative (structure 28) and 2,4,6-triaminopyrimidine derivative (structure 29).[79,93] Similar open associations of 1:1 complexes of two kinds of molecules having complementarity were reported for bis-sufonate compounds with guadinium ion into clathratable nanoporous two-dimensional associations,[94] and isophthalic acid derivative (which can form its own open association) with pyrazine or dimethylpyrazine.[95]

As freedom of the molecular motion in a stable open association is extremely limited and molecular weight of the association may be infinite, open associations might have difficulty for existing in a solution or liquid state having dynamic character. Lehn and coworkers reported liquid-crystalline open associations (Figure 3.24).[96-99] Equimolar mixture of nonmesogenic complementary components (TP_2) and (TU_2) (structures 32 and 33) produces the hydrogen-bonded open association $(TP_2, TU_2)_n$ (structure 34) that displays liquid-crystalline behavior in the temperature range from 25°C to 200°C. The stereochemistry of the components has almost no effect on the formation of the liquid-crystalline polyassembly; all of the D, L, and *meso* isomers of structures 32 and 33 give thermotropic mesophases. However, the internal structures of the mesophases formed by the stereoisomeric pairs are quite different (Figure 3.25).[97] This system shows the self-assembly process can lead to drastic changes in the physical properties of the system through molecular recognition directed by hydrogen bonding. Microscopic intermolecular recognition determines the macroscopic structure of the mesophase. Meijer et al. reported hydrogen-bonded soluble polyassembly using bis-(2-ureido-4-pyrimidone) compound 35 in $CHCl_3$

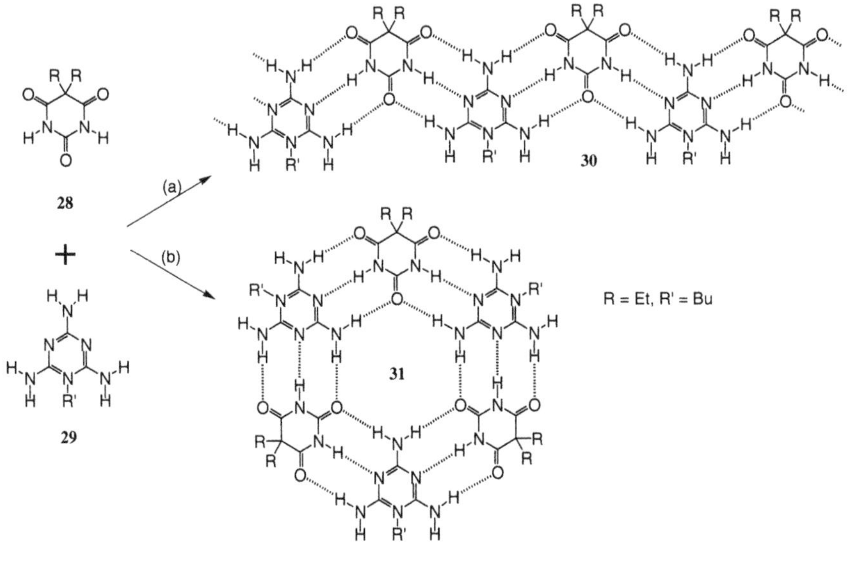

FIGURE 3.23 (a) Tape-type open (30) and (b) cyclic closed (31) associations by complementary 1:1 complexes of barbituric acid derivative (28) and 2,4,6-triaminopyrimidine derivative (29).[79]

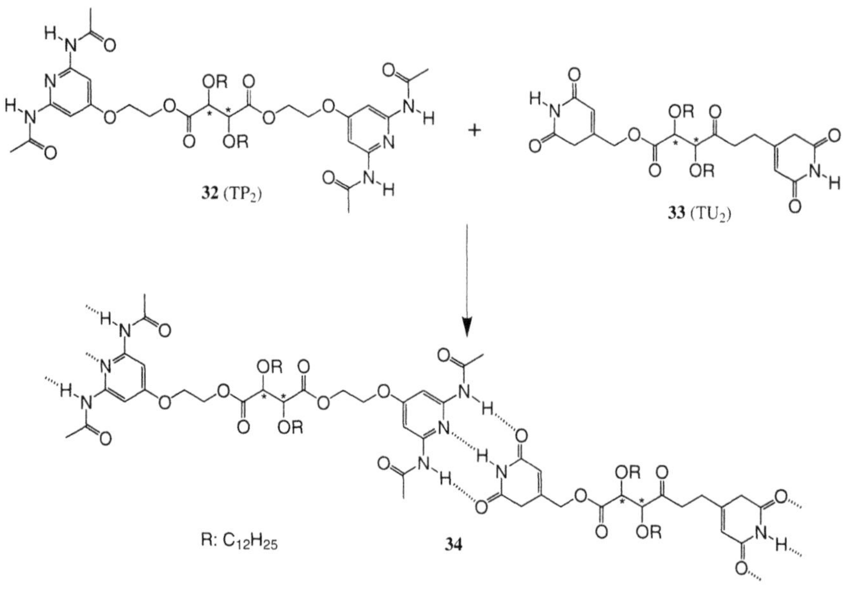

FIGURE 3.24 The formation of thermotropic liquid crystalline polyassembly $(TP_2, TU_2)_n$ (34) by hydrogen bonding-directed molecular recognition of compounds TP_2 (32) and TU_2 (33).[97] T represents L- (L), D- (D) , or *meso*- (M) tartaric acid.

(Figure 3.26).[100] Compound 35 showed temperature-dependent specific viscosity, which was reduced by the addition of monomeric compound 36. They also demonstrated the formation of a hydrogen-bonded three-dimensional polymer network by using polymers having three units of the terminal 2-ureido-4-pyrimidone group.[100]

Most artificially synthesized supramolecular architectures in open and closed associations were stable only in the solid state, liquid–crystalline state, or in nonpolar solvents. It might be difficult to construct a hydrogen-bonded open association in aqueous solution; however, a combination of enough free energy change, freedom of conformation (flexibility), and highly hydrophilic solubilizing groups might produce soluble open association in aqueous phase. Oligonucleotides are good candidates because they have highly hydrophilic phosphate groups and bind specifically with complementary counterparts by multiple hydrogen bonding and stacking of base pairs (Figure 3.27). Equimolar mixture of the *Janus* oligonucleotide derivatives (structures 37 and 38), which are semisymmetric oligo-DNA dimers having two strands of adenine tetramers or thymine tetramers attached to central cores (benzene) in the opposite direction, was reported to form a high molecular-weight open association (structure 39) in aqueous solution by corresponding complementarity[101] (Figure 3.27a). A similar approach was reported for bipyridines attached to oligonucleotides (20-mer, dA_{20} and dT_{20}) at their termini.[102] Using the 1:3 complex formation of ferrous and the bipyridinyl oligonucleotides, construction of two- or three-dimensional

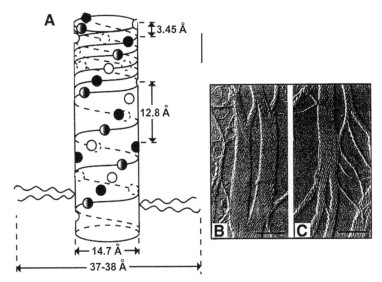

FIGURE 3.25 A: The columnar superstructure suggested by x-ray data for $(LP_2, LU_2)_n$;[97] each spot represents a PU or UP base pair; spots of the same type belong to the same strand of the triple helix; the aliphatic chains stick out of the cylinder more or less perpendicularly to its axis. For $(LP_2, LU_2)_n$, a single helical strand and the full triplex are represented on the bottom and at the top of the column, respectively. B and C: Scanning electron microscopic observation of the $(DP_2 + LU_2)$ mixture (B) and the $(LP_2 + DU_2)$ mixture (C).[97] Bars = 0.2 μm.

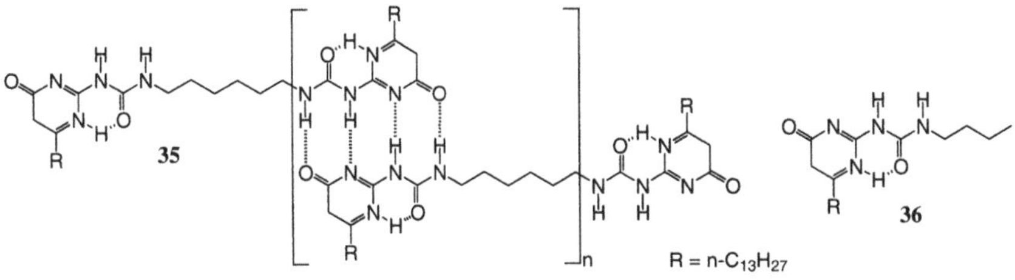

FIGURE 3.26 The formation of a soluble polyassembly by bifunctional 2-ureido-pyrimidone derivative (35) and the structure of the monofunctional derivative (36).[100]

DNA networks was reported. The great advantages of these systems using oligonucleotides are their solubilities in aqueous media and also that sequential arrangements of core groups may be possible. Asymmetric *Janus* oligonucleotide molecules having different sequences of oligo-DNAs attached to various kinds of functional core groups are expected to form programmed sequential arrangements of the core groups (Figure 3.27b). This is a special feature of the assembly system using oligonucleotides in contrast to the open associations described above.

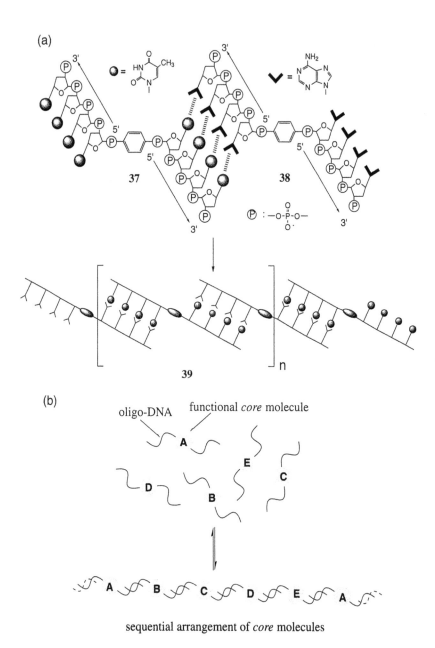

FIGURE 3.27 (a) The formation of polyassembly (39) by equivalent mixture of the oligo-DNA dimer conjugates (T4)₂Bz (37) and (A4)₂Bz (38) in aqueous solution.[101] (b) Construction of the sequential arrangement of functional *core* molecules by using oligo-DNA heterodimer conjugates.

3.4.3 HYDROGEN-BONDED CLOSED ASSOCIATION SYSTEMS

Closed association systems may represent significant expansion of host–guest chemistry. There are many examples of hydrogen-bonded closed association systems,[7,15,16,103-107] but only a few representative examples are introduced in this text.

Rebek and coworkers reported the construction of a molecular "tennis ball" by hydrogen bonding-directed self-assembly (Figure 3.28).[108] Molecule 40 is self-complementary and associates in organic solvent via eight hydrogen bonds to form a stable dimer with an internal cavity. They also reported cylindrical,[109] pseudospherical,[110] and enatiometric[111] molecular capsules having larger and/or chiral cavities and their encapsulation behavior against small molecules. Reinhoudt et al. reported the construction of D_3 symmetrical hydrogen-bonded molecular assemblies (Figure 3.29) of three equivalent calyx[4]arene bismelamine (structure 41) and six equivalents of barbiturate derivatives (structure 42 or 43).[112] They also reported the construction of enatiometrically pure hydrogen-bonded molecular assemblies having basically the same structure and "chiral memory" effect of the hydrogen bonding.[113-114] Chiral spherical molecular assembly was also reported by MacGillivray and Atwood.[115]

Oligonucleotides are useful for construction of supramolecular assemblies. Seeman and coworkers reported topological closed associations, cube and truncated octahedron (Figure 3.30) of DNA using DNA ligases and branched junction structures of DNA.[116-118] They also demonstrated the construction of sheet-like two-dimensional open association of DNA.[119,120]

3.4.4 POLYMERIC SYSTEMS

Many types of polymers have been used for biomaterials such as medical devices. Understanding the morphology and phase separation behavior of block- or graft-copolymers or polymer blends is essential for the design of polymeric materials including biomaterials. Hydrogen bonding may play important roles in such cases. Polymer–polymer interaction by hydrogen bonding has been studied since the late 1960s. Polycarboxylates, such as poly(acrylic acid) (PAA) and poly(methacrylic

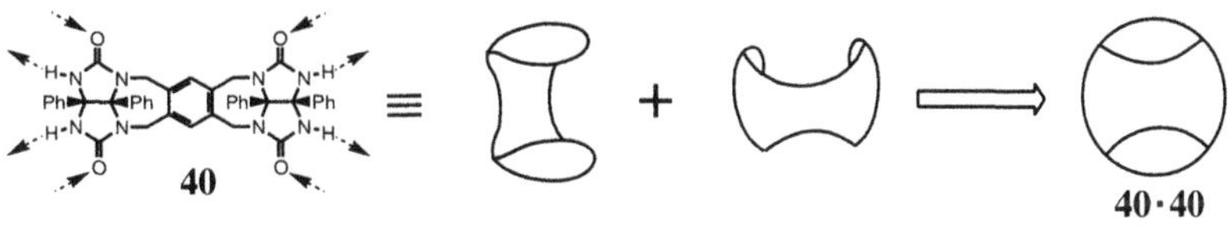

FIGURE 3. 28 "Tennis ball"-forming molecule.[108] Two-cyclic *bis* (urea) derivative (40) forms "tennis ball"-like self-association (40•40).

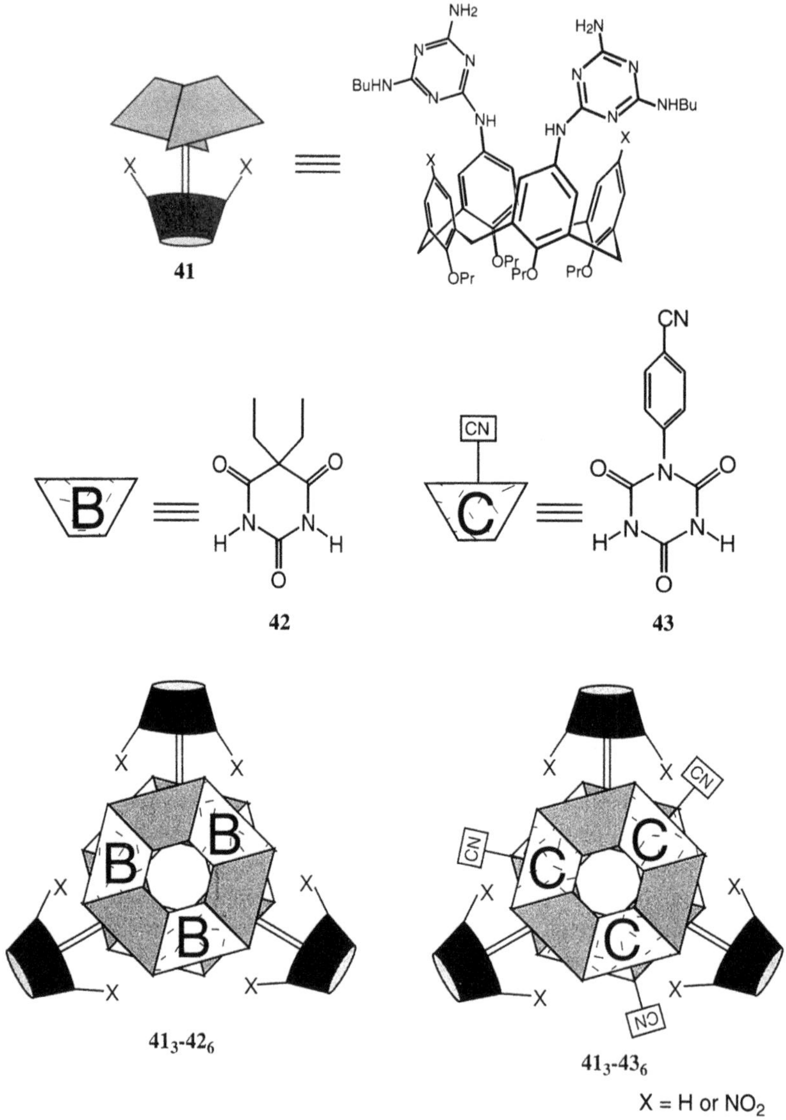

X = H or NO$_2$

FIGURE 3.29 Hydrogen-bonded assemblies resulting from the mixture of three equivalent calyx[4]arene bismelamine (41) and six equivalent barbiturate derivatives (42) and (43).[112]

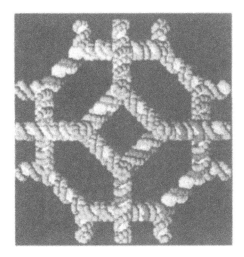 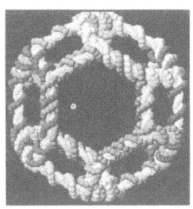

FIGURE 3.30 Left: double-helical representation of an ideal truncated octahedron of DNA. Right: octacatenane formed by the strands that correspond to the hexagons.[118] For detailed information, see References 116–118.

acid) (PMAA), form self-aggregates and also form complexes with other polymers by hydrogen bonding.[121-126] The interactions of PAA and PMAA with poly(N-vinyl-2-pyrrolidone) (PVP),[122,123] poly(acrylamide) (PAAm)[124] and poly(ethylene glycol) (PEG)[125,126] are well studied. Basic phenomena of such complexation processes and the properties of the polymer complexes were described by Bekturov et al.[121] In some polymeric complex systems derived from hydrogen bonding, interesting phase transition behavior can be observed. For example, the PEG–PMAA complex is known as a chemomechanical system in which chemical energy can be converted into kinetic energy.[126] The addition of PEG to PMAA gel membrane leads to a change in permeation rate through the membrane that acts as chemical valve. Gels and polymer networks are described in Chapters 6, 9, and 10. Other types of polymeric supramolecular architectures are described in a review by Beginn and Möller.[127]

Hydrogen bonding in polymeric systems is useful for memorization of molecular or macromolecular shapes. Molecular imprinting developed by Wulff's group and Shea's group is an approach to construct a cavity complementary to a desired template molecule in a polymeric solid support[128-130] (Figure 3.31). A rigid binding site for a target template molecule can be prepared by copolymerization of a monomer having suitable functional groups complementary to the template in the presence of cross-linking agents (and co-monomer) after preorganization of the monomers with the templates by intermolecular interaction including hydrogen bonding.[128-130] The polymerization fixes the optimum three-dimensional arrangement of functional groups on the polymeric solid support that provides a complementary cavity for the template molecule, thus enhancing binding selectivity. The imprinted

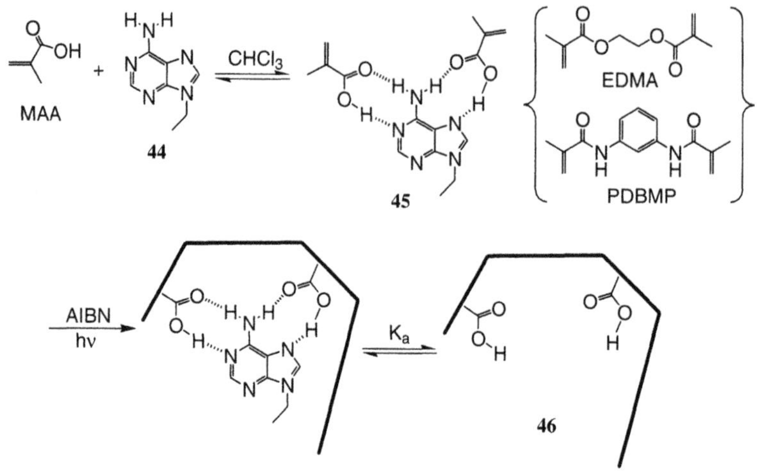

FIGURE 3.31 Molecular imprinting by methacrylic acid (MAA). MAA and adenine derivative (44) were preorganized to form complex (45) and polymerization was carried out in the
presence of cross-linking agents, ethylene glycol dimethacrylate (EDMA) and *N,N′*-1,3-
phenylenebis(2-propenamide) (PDBMP) to produce a binding cavity (46) for (44) on the solid
support.[129]

polymer matrixes can be used as selective absorbents for separation or chromatography and as catalysts.[129] In rare cases polymerization of preorganized monomers is not
needed; already-polymerized polymers having functional groups can be used as
polymeric hosts in molecular imprinting. Moreover, natural polymers can also be
used. Protein, such as albumin, can be regarded as a random copolymer of various
amino acids. It can be used, like a catalytic antibody, as a polymeric host of molecular imprinting for a transition state analogue of a reaction to show catalytic activity
of the reaction[131] (Figure 3.32).

Miyata et al. also reported a "shape-memory-like effect" as a soft molecular imprinting was observed in hydrogel systems using antigen–antibody recognition[132]
(see Chapter 9). Yashima and coworkers reported a memorization phenomenon on
the helicity of a helix-forming polymer by hydrogen bonding[133] (Figure 3.33). *Cis-
transoidal* poly[(4-carboxyphenyl)acetylene] (structure 47) forms a stable
left-handed helix in the presence of a chiral amine *(R)*-48. The addition of an excess
amount of another chiral amine *(S)*-49 to the 47–*(R)*-48 complex induced dynamic
transition into a right-handed helix. The left-handed helical conformation was still
observed after the addition of an excess amount of achiral amine 50 to the complex.
The one-handed helical conformation of 47 induced by *(R)*-48 was memorized even
after the *(R)*-48 was replaced by achiral 50. Thus, they succeeded in producing one-
handed helicity from achiral molecules.

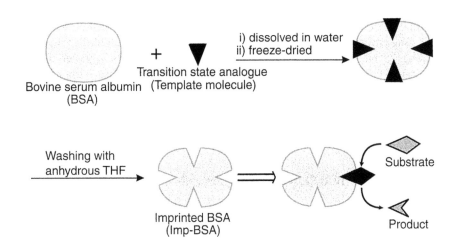

FIGURE 3.32 The preparation of imprinted bovine serum albumin (Imp-BSA) and the reaction catalyzed by it.[131]

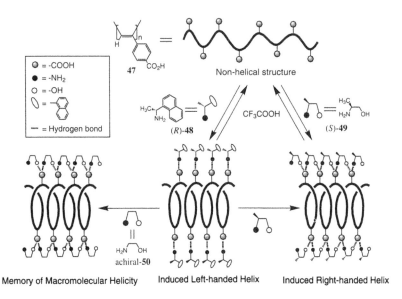

FIGURE 3.33 Induced one-handed helicity in polymer (47) and the memory of macromolecular helicity (see text).[133]

A hydrogen bonded closed association in a polymeric system was also reported.[134,135] Chitosan, a deacetylated derivative of chitin, is insoluble in water and organic solvents because of the formation of strong intermolecular hydrogen bonding.[136] Chitosan grafted with highly water-soluble PEG, PEG-grafted chitosan (chitosan-g-PEG), formed a nanometer scale aggregate in aqueous solution through interchain hydrogen bonding[134] (Figure 3.34). As an aggregate constructed by hydrogen bonding, it is expected to incorporate water-soluble polar substances. Indeed, the possibility of using such an aggregate as a carrier for a peptide drug delivery system was also reported using insulin as a model peptide drug.[135]

3.5 TOWARD BIOLOGICAL FUNCTIONS

3.5.1 BIOLOGICAL FUNCTIONS

Most biological processes are performed by noncovalent molecular organization and proteins having specific three-dimensional structures. Accordingly, artificial supramolecular architectures constructed by noncovalent interactions including hydrogen bonding have great potential to achieve various biological functions.

Biological functions in a biological system are catalytic activities, including transportation of chemicals, transmission of information, and energy conversions. From the standpoint of biomaterials science, typical examples of biological functions are biocompatibility, blood compatibility, pharmaceutical activity (e.g., inhibition or acceleration of specific enzymes), and drug delivery system. A small number of biological functions in the biomaterials science field have been achieved by supramolecular approaches.

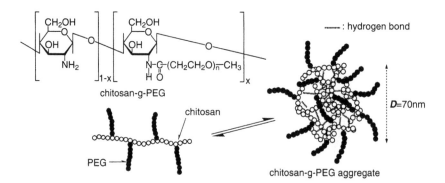

FIGURE 3.34 Structure of PEG-grafted chitosan (chitosan-g-PEG) and its formation of hydrogen bonding-directed aggregate in aqueous solution.[134] Molecular weights of chitosan and PEG are 1.5×10^5 and 5.0×10^3, respectively. The degree of introduction of PEG was 25 mol%/sugar unit. The diameter of the aggregate (D) was estimated to be about 70 nm by dynamic light scattering.

Many hydrogen bonding-directed supramolecular assembly systems have been studied as biomimetic systems such as artificial receptors and enzyme-like catalysis.[7,15,16,103-106] Some examples, such as artificial proteins,[38-48] artificial ion channels,[82] and self-assembled clathrate compounds[94,108-111] have already been introduced. Self-replication systems as special catalytic reaction systems and photo-induced energy/electron transfer systems as energy transmission/conversion systems aiming at an artificial photosynthetic system are introduced as two more examples of hydrogen bonding-directed supramolecular assemblies.

3.5.2 SELF-REPLICATION

The most important feature of life is its ability to replicate itself. While the "primordial soup" of prebiotic earth may have been the origin of life, synthetic designs of self-replicating molecules have been researched. Template effects, as observed in the autocatalytic process of nucleic acid replication, lead to reduced activation entropies or stabilized intermediates. In 1986, von Kiedrowski showed that self-complementary oligo-DNA could act as a template for its own formation, even without the aid of enzymes, as the first abiotic self-replication system.[137] The complementary trideoxynucleotides CCG and CGG were coupled in the presence of a water-soluble condensation reagent to form the self-complementary hexadeoxynucleotide by an autocatalytic process through the template effect with complementary hydrogen bonding. Although this approach to self-replication system uses a part of biological molecules, von Kiedrowski also reported another self-replication system using totally synthetic molecules.[138]

Rebek and coworkers reported a series of studies on self-replication systems[139-144] (Figure 3.35). Kemp's triacid derivative (structure 51) can recognize and bind the adenine derivative (structure 52) to give the complex (structure 53). This complex is stabilized by the hydrogen bonding and π–π stacking interaction of the adenine residue of 52 with the imide and naphthalene groups of 51. The arrangement in the complex 53 allows access of the activated ester of 51 to the amino group of 52, and formation of a *cis* amide bond between 51 and 52 occurs to produce 54. Compound 54, having *cis* amide linkage, spontaneously isomerizes into a more stable *trans* isomer 55. The isomerization provides two new binding sites on 55 for 51 and 52. Compound 55 must be the bisubstrate reaction template for 51 and 52 in the ternary complex. Since the product of the reaction between 51 and 52 is 55, the formation of 55 is autocatalytic and self-replicating. The kinetics (competition, inhibition, and reciprocal template effects) of this system have been well studied.[142-144]

3.5.3 ELECTRON AND ENERGY TRANSFER SYSTEMS

The construction of an artificial photosynthetic system is one of the ultimate goals in supramolecular biomimetic chemistry. The structure of a light-harvesting complex of photosynthetic bacteria was revealed in 1995.[145] In such natural photosynthetic systems, chlorophyll molecules are arranged noncovalently with suitable distances and geometries, and they enable highly efficient photo-induced energy and

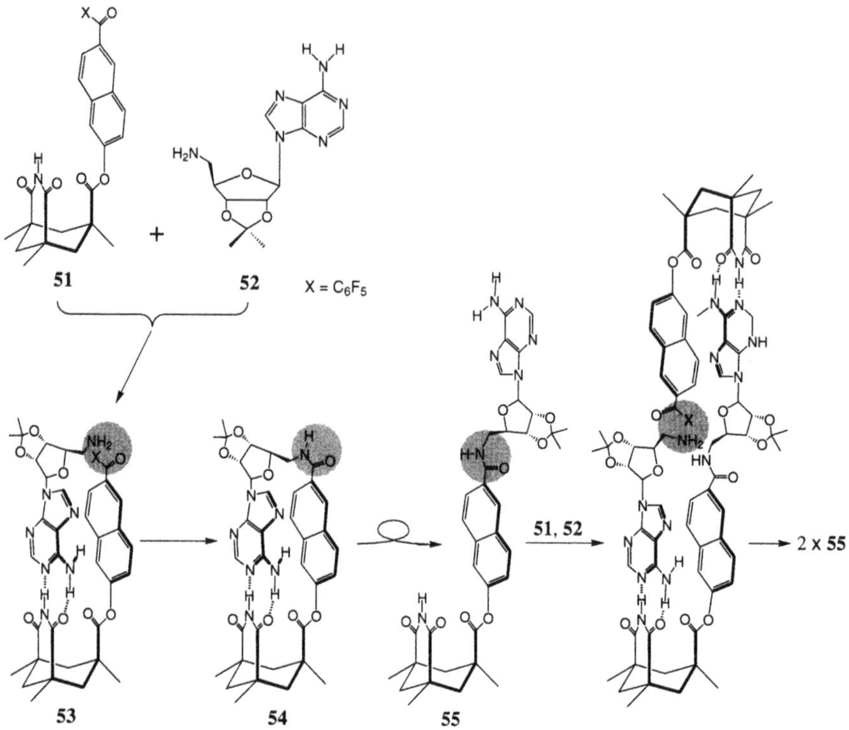

FIGURE 3.35 The construction of a self-replicating system based on adenine recognition through hydrogen bonding and amide formation.[141]

electron transfer reactions. Light trapped by chlorophyll molecules in an extensive antenna system is channeled via singlet excitation energy transfer to a reaction center containing a "special pair" of chlorophylls, in which a charge separation state is produced by a series of electron transfers. Many researchers have investigated energy and electron transfer behaviors between photo-energy donors and acceptors or electron donors and acceptors assembled via hydrogen bonding as models of photosynthetic systems.[146-152] Sessler and coworkers studied photo-induced electron transfer behaviors in porphyrin–porphyrin and porphyrin–quinone systems assembled via hydrogen bonding using nucleotide base analogues in an organic solvent.[147-150] A guanosine-substituted Zn–porphyrin donor (structure 56) and a cytidine-substituted quinone acceptor (structure 57) form the assembly and photo-induced electron transfer can be observed (Figure 3.36).

Since the DNA duplex has a rich π-electron system of bases stacked upon each other, there has been an argument for the kinetics of electron transfer through the DNA duplex and the conductivity of the DNA duplex.[153-157] The labeling of DNAs with fluorescent probes and the measurements of energy transfer behavior between

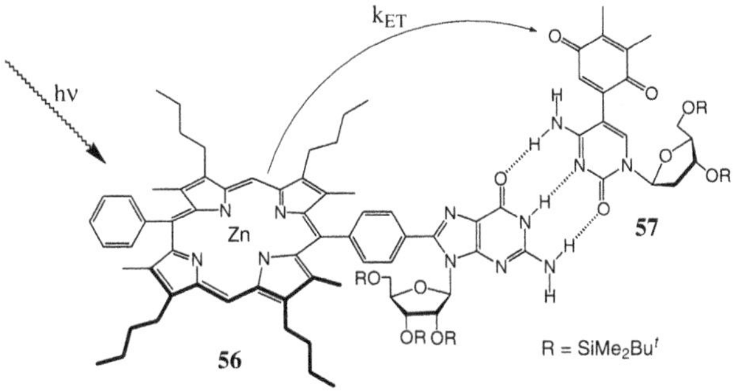

FIGURE 3.36 Photo-induced electron transfer from Zn–porphyrin to quinone assembled by hydrogen bonds using a guanosine-substituted porphyrin donor (56) and a cytidine-substituted quinone acceptor (57).[147]

the probes have been investigated[158-163] for detection of specific genes by duplex or triplex formulation of DNAs. As mentioned in section 3.4.2, oligonucleotides are useful for construction of programmed sequential arrangements of functional groups or molecules in aqueous media. Using oligo-DNAs, a variety of noncovalent binding pairs (binding donors and binding acceptors) with high specificity can easily be provided by varying the sequences of the oligo-DNAs. Multistep fluorescence resonance energy transfer (FRET) in aqueous media has been investigated in noncovalent supramolecular assembly systems using oligo-DNA as a specific molecular glue[164,165] (Figure 3.37). Three kinds of chromophores (photo-energy donor, mediator, and acceptor), were attached to 5′-terminals of 10 residues of oligo-DNAs to yield chromophore/oligo-DNA conjugates (structures 58, 59, and 60). The sequential arrays of chromophores in the donor–(mediator)$_n$–acceptor (n = 1,2) arrangement along the DNA duplexes 61 and 62 were constructed by mixing the oligo-DNA/chromophore conjugates with complementary matrix oligo-DNA in aqueous solution (Figure 3.37). In the chromophore arrays, chromophores were aligned on the same side of the DNA duplex (because 10 residues = 1 pitch of helix) in the energy level order. Multistep and long-distance photo-induced energy transfer behavior from the donor to the acceptor through n mediators was observed. Such a system can be a good model for an artificial photo-harvesting system.

3.6   SUMMARY AND PERSPECTIVES

Hydrogen bonding is one of the most important interactions required to construct functional supramolecular architectures. The control of open and closed self-assemblies via hydrogen bonding has been achieved to an extent. The geometrically strict arrangement of hydrogen bonds is useful for the construction of well-organized architectures having programmed structures; however, we must consider the other interactions involvd in the architectures. Although the functions of the self-organized

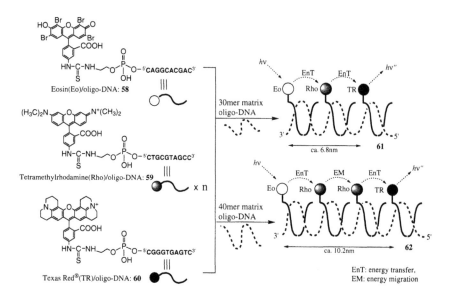

FIGURE 3.37 The construction of sequential chromophore arrays by using chromophore/oligo-DNA conjugates and complementary matrix oligo-DNAs, and their multistep and long-range photo-induced energy transfers.[164,165] Eosin (Eo), tetramethylrhodamine (Rho), and Texas Red® (TR) were employed as energy donor, mediator, and acceptor, respectively, and attached to the 5′-terminals of 10 residues of oligo-DNAs to yield conjugates (58), (59), and (60). Sequential chromophore arrays (61) and (62) were constructed by mixing these conjugates with 30 or 40 residues of matrix oligo-DNA having complementarity with the conjugates.

supramolecular architectures obtained here may still be primitive in contrast to natural biological systems, such as photosynthetic systems, cells, and organs, we succeeded in simulating some essential functions of biological systems.

The next step of hydrogen bonding-directed supramolecular architecture in research should be to take the systems out of the laboratory. At present, small numbers of hydrogen bonding-directed supramolecular architectures are applied in industrial uses. A system that detects specific genes or single nucleotide polymorphisms (SNPs) of DNAs[161-163,166-168] is one of the few examples (see Chapter 13). Hydrogen bonding-directed supramolecular architecture has expanded from the solid state to the liquid and liquid–crystalline states, and from nonaqueous solutions to aqueous solutions, and approaches biological activity. The author strongly believes that supramolecular architectures constructed by intermolecular forces including hydrogen bonding will be used in biological, medical, and industrial situations in the near future.

REFERENCES

1. Pauling, L.C., *The Nature of the Chemical Bond*, Cornell University Press, Ithaca, 1939.
2. Pimentel, G.C. and McClellan, A.L., *The Hydrogen Bond*, Freeman, San Francisco, 1960.
3. Schuster, P., Ed., *The Hydrogen Bond — Recent Developments in Theory and Experiments*, Vols. I–III, North-Holland, Amsterdam, 1976.
4. Jeffrey, G.A. and Saenger, W., *Hydrogen Bonding in Biological Structures*, Springer, Berlin, 1994.
5. Jeffrey, G.A., *An Introduction to Hydrogen Bonding*, Oxford University Press, New York, 1997.
6. Huyskens, P.C., Luck, W.A., and Zeegers-Huyskens, T., Eds., *Intermolecular Forces,* Springer, Berlin, 1991, 31.
7. Lehn, J.-M., *Supramolecular Chemistry — Concepts and Perspectives*, VCH, Weinheim, 1995.
8. Vögtle, F., Ed., Comprehensive *Supramolecular Chemistry*, Vol. 2, *Molecular Recognition: Receptors for Molecular Guests,* Pergamon, New York, 1996.
9. Murakami, Y., Ed., *Comprehensive Supramolecular Chemistry*, Vol. 4, *Supramolecular Reactivity and Transport: Bioorganic Systems*, Pergamon, New York, 1996.
10. MacNicol, D.D., Toda, F., and Bishop, R., Eds., *Comprehensive Supramolecular Chemistry,* Vol. 6, *Solid-State Supramolecular Chemistry: Crystal Engineering*, Pergamon, New York, 1996.
11. Sauvage, J.-P. and Hosseini, M. W., Eds., *Comprehensive Supramolecular Chemistry,* Vol. 9, *Templating, Self-Assembly, and Self-Organization*, Pergamon, New York, 1996.
12. Desiraju, G.R., Ed., *The Crystal as a Supramolecular Entity,* John Wiley & Sons, Chichester, 1996.
13. Hamilton A.D., Ed., *Supramolecular Control of Structure and Reactivity*, John Wiley & Sons, Chichester, 1996.
14. Reinhoudt, D.N., Ed., *Supramolecular Materials and Technologies*, John Wiley & Sons, Chichester, 1996.
15. Schneider H.J. and Yatsimirsky, A., *Principles and Methods in Supramolecular Chemistry,* John Wiley & Sons, Chichester, 2000, 79.
16. Philip, D. and Stoddart, J.F., Self-assembly on natural and unnatural systems, *Angew. Chem. Int. Ed. Engl.*, 35, 1154, 1996.
17. Hamilton, W.C. and Ibers, J.A., *Hydrogen Bonding in Solids*, Benjamin, New York, 1968.
18. Newton, M.D., Jeffrey, G.A., and Takagi, S., Application of *ab-initio* molecular orbital calculation to the structure moieties of carbohydrates. 5. The geometry of the hydrogen bond, *J. Am. Chem. Soc.*, 101, 1997, 1979.
19. Marsh, R.E., Refinement of the crystal structure of glycin, *Acta Cryst.*, 11, 654, 1958.
20. Etter, M.C., Encoding and decoding hydrogen-bond patterns of organic compounds, *Acc. Chem. Res.*, 23, 120, 1990.
21. Aakeröy, C.B. and Seddon, K.R., The hydrogen bond and crystal engineering, *Chem. Soc. Rev.*, 23, 397, 1993.
22. Amabilino, D.B., Stoddart, J.F., and Williams, D.J., From solid-state structures and superstructures to self-assembly processes, *Chem. Mater.,* 6, 1159, 1994.

23. Bernstein, J. et al., Patterns in hydrogen bonding: functionality and graph set analysis in crystals, *Angew. Chem. Int. Ed. Engl.*, 34, 1555, 1995.
24. Desiraju, G.R., Supramolecular synthons in crystal engineering — a new organic synthesis, *Angew. Chem. Int. Ed. Engl.*, 34, 2311, 1995.
25. Weber, P.C. et al., Crystallographic and thermodynamic comparison of natural and synthetic ligands bound to streptavidin, *J. Am. Chem. Soc.*, 114, 3197, 1992.
26. Cantor, C.R. and Schimmel, P.R., *Biophysical Chemistry Part I: The Conformation of Biological Macromolecules*, Freeman, San Francisco, 1980.
27. Branden, C. and Tooze, J., *Introduction to Protein Structure*, Garland, New York, 1991.
28. Wada, A., α-Helix as an electric macro-dipole, *Adv. Biophys.*, 9, 1, 1976.
29. Shoemaker, K.R. et al., Test of the helix dipole model for stabilization of α helices, *Nature*, 326, 563, 1987.
30. Blagdon, D.E. and Goodman, M., Mechanisms of protein and polypeptide helix initiation, *Biopolymers*, 14, 241, 1975.
31. Ihara, S., Ooi, T., and Takahashi, S., Effects of salts on the nonequivalent stability of the α-helixes of isomeric block copolypeptides, *Biopolymers*, 21, 131, 1982.
32. Chou, P.Y. and Fasman, G.D., Conformational parameters for amino acids in helical, β-sheet, and random coil regions calculated from proteins, *Biochemistry*, 13, 211, 1974.
33. Hol, W.G.J., The role of the α-helix dipole in protein function and structure., *Prog. Biophys. Mol. Biol.*, 45, 149, 1985.
34. Hol, W.G.J., Van Duijnen, P.T., and Berendsen, H.J.C., The α-helix dipole and the properties of proteins, *Nature*, 273, 443, 1978.
35. Salemme, E.R. and Weatherford D.W., Conformational and geometrical properties of β-sheets in proteins. I. Parallel β-sheets, *J. Mol. Biol.*, 146, 101, 1981.
36. Salemme, E.R. and Weatherford D.W., Conformational and geometrical properties of β-sheets in proteins. II. Antiparallel and mixed β-sheets, *J. Mol. Biol.*, 146, 119, 1981.
37. Chou, K.-C. et al., Structure of β-sheets. Origin of the right-handed twist and the increased stability of antiparallel over parallel sheets, *J. Mol. Biol.*, 162, 89, 1982.
38. Sasaki, T. and Lieberman, M., Protein mimetics, in ref. 9, chap. 5.
39. Lee, D.H. and Ghadiri, M.R., Control of peptide architecture via self-assembly and self-organization processes, in ref. 11, chap. 12.
40. Tanaka, T. et al., *De novo* design and the synthesis of TIM barrel proteins, *J. Cell. Biochem.*, 14C, 233, 1990.
41. DeGrado, W.F., Wasserman, Z.R., and Lear, J.D., Protein design, a minimalist approach, *Science*, 243, 622, 1989.
42. Regan, L. and DeGrado, W.F., Characterization of a helical protein designed from first principles, *Science*, 241, 976, 1988.
43. Mutter, M. et al., Strategies for the *de novo* design of proteins, *Tetrahedron*, 44, 771, 1988.
44. Mutter, M. and Vuilleumier, S., A chemical approach to protein design — template-assembled synthetic proteins (TASP), *Angew. Chem. Int. Ed. Engl.*, 28, 535, 1989.
45. Tuchscherer, G. and Mutter, M., Template-assembled synthetic proteins, in ref. 9, chap. 6.
46. Sasaki, T. and Kaiser, E.T., Helichrome: synthesis and enzymatic activity of a designed hemeprotein, *J. Am. Chem. Soc.*, 111, 380, 1989.
47. Sasaki, T. and Kaiser, E.T., Synthesis and structural stability of helichrome as an artificial hemeprotein, *Biopolymers*, 29, 79, 1990.

48. Hahn, K.W., Klis, W.A., and Stewart, J.M., Design and synthesis of a peptide having chymotrypsin-like esterase activity, *Science*, 248, 1544, 1990.

49. Watson, J.D. and Crick, F.H.C., A structure for deoxyribose nucleic acid, *Nature*, 171, 737, 1953.

50. Saenger, W., *Principles of Nucleic Acid Structures*, Springer, New York, 1984.

51. Jonson, D.S. and Boger, D.L., DNA binding agents, in ref. 9, chap. 3.

52. Hoogsteen, K., The structure of crystals containing a hydrogen-bonded complex of 1-methylthymine and 9-methyladenine, *Acta Cryst.*, 12, 822, 1959.

53. Moser, H.E. and Dervan, P.B., Sequence-specific cleavage of double helical DNA by triple helix formation, *Science*, 238, 645, 1987.

54. Cooney, M. et al., Site-specific oligonucleotide binding represses transcription of the human c-*myc* gene *in vitro*, *Science*, 241, 456, 1988.

55. Beal, P.A. and Dervan, P.B., Second structural motif for recognition of DNA by oligonucleotide-directed triple-helix formation, *Science*, 251, 1360, 1991.

56. Helene, C., The antigene strategy: control of gene expression by triplex-forming-oligonucleotides, *Anticancer Drug Des.*, 6, 569, 1991.

57. Allsopp, R.C. et al., Telomere length predicts replicative capacity of human fibro-blasts, *Proc. Natl. Acad. Sci. U.S.A.*, 89, 10114, 1992.

58. Gottarelli, G., Masiero, S., and Spada, G.P., Self-assembly in organic solvents of a de-oxyguanosine derivative induced by alkali metal picrates, *J. Chem. Soc., Chem. Commun.*, 2555, 1995.

59. Tirumala, S. and Davis, J.T., Self-assembled ionophores. An isoguanosine-K^+ oc-tamer, *J. Am. Chem. Soc.*, 119, 2769, 1997.

60. Gottarelli, G. and Spada, G.P., Self-assembled columnar mesophases based on gua-nine-related molecules, in ref. 11, chap. 13.

61. Haseloff, J. and Gerlach, W.L., Simple RNA emzymes with new and highly specific endoribonuclease activities, *Nature*, 334, 585, 1988.

62. Giovannangeli, C., Sun, J.-S., and Helene, C., Nucleic acids: supramolecular struc-tures and rational design of sequence-specific ligands, in ref. 9, chap. 4.

63. French, A.D., Roughhead, W.A., and Miller, D.P., The structure of cellulose: charac-terization of the solid state, *ACS Symposium Series*, 340, 15, 1986.

64. Franks, F., Ed., *The Chemistry and Physics of Water, Complehensive Treatise*, Vols. 1–7, Plenum Press, New York, 1972–1980.

65. Kavanau, J.L., *Water and Solute–Water Interactions*, Holden-Day, San Francisco, 1964.

66. Jeffrey, G.A. and Saenger, W., Hydrogen bonding by the water molecule, in ref. 4, part IV.

67. Lu, D.R., Lee, S.J., and Park, K., Calculation of solvation interaction energies for pro-tein adsorption on polymer surfaces, *J. Biomat. Sci. Polym. Edn.*, 3, 127, 1991.

68. Sim, G.A., Robertson, J.M., and Goodwin, T.H., The crystal and molecular structure of benzoic acid, *Acta Cryst.*, 8, 157, 1955.

69. Bailey, M. and Brown, C.J., The crystal structure of terephthalic acid, *Acta Cryst.*, 22, 387, 1967.

70. Alcala, R. and Martinez-Carrera, S., Crystal structure of isophthalic acid, *Acta Cryst.*, B28, 1671, 1972.

71. Yang, J. et al., Hydrogen bonding control of self-assembly: simple isophthalic acid de-rivatives form cyclic hexameric aggregates, *Tetrahedr. Lett.*, 35, 3665, 1994.

72. Duchamp, D.J. and Marsh, R.E., Crystal structure of trimesic acid (benzene-1,3,5-tri-carboxylic acid), *Acta Cryst.*, B25, 5, 1969.

73. Herbstein, F.H., 1,3,5-Benzenetricarboxylic acid (trimesic acid) and some analogues, in ref. 10, chap. 3.

74. Mak, T.C.W. and Bracke, B.R.F., Hydroquinone clathrates and diamondoid host lattice, in ref. 10, chap. 2.

75. Fredericks, J.R. and Hamilton A.D., Hydrogen bonding control of molecular self-assembly: recent advances in design, synthesis, and analysis, in ref. 11, chap. 16.

76. Ermer, O., Fivefold-diamond structure of adamantane-1,3,5,7-tetracarboxylic acid, *J. Am. Chem. Soc.*, 110, 3747, 1988.

77. Copp, S.B., Subramanian, S., and Zaworotko, M.J., Supramolecular chemistry of [Mn(CO)$_3$(μ_3-OH)]$_4$: assembly of a cubic hydrogen-bonded diamondoid network with 1,2-diaminoethane, *J. Am. Chem. Soc.*, 114, 8719, 1992.

78. Copp, S.B., Subramanian, S., and Zaworotko, M.J., Supramolecular chemistry of [Mn(CO)$_3$(μ_3-OH)]$_4$ (M = manganese, rhenium): spontaneous strict self-assembly of distorted super-diamondoid networks that are capable of enclathrating acetonitrile, *J. Chem. Soc. Chem. Commun.*, 1078, 1993.

79. Lehn, J.-M. et al., Molecular ribbons from molecular recognition directed self-assembly of self-complementary molecular components, *J. Chem. Soc., Perkin Trans.*, 2, 461, 1992.

80. Ghadiri, M. R. et al., N.,Self-assembling organic nanotubes based on a cyclic peptide architecture, *Nature*, 366, 324, 1993.

81. Khazanovich, N. et al., Nanoscale tubular ensembles with specified internal diameters. Design of a self assembled nanotube with 13-Å pore, *J. Am. Chem. Soc.*, 116, 6011, 1994.

82. Ghadiri, M. R., Granja, J. R., and Buehler, L. K., Artificial transmembrane ion channels from self-assembling peptide nanotubes, *Nature*, 369, 301, 1994.

83. Fan, E. et al., Hydrogen-bonding control of molecular aggregation: self-complementary subunits lead to rod-shaped structures in the solid state, *J. Chem. Soc. Chem. Commun.*, 1251, 1995.

84. Seto, C.T. and Whitesides, G.M., Self-assembly based on the cyanuric acid-melamine lattice, *J. Am. Chem. Soc.*, 112, 6409, 1990.

85. Seto, C.T. and Whitesides, G.M., Self-assembly of hydrogen-bonded 2 + 3 supramolecular complex, *J. Am. Chem. Soc.*, 113, 712, 1991.

86. Mathias, J.P., Simanek, E.E., and Whitesides, G.M., Self-assembly through hydrogen bonding: peripheral crowing — a new strategy for the preparation of stable supramolecular aggregates based on parallel, connected CA$_3$•M$_3$ rosettes, *J. Am. Chem. Soc.*, 116, 4326, 1994.

87. Seto, C.T., Mathias, J.P., and Whitesides, G.M., Molecular self-assembly through hydrogen bonding: aggregation of five molecules to form a discrete supramolecular structure, *J. Am. Chem. Soc.*, 115, 1321, 1993.

88. Seto, C.T. and Whitesides, G.M., Molecular self-assembly through hydrogen bonding: supramolecular aggregates based on the cyanuric acid-melamine lattice, *J. Am. Chem. Soc.*, 115, 905, 1993.

89. Seto, C.T. and Whitesides, G.M., Synthesis, characterization, and thermodynamic analysis of a 1 + 1 self-assembling structure based on the cyanuric acid-melamine lattice, *J. Am. Chem. Soc.*, 115, 1330, 1993.

90. Mathias, J. P. et al., Self-assembly through hydrogen bonding: preparation of a supramolecular aggregate composed of ten molecules, *Angew. Chem. Int. Ed. Engl.*, 32, 1766, 1993.

91. Isaacs, L. et al., Self-assembling systems on scales from nanometers to millimeters: design and discovery, in ref. 14, chap. 1.

92. Simanek, E.E. et al., Cyanuric acid and melamine: a platform for the construction of soluble aggregates and crystalline materials, in ref. 11, chap. 17.

93. Lehn, J.-M. et al., Molecular recognition directed self-assembly of ordered supramolecular strands by cocrystallization of complementary molecular components, *J. Chem. Soc., Chem. Commun.,* 479, 1990.

94. Russell, V.A. et al., Nanoporous molecular sandwiches: pillared two-dimensional hydrogen-bonded networks with adjustable porosity, *Science,* 276, 575, 1997.

95. Eichhorst-Gerneer, K. et al., Self-assembly of a two-component hydrogen-bonded network: comparison of the two-dimensional structure observed by scanning tunneling microscopy and the three-dimensional crystal lattice, *Angew. Chem. Int. Ed. Engl.,* 35, 1493, 1996.

96. Fouquey, C., Lehn, J.-M., and Levelut, A.-M., Molecular recognition directed self-assembly of supramolecular liquid crystalline polymers from complementary chiral components, *Adv. Mater.,* 2, 254, 1990.

97. Gulik-Krzywicki, T., Fouquey, C., and Lehn, J.-M., Electron microscopic study of supramolecular liquid crystalline polymers formed by molecular-recognition-directed self-assembly from complementary chiral components, *Proc. Natl. Acad. Sci. U.S.A.,* 90, 163, 1993.

98. Yang, W. S. et al., Formation of mesophase by hydrogen bond-directed self-assembly between barbituric acid and melamine derivatives, *Synth. Metals,* 71, 2107, 1995.

99. Kotera, M., Lehn, J.-M., and Vigneron, J. P., Self-assembled supramolecular rigid rods, *Chem. Commun.,* 197, 1994.

100. Sijbesma, R.P. et al., Reversible polymers formed from self-complementary monomers using quadruple hydrogen bonding, *Science,* 278, 1601, 1997.

101. Ohya, Y. et al., Synthesis of symmetric oligo-DNA dimers and their formation of polymeric supramolecular assembly, *Chem. Lett.,* 447, 1996.

102. Takenaka, S., Funatsu, Y., and Kondo, H., Spontaneous formation of a molecular net assembly by using nucleotide complementarity, *Chem. Lett.,* 891, 1996.

103. Weber, E. and Vögtle, F., Introduction and historical perspective, in ref. 8, chap.1.

104. Schneider, H.-J. and Mohammad-Ari, A.K., Receptors for organic guest molecules: general principles, in ref. 8, chap. 3.

105. Bell, D.A. and Anslyn, E.V., Hydrogen-bonding receptors: open chain catalytic systems, in ref. 8, chap. 14.

106. Seel, C. and De Mendoza, J., From chloride katapinates to trinucleotide complexes: developments in molecular recognition of anionic species, in ref. 8, chap. 17.

107. Bruckner, D., Xie, L.Y., and Dolphin, D., Historical perspectives and general introduction, in ref. 9, chap. 1.

108. Wyler, R., de Mendoza, J., and Rebek, J., Jr., A synthetic cavity assembles through self-complementary hydrogen bonds, *Angew. Chem. Int. Ed. Engl.,* 32, 1699, 1993.

109. Heinz, T., Rudkevich, D.M., and Rebek. J., Jr., Pairwise selection of guests in a cylindrical molecular capsule of nanometer dimensions, *Nature,* 394, 764, 1998.

110. Martin, T., Obst, U., and Rebek, J., Jr., Molecular assembly and encapsulation directed by hydrogen bonding preferences and the filling of space, *Science,* 281, 1842, 1998.

111. Rivera, J.M., Martin, T., and Rebek. J., Jr., Chiral spaces: dissymmetric capsules through self-assembly, *Science,* 279, 1021, 1998.

112. Calama, M.C. et al., Libraries of non-covalent hydrogen bonded assemblies; combinational synthesis of supramolecular systems, *Chem. Commun.*, 1021, 1998.

113. Prins, L. J. et al., Complete asymmetric induction of supramolecular chirality in a hydrogen-bonded assembly, *Nature*, 398, 498, 1999.

114. Prins, L. J. et al., An enantiometrically pure hydrogen-bonded assembly, *Nature*, 408, 181, 2000.

115. MacGillivray, L.R. and Atwood, J.L., A chiral spherical molecular assembly held together by 60 hydrogen bonds, *Nature*, 389, 469, 1997.

116. Chen, J. and Seeman, N.C., Synthesis from DNA of a molecule with the connectivity of a cube, *Nature*, 350, 631, 1991.

117. Seeman, N.C., Construction of three-dimensional stick figures from branched DNA, *DNA Cell Biol.*, 10, 475, 1991.

118. Zhang, Y. and Seeman, N.C., Construction of a DNA-truncated octahedron, *J. Am. Chem. Soc.*, 116, 1661, 1994.

119. Winfree, E. et al., Design and self-assembly of two-dimensional DNA crystals, *Nature*, 394, 539, 1998.

120. Mao, C., Sun, W., and Seeman, N.C., Designed two-dimensional DNA holiday junction arrays visualized by atomic force microscopy, *J. Am. Chem. Soc.*, 121, 5437, 1999.

121. Bekturov, E.A. and Bimendina, L.A., Interpolymer complexes, *Adv. Polym. Sci.*, 41, 99, 1981.

122. Ohno, H., Abe, K., and Tsuchida, E., Solvent effect on the formation of poly (methacrylic acid)-poly(N-vinyl-2-pyrrolidone) complex through hydrogen bonding, *Macromol. Chem.*, 179, 755, 1978.

123. Bimendina, L.A., Roganov, V.V., and Bekturov, E.A., Hydrodynamic properties of complexes of polymethacrylic acid-polyvinylpyrrolidone, *J. Polym. Sci. Polym. Symp.*, 44, 65, 1974.

124. Nikolaev, A. F. et al., Interaction of polyacrylamide with polyacrylic acid, *Vysokomol. Soedin. Ser. B*, 21, 723, 1979.

125. Antipina, A. D. et al., Equilibrium during complexing of polymeric acids with polyethylene glycols, *Vysokomol. Soedin. Ser. A*, 14, 941, 1972.

126. Osada, Y. and Takeuchi, Y., Water and protein permeation through polymeric membrane having mechanochemically expanding and contracting pores. Function of chemical valve. I., *J. Polym. Sci. Polym. Lett. Ed.*, 19, 303, 1981.

127. Beginn, U. and Möller M., Supramolecular structures with macromolecules, in ref. 14, chap. 3.

128. Wulff, G., Molecular imprinting in cross-linked materials with the aid of molecular templates — a way towards artificial antibodies, *Angew. Chem. Int. Ed. Engl.*, 34, 1812, 1995.

129. Shea, K.J., Spivak, D.A., and Sellergren, B., Polymer complements to nucleotide bases, selective binding of adenine derivatives to imprinted polymers, *J. Am. Chem. Soc.*, 115, 3368, 1993.

130. Spivak, D., Gilmore, M.A., and Shea, K.J., Evaluation of binding and origins of specificity of 9-ethyladenine imprinted polymers, *J. Am. Chem. Soc.*, 119, 4388, 1997.

131. Ohya, Y., Miyaoka, J., and Ouchi, T., Recruitment of enzyme activity in albumin by molecular imprinting, *Macromol. Rapid Commun.*, 17, 871, 1996.

132. Miyata, T., Asami, N., and Uragami, T., A reversibly antigen-responsive hydrogel, *Nature*, 399, 766, 1999.

133. Yashima, E., Maeda, K., and Okamoto, Y., Memory of macromolecular helicity assisted by interaction with achiral small molecules, *Nature*, 399, 449, 1999.

134. Ohya, Y., Nishizawa, H., and Ouchi, T., Aggregation phenomenon of PEG-grafted chitosan in aqueous solution, *Polymer*, 39, 235, 1998.

135. Ohya, Y. et al., Preparation of PEG-grafted chitosan nanoparticles as peptide drug carriers, *STP Pharma Sci.*, 10, 77, 2000.

136. Ogawa, K. et al., A new polymorph of chitosan, *Macromolecules*, 17, 973, 1984.

137. von Kiedrowski, G., A self-replicating hexadeoxynucleotide, *Angew. Chem. Int. Ed. Engl.*, 25, 932, 1986.

138. Terfort, A. and von Kiedrowski, G., Self-replication by condensation of 3-amino-benzamidines and 2-formylphenoxyacetic acids, *Angew. Chem. Int. Ed. Engl.*, 31, 654, 1992.

139. Rebek, J., Jr., Molecular recognition with model systems, *Angew. Chem. Int. Ed. Engl.*, 29, 245, 1990.

140. Famulok, M., Nowick, J.S., and Rebek, J., Jr., Self-replicating systems, *Acta Chem. Scand.*, 46, 315, 1992.

141. Tjivikua, T., Ballester, P., and Rebek, J., Jr., A self-replicating system, *J. Am. Chem. Soc.*, 112, 1249, 1990.

142. Nowick, J.S. et al., Kinetic studies and modeling of a self-replicating system, *J. Am. Chem. Soc.*, 113, 8831, 1991.

143. Wintner, E.A., Conn, M.M., and Rebek, J., Jr., Studies in molecular replication, *Acc. Chem. Res.*, 27, 198, 1994.

144. Winter, E.A. and Rebek, J., Jr., Recent developments in the design of self-replicating systems, in ref. 13, chap. 5.

145. McDermott, G. et al., Crystal structure of an integral membrane light-harvesting complex from photosynthetic bacteria, *Nature*, 374, 517, 1995.

146. Sessler, J.L. et al., Electron and energy transfer reactions in noncovalently linked supramolecular model system, in ref. 9, chap.9.

147. Harriman, A., Kubo, Y., and Sessler, J.L., Molecular recognition via base pairing: photoinduced electron transfer in hydrogen-bonded zinc porphyrin-benzoquinone conjugates, *J. Am. Chem. Soc.*, 114, 388, 1992.

148. Sessler, J.L., Wang, B., and Harriman, A., Long-range photoinduced electron transfer in an associated but noncovalently linked photosynthetic model system, *J. Am. Chem. Soc.*, 115, 10418, 1993.

149. Sessler, J.L., Wang, B., and Harriman, A., Photoinduced energy transfer in associated but non-covalently linked photosynthetic model systems, *J. Am. Chem. Soc.*, 117, 704, 1995.

150. Berman, A. et al., Photoinduced intra-ensemble electron transfer in a base-paired porphyrin–quinone system. Time-resolved EPR spectroscopy, *J. Am. Chem. Soc.*, 117, 8252, 1995.

151. Osuka, A., et al., Electron transfer in a hydrogen-bonded assembly consisting of porphyrin-diimide, *Chem. Commun.*, 1567, 1998.

152. Pecilla, P. et al., Hydrogen-bonding self-assembly of multichromophore structures, *J. Am. Chem. Soc.*, 112, 9408, 1990.

153. Ratner, M., Electronic motion in DNA, *Nature*, 397, 480, 1999.

154. Wilson, E.K., DNA's conductance still confounds, *Chem. Eng. News,* 76, 51, 1998.

155. Murphy, C.J. et al., Long-range photoinduced electron transfer through a DNA helix, *Science*, 262, 1025, 1993.

156. Fukui, K. and Tanaka, K., Distance dependence of photoinduced electron transfer in DNA, *Angew. Chem. Int. Engl. Ed.*, 37, 158, 1998.

157. Meggers, E., Michael-Beyerle, M.E., and Giese, B., Sequence dependent long range hole transport in DNA, *J. Am. Chem. Soc.*, 120, 12950, 1998.

158. Cardullo, R.A. et al., Detection of nucleic acid hybridization by nonradiative fluorescence resonance energy transfer, *Proc. Natl. Acad. Soc. U.S.A.*, 85, 8790, 1988.

159. Mergny, J.L. et al., Fluorescence energy transfer between two triple helix-forming oligonucleotides bound to duplex DNA, *Biochemistry*, 33, 15321, 1994.

160. Magda, D. et al., Energy transfer assemblies composed of expanded porphyrin-oligonucleotide conjugates, *Tetrahedr. Lett.*, 38, 5759, 1997.

161. Morrison, L.E., Hadler, T.C., and Stols, L.M., Solution-phase detection of polynucleotides using interacting fluorescent labels and competitive hybridization, *Anal. Biochem.*, 183, 231, 1989.

162. Tyagi, S. and Kramer, F.R., Molecular beacons: probes that fluoresce upon hybridization, *Nature Biotech.*, 14, 303, 1996.

163. Horsey, I. et al., Double fluorescence resonance energy transfer to explore multicomponent binding interaction: a case study of DNA mismatches, *Chem. Commun.*, 1043, 2000.

164. Ohya, Y. et al., Sequential arrangement of chromophores and energy transfer behavior on oligonucleotides assemblies, *Polym. Adv. Technol.*, 11, 845, 2000.

165. Ohya, Y. et al., Sequential arrangement of chromophores and their energy transfer behavior on oligonucleotides assemblies, Paper PL-38b, in *Proc. 5th Int. Symp. Polym. Adv. Technol.*, Tokyo, 1999.

166. Elghanian, R. et al., Selective colorimetric detection of polynucleotides based on the distance-dependent optical properties of gold nanoparticles, *Science*, 277, 1078, 1997.

167. Taron, T.A., Mirkin, C.A., and Letsinger, R.L., Scanometric DNA array detection with nanoparticle probes, *Science*, 289, 1757, 2000.

168. Schena, M., Ed., *DNA Microarrays. A Practical Approach,* Oxford University Press, Oxford, 1999.

4 Electrostatic Interaction

Atsushi Maruyama

CONTENTS

4.1 INTRODUCTION

The electrostatic interaction involves ions, dipoles, and induced dipoles. Electrostatic interactions together with hydrophobic and hydrogen bonding interactions play pivotal roles in folding and molecular recognition of natural biomolecules. Even weak electrostatic interactions such as dipole/dipole and dipole/induced dipole interactions significantly contribute to these processes when overall contact area between the groups is considerable. The electrostatic interactions seen in the supramolecular formation and functional generation of natural biomolecules can offer guidance for the artificial design of biomaterials. Electrostatic interactions should be considered also when artificial biomaterials come in contact with natural biomolecules or biological systems.

Some electrostatic interactions are useful for artificial construction of biomaterials with supramolecular structures. While weak electrostatic interactions are hard to control, strong electrostatic interaction between ions, especially interactions between polyions, are relatively easy to manipulate. These interactions enable us to construct artificial materials having desirable structures and may control interactions of natural biomolecules and artificial biomaterials.

This chapter briefly describes the fundamentals of electrostatic interaction. Special attention is given to electrostatic interactions of multivalent ions (polyions and polyelectrolytes). Supramolecular formation of nucleic acids that are highly charged biomaterials is cited. The assembling of a polyion with an oppositely charged polyion is also described.

4.2 ELECTROSTATIC INTERACTIONS AND THEIR ROLES UPON NATURAL BIOMOLECULAR ASSEMBLING

The categories of electrostatic interactions are depicted in Figure 4.1. Coulomb's law describes the electrostatic interaction. The interaction (binding energy, $w(r)$) between two ions is expressed as:

$$w(r) = \frac{q_1 q_2}{4\pi\varepsilon_0\varepsilon_r r}$$

$$(1)$$

a)

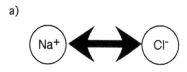

b)

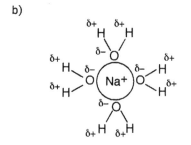

c)

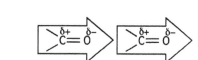

FIGURE 4.1 The electrostatic interactions between molecules/groups: (a) ion/ion interaction, (b) ion/dipole interaction, (c) dipole/dipole interaction, (d) dipole/induced dipole interaction, and (e) London force.

d)

e)

where q_1, q_2, are electric charges, r is the distance between the charges, ε_0 is the dielectric constant in vacuum, and ε is the relative dielectric constant of the medium. Ion/ion interaction is strong and long ranging. Since water has a considerably higher dielectric constant ($\varepsilon_{water}/\varepsilon_0 = 78.5$) than other solvents (e.g., $\varepsilon_{hexane}/\varepsilon_0 = 1.9$, $\varepsilon_{methanol}/\varepsilon_0 = 32.6$), the ion/ion interaction in a biological medium is weakened. Further, the electrostatic interactions of the ions are reduced by the dipoles of water molecules in biological media. The interior of a protein has a dielectric constant ranging $\varepsilon_{proteinr, in}/\varepsilon_0 = 2$ to 3 and this allows strong ion/ion interactions. The contribution made by ion/ion interactions to protein folding is not large, however, because ion/ion interaction energy compensates for the dehydration energy of the ionic groups. Thus, ionic groups of proteins rarely form ion pairs in protein cores, and most ionic groups are preferentially located on the surfaces of proteins.[1,2]

The ion/dipole interaction between charge 1 and dipole 2 is:

$$w(r) = -\frac{q_1^2 \mu_2^2}{4\pi\varepsilon_0\varepsilon_r r^2}$$

(2)

where, $\mu 2$ is the dipole moment of dipole 2. This interaction is commonly involved in ion/solvent interaction. Water is a good solvent for a variety of salts due to the strong electrostatic interaction between ionic charges and dipoles of water. The ion/dipole interaction accounts for a major part of the hydration enthalpy of cations such as Li^+ and Na^+, while other interactions are involved in hydration enthalpy of proton and anions.

The electrostatic interaction between permanent dipoles is:

$$w(r) = -\frac{\mu_1\mu_2}{4\pi\varepsilon_0\varepsilon_r r^3}$$

(3)

The dipole/dipole interaction is much weaker than the ion/ion interaction and is strongly affected by the distance between dipoles which is inversely proportional to r^3. The interaction, however, is capable of contributing to the assembling structures of proteins when a segment of the protein takes an α-helical conformation.[1] All consecutive peptide bonds and all hydrogen interactions point in the same direction in α helices. A strong dipole moment, a macrodipole, builds up along the helix axis, with a positive pole at the N terminus (Figure 4.2). The interaction of the macrodipoles becomes considerable in the protein core where the dielectric constant is low. The macrodipoles of helical peptides also contribute to the specific interactions of DNA-binding proteins.[3] Binding of a macrodipole with a single negative charge (a phosphate) contributes an attractive energy of about 12 kcal/mol. Assuming that water molecules that must be replaced consume about 0.2 kcal/mole, the net attraction is still considerable.[4]

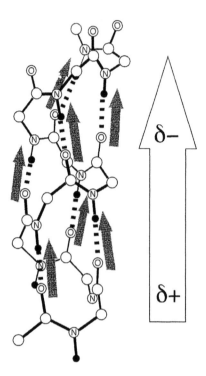

FIGURE 4.2 Macrodipole generation on a helical peptide.

Very weak electrostatic interaction takes place even with nonpolar groups or molecules owing to induced dipole interaction or London dispersion force. Nonpolar groups are weakly polarized in the electric field from adjacent ionic charges or dipoles, leading to electrostatic interaction between them.

The London dispersion force is an electrostatic interaction observed between nonpolar groups. Heterogeneous or wobble distribution of an electron causes instantaneous dipole formation of nonpolar groups. The instantaneous dipole induces polarization of adjacent molecules, leading to a very weak dipole/dipole interaction. The London dispersion force is inversely proportional to r^6, so that it only acts on groups contacting each other. The interaction is, hence, an influential factor determining protein conformations because a number of groups are in contact in folded protein structures. Similarly, assembling and recognition of macromolecules largely rely on the London dispersion forces. The interactions between uncharged molecules such as dipole/dipole, dipole/induced dipole, and London dispersion forces construct the van der Waals interaction between molecules.

4.3   COUNTERION CONDENSATION ON POLYIONS

Polyions (or polyelectrolytes) that have multivalent ionic groups along their polymer chains show inherent characteristics different from noncharged or low charged polymers. Polyions are classified into three categories: polycations, polyanions, and polyampholytes. Polyampholytes are ionic polymers having both positive and negatively charged groups, whereas polycations and polyanions have positively and negatively charged groups, respectively. Polycations and polyanions have extended chain conformations owing to repulsive forces among homologously charged groups; polyampholytes have compact conformations due to attractive forces between the opposite charges. High charge density is another intrinsic characteristic of polyions. The high density of charged groups along the backbones of polyions (polycations or polyanions) attracts many counterions to its immediate neighborhood (counterion condensation).[5-8] The fraction (ψ) of counterion condensed per polyion charge is:

$$\psi = 1\frac{1}{\xi} \quad \left(\xi = \frac{e^2}{\varepsilon kTb}, 0 \le \psi \ge 1 \right)$$

(4)

where e is the magnitude of the electronic charge, k is Boltzmann's constant, T is the absolute temperature, ε ($= \varepsilon_0\varepsilon_r$) is the bulk dielectric constant, and b is the axial ionic group distance along the polyion and equal to L/P (L is the contour length, end-to-end distance in the state of maximum extension, of the polyion; P is the number of charged groups). Therefore, ψ is a function of the linear charge densities of the polyions. The calculated values of ψ for polyions are 0.46 for sodium [poly(vinyl sulfate)] in aqueous NaBr; 0.65 for potassium [poly(styrenesulfonate)] in aqueous KBr; 0.56 and 0 for sodium [poly(acrylate)] with a (fraction of ionized groups = 0.8 and 0.3, respectively).

The condensation of counterions affects the free energy changes accompanying the assembling and supramolecular formation of polyions. For example, supramolecular formation, i.e., order–disorder transition, of nucleotides is strongly influenced by the counterion condensation effect. As shown in Figure 4.3, double-stranded (ds) DNAs have higher linear density of phosphate groups than single-stranded (ss) DNAs. Hence, ψ for ds DNA ($\psi = 0.76$) is higher than that for ss DNA ($\psi = 0.42$),[9] indicating that accumulation of counterions is accompanied by coil-to-helix transition of DNAs. The accumulation of the counterions in medium with low or physiologic ionic strength is an entropy-consuming process that is thermodynamically unfavorable for ds DNA formation (Figure 4.4). Conversely, the ds DNA with high counter-ion condensation can be stabilized by an increase in the ionic strength of the medium.

The helix-coil transitions of DNAs as well as other transition of supramolecular assemblies can be featured by transition temperature Tm, which denotes thermal stability of the assemblies. The Tm of DNA increased with increasing the ionic strenth of the medium. Values of the Tm of T4 DNA are 42.6, 61.6, and 81.2°C, respectively, at NaCl concentrations of 10^{-3}, 10^{-2}, and 10^{-1} M.[9]

Counterion Condensation (CC) Theories:
The high electrostatic potential from a polyion results in the accumulation of counterions in the immediate vicinity of the polyion

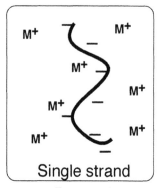

Single strand

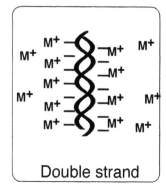

Double strand

ψ : Fraction of counterion thermodynamically associated
per phosphate and function of linear charge density;

$$\psi_{ss} < \psi_{ds}$$

FIGURE 4.3 The counterion condensation effect in supramolecular formation involving polyion components. Change in counterion condensation accompanying helix-coil transition is depicted. Counterion condensation affects assembling and/or conformational changes of polyion.

State with higher counterion condensation is unstable under lower ionic strength condition

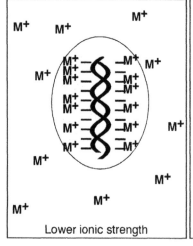

Lower ionic strength

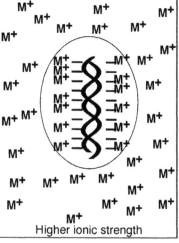

Higher ionic strength

FIGURE 4.4 Salt effects on polyionic supermolecules. Medium with higher ionic strength stabilizes a state with higher counterion condensation.

The ionic strength dependency of the helix-coil transition of DNA is described as:

$$dTm/dlog[Na^+] = 0.9\ (2.303RTm^2/\Delta H)\ (Nu\Delta\psi) \qquad (5)$$

where ΔH is the transition enthalpy, R is the gas constant (cal/mol•K), and Nu is the number of phosphates per cooperative transition unit.[10] The ratio $RTm^2/\Delta H$ has been found experimentally to be constant.[10] Thus, the linear relationship between Tm and log[Na$^+$] is expected. Indeed, thermal melting behavior of a variety of DNAs and RNAs obeys the relation expressed by Equation (5). The difference ($\Delta\psi$) in the counterion condensation between two states could be estimated from a slope of the plot of Tm vs. log[Na$^+$].

As described above, the counterion condensation effect is an obstacle for double helix formation. Alleviation of the counterion condensation effect has been indicated as a strategy to achieve stable double helix formation. For example, several types of nucleic acid mimics with lower charge densities or without charged groups have been prepared and examined for hybrid formation. Among such mimics, peptide nucleic acid (PNA) was demonstrated to form stable double helical and triple helical structures.[11,12] The effect of the counterion condensation upon double helical formation involving PNA was estimated by following the salt dependency of Tm.[13] While a native DNA/DNA duplex resulted in a positive slope in Tm vs. log[Na$^+$] plot for helix-coil transition, the DNA/PNA duplex showed a slightly negative slope. The positive slope obtained for DNA/DNA is characteristic of the counterion association process that takes place upon DNA helix formation (see Figure 4.8). Conversely, the slight slope observed for DNA/PNA indicates scarce involvement of the counterion condensation effect in helix formation. This is reasonable because helix formation with uncharged PNA does not cause considerable change in charge density between the coil and helix states.

The theoretical model describing order-disorder transition of polyions was further elaborated by Record et al. Their model takes into account two structural quantities: b, the average spacing between polyion charges projected onto the axis of the cylindrical polyion; and a, the distance of closest approach between the center of a small ion and the polyion axis.[14]

4.4 PROPERTIES OF POLYION COMPLEXES (INTERPOLYELECTROLYTE COMPLEXES)

Mixing solutions containing two oppositely charged polyions results in polyion (interpolyelectrolyte) complex formation. The complexes are separated out of the solution as precipitates, hydrogels, and coacervates (droplets separated out of solution). The coacervates consisting of polyion complexes are termed *complex coacervates*, to distinguish them from *simple coacervates* consisting of single polymers due to solubility limits. Polyion complexes in the form of complex coacervation can be prepared by mixing very diluted polyion solutions.

The pioneering observation of polyion complex formation βs was made by Bungenberg and coworkers in the 1930s.[15] During exhaustive studies on the interactions between several natural hydrophilic polymers in aqueous media, they found that certain water-soluble polymers containing ionizable groups were capable of co-reacting with one another in water solution to form complex coacervates. The nature and extent of the reactions were found to be sensitive to temperature, pH, and the ionic strength of the media. The interaction between a strongly acidic polyanion sodium [poly(styrenesulfonate)] and a strongly basic polycation [poly(N-methyl-4-vinylpyridinium chloride)] was reported by Fuoss and Sadek in 1949.[17] They found that the interaction between these two polyions yielded a colloidal precipitate rather than a coacervate. The complex formed rapidly and yielded a product containing essentially stoichiometric equivalents of the consisting polyions.

Michaels et al. studied the interaction between sodium [poly(styrenesulfonate)] and poly(vinylbenzyl trimethylammonium chloride) and the nature of the resulting complexes.[18] The exact stoichiometry was further confirmed in their study. The complex contained virtually no counterions (Na$^+$ and Cl$^-$) initially associated with the polyions (if the ionic strength of medium was very low). Nonstoichiometric and soluble polyion complexes were reported later.[19,20] The soluble complex can be obtained when one of the constituting polyions (host polyion, HP) has a higher degree of polymerization than the other (guest polyion, GP), and the former is added in excess ($\varphi = $ [GP]/[HP] based on charged units < 1).[21] Under conditions of critical composition ($\varphi_c < 1$), water soluble nonstoichiometric complexes in which the content of GP units is lower than that of HP form (Figure 4.5). Under these conditions, the guest polyions are evenly distributed among the host polyions.

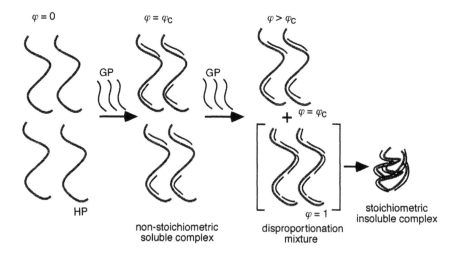

FIGURE 4.5 Formation of nonstoichiometric soluble and stoichiometric insoluble polyion complexes between host (HP) and guest (GP) polyions.

TABLE 4.1
General Properties of Interpolyelectrolyte Complex

Physicochemical properties

Insolubility in common solvents
Infusibility
Plasticizability by water and electrolytes
Highly specific; limited water absorption
Transparency of flexible solid when wet
Selectivity of ion sorption and ion exchange properties

Electrical properties

High dielectric constant and loss factor when wet and ion doped
Dielectric properties very sensitive to moisture and ion content

Transport properties

Highly permeable to water
Highly permeable to electrolytes and other water-soluble microsolutes
Impermeable to macrosolutes

When the composition φ exceeds φ_c, two populations of nonstoichiometric and stoichiometric complexes that differ in composition and solubility present simultaneously (disproportionation mixture). The nonstoichiometric polyion complex with the critical composition ($\varphi = \varphi_c$) remains in solution, while the stoichiometric complex precipitates. As the concentration of GP further increases, additional GP molecules result in an increase in the insoluble stoichiometric complex. The portion of the stoichiometric complex increases, while that of the nonstoichiometric complex decreases. When the unit molar concentrations of HP and GP in the system become equal ($\varphi = 1$), all the HPs are involved in formation of the stoichiometric complex. Further increase in the concentration of the GP may lead to recharging of the complex and its dissolution. Under these conditions, the polyion complex particles are stabilized in solution because of the excess charges of GP bound to HP. The critical composition φ_c relies on the ionic strength of the medium, species of salt, and properties, especially hydrophobicity, of both polycations and polyanions. The general properties of polyion complexes are summarized in Table 4.1.[16]

4.5 EFFECT OF COUNTERION CONDENSATION ON POLYION COMPLEX FORMATION

The polyion complex formation is rarely driven by enthalpy change. Formation and stability of polyion complexes are closely related to the release of counterions from polyions. As shown in Figure 4.3, the high electrostatic potential from the polyions results in the accumulation of counterions in the immediate vicinity of the polyions to partially neutralize the backbone charge. Even after condensation of the counterions, relatively high electropotential remains around the polyions. The remaining electropotential causes further association of additional counterions (screening ions) that screen remaining unneutralized charges.[5]

The interaction of oppositely charged ligands causes a perturbation of the electrostatic potential surrounding the polyions. This perturbation leads to release of a fraction of the thermodynamically associated counterions, condensed and screening ions, into the bulk solution. The release of these counterions into a solution of low salt concentration causes a net increase in the entropy of the system, thus providing a major favorable component to interaction free energy (Figure 4.6). Thus, release of both condensation and screening ions contribute to binding of the oppositely charged ligand to the polyion. This explanation is supported by the fact that the polyion complex is destabilized markedly with increasing ionic strength of the medium.

The interaction between DNA and oligomeric cations such as oligomers of lysine and arginine were documented in detail as a model of DNA/nuclear protein interaction,[22-24] and may be a good example for considering the fundamentals of polyion complex formation. Consider the interaction of a small cationic ligand (L) with a nucleic acid (P) in which association involves the formation of z ion pairs. We neglect anion binding to the ligand (Figure 4.6). The binding reaction of L to P is written as:

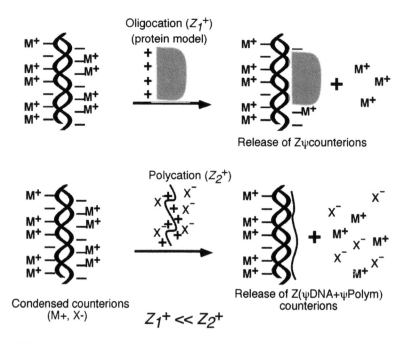

FIGURE 4.6 Complex formation of a polyanion and small or large cationic molecules. Release of counterions thermodynamically associated with the polyion(s) is the major driving force for complex formation.

$$L + P \, (z \, \text{sites}) \xrightleftharpoons{K} LP + z\psi_{c+s}M^+$$

(6)

where K is a thermodynamic equilibrium constant that is a function of temperature and pressure only and not of ion concentrations, ψ_{c+s} is the fraction of a counterion (bound in the thermodynamic sense) per polyanion charge and the sum of condensed and screening effects, and M^+ is the counterion of P.[25] ψ_{c+s}, like ψ_c, is also a function of the linear charge densities of the polyions and is expressed as:

$$\psi_{c+s} = 1 - \frac{1}{2\xi}$$

(7)

For example, the magnitudes of ψ_{c+s} are 0.88 and 0.71, respectively, for ds DNA and ss DNA.

As experimentally determined, the observed equilibrium constant K_{obs} is written as:

$$K_{obs} = \frac{[LP]}{[L][P]}$$

(8)

The variation of K_{obs} with M^+ concentration is expressed as:

$$-\frac{\partial \log K_{obs}}{\partial \log[M^+]} = z\psi_{c+s}$$

(9)

Experimental data coincided well with the relationship expressed by Equation (9). The ionic strength dependency, K_{obs} vs. $\log[Na^+]$, of oligolysine binding to DNA [poly(A)•poly(U)] appears as a family of straight lines (Figure 4.7). The slopes of these lines increase in magnitude in direct proportion to the chain length N of the oligolysines:[25]

$$-\frac{\partial \log K_{obs}}{\partial \log[M^+]} = (0.9 \pm 0.05)N$$

(10)

The proportional constant in Equation (10) was close to the ψ_{c+s} value for poly(A)•poly(U) ($\psi_{c+s} = 0.89$). The entropic effect of counterion release therefore makes a major contribution to the overall free energy of the formation of complexes between polynucleotides (RNA and DNA in ds or ss state) and the oligolysine model ligands of the multivalent cations. It is possible to estimate the number of ion pairs participating in ligand binding if the ψ values of the polyion are known. A linear

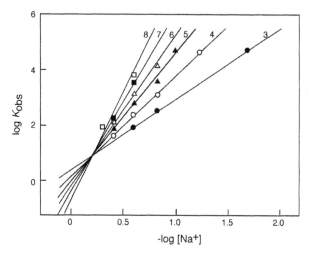

FIGURE 4.7 Log–log plot of apparent association constants K_{obs} for the interaction of poly(A)•poly(U) with oligolysines of the type of ε-dinitrophenyllysine(lys)n as functions of Na^+ concentration. Values of n are indicated on the figure. Reproduced from Reference 25 (Record, M.T., Jr., Lohman, T.M., and Haseth, P.D., *J. Mol. Biol.,* 107, 145, 1976, with permission).

function of log K_{obs} vs. log[M^+] was also reported for the binding of charged oligopeptides to heparin.[26]

In the case of a polycationic ligand such as polylysine, release of counterions from the polycation ligand should be considered (Figure 4.6), and Equation (8) is rewritten as:

$$-\frac{\partial \log K_{obs}}{\partial \log[M^+]} = z(\Psi_{c+s,\,PC} + \Psi_{c+s,\,PA})$$

(11)

where $\Psi_{c+s,PC}$ and $\Psi_{c+s,PA}$, respectively, indicate contribution from the polycation (PC) and polyanion (PA). Consequently, the complex of polyanion and polycation is further stabilized by the release of counterions from both components (Figure 4.6). However, binding constants for these complexes are only estimated because of the extraordinarily high binding affinities and insolubilities of the complexes. In the case of polyion/polyion complexes, other factors such as the release of water molecules from the polyions and conformational change of the complexes should be involved in overall free energy change of the system.

The interaction of DNA with polylysine was initially studied by observing the melting behavior of ds DNA.[27] A dilute salt solution containing polylysine and DNA produced a bimodal transition when the lysine/nucleotide ratio was less than one. The first transition was identical to that of free DNA, and the second transition at a higher temperature corresponded to the melting of a polylysine/polynucleotide complex. As the polylysine concentration in the mixture increases, the magnitude of the first transition decreases proportionally, along with a corresponding increase of the magnitude of the second transition. In combination with the results of density-gradient electrophoresis, it was concluded that at room temperature and in a dilute salt solution, polylysine polynucleotide binding is quantitative, irreversible, and has a definite stoichiometric ratio.

4.6   USE OF POLYION COMPLEX TO PROMOTE NUCLEIC ACID HYBRID FORMATION

As described above, supramolecular formation or assembling of polyions, such as DNAs and RNAs, usually suffers from counterion condensation effect in a physiologic medium. Polyion complex formation, on the other hand, is driven by the release of physicochemically condensed counterions. Hence, polyion complex formation can alleviate the counterion condensation effect accompanying supramolecular formation of polyions. A state with higher counterion condensation can be stabilized through polyion complex formation. This accounts for the increase in Tm, i.e., the thermal stabilization of ds DNA observed for DNA/polylysine complexes.

Using a series of polyamines such as spermine and spermidine, stabilization of DNA hybrids, especially triple helical DNA, has been examined.[28-30] Triple helical DNA is a structure consisting of three DNA strands. The third strand aligns into the major groove of ds DNA without changing helical pitch and diameter, thus generating considerably higher linear charge density along the helical axis. This higher charge density makes triple helical DNA hard to produce under physiological conditions, because of massive counterion condensation.

A physiological role for triple helical DNAs is questionable, although several lines of evidence suggest their presence in eucaryotic cells. Polyamines are ubiquitous in living cells, and thus considered to stabilize triple helical DNAs. Spermine (tetravalent oligocation), and spermidine (trivalent oligocation), indeed show profound effects on the stability of triple helical DNA at lower ionic strength.[28-30] The effect is significantly reduced as ionic strength increases up to physiological level. At lower ionic strengths, polyamines sufficiently bind to DNAs, leading to release of counterions and consequent alleviation of counterion condensation effects. As described by Equation (9), however, the binding affinity is reduced with increasing ionic strength, resulting in the loss of the stabilization effect.

The physiological role of polyamines on triple helical DNA remains obscure, but tailor-made polyion complexes may represent a technique to promote supramolecular formation of DNAs. A polycationic stabilizer that takes advantage of the strong association between polycation and DNA is studied. The graft copolymers consisting of polycation backbones and hydrophilic side chains exhibit unique properties upon complexes formation with DNAs. The copolymers stably associate with DNA to form soluble complex even at physiological ionic strength.[31-32] The secondary and higher ordered structures of DNAs are preserved in the complex. The effect of the copolymer on ds and triple helical DNA formation was evaluated.[31,33,34] The copolymer at very low concentration (electrostatically equivalent to DNA) significantly in-

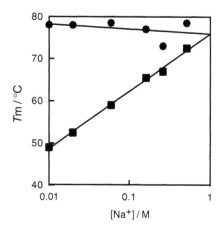

FIGURE 4.8 Salt concentration dependency of T_m of 15 bp DNA measured in the absence (square) and presence (circle) of polylysine-*graft*-dextran copolymer. (From Maruyama, A. et al., *Colloids Surf. B,* 16, 273, 1999, with permission.)

creases stability of both ds and triple-helical DNAs. The stabilization mechanism of the copolymer was investigated by assessing salt concentration dependency. The plots of the logarithm of [NaCl] vs. the T_m of 15 base pairs ds DNA in the presence and absence of the copolymer are shown in Figure 4.8.[35]

The straight relationship with a positive slope is observed in the absence of the copolymer. The positive slope is characteristic of the counterion association process that takes place upon DNA helix formation. On the other hand, the [NaCl] dependency of the T_m of the ds DNA in the presence of the copolymer was not significant, indicating that the extent of counterion condensation is unchanged ($\Delta\psi = 0$) between the ds form and the single-stranded form. The association of the polycationic copolymer to DNA causes perturbation of the electrostatic potential surrounding the DNA and releases the condensed counterions. The result allows us to conclude that the copolymer stabilizes the ds DNA by abolishing the counterion condensation effect.

Since the salt dependency in the presence of the copolymer is similar to that observed for uncharged peptide nucleic acid, it seems that the copolymer makes native DNAs behave as uncharged nucleotides upon hybrid formation. Unlike the polylysine homopolymer, the copolymer does not disturb ss DNAs to form ds and triple-helical DNAs. Figure 4.9 shows thermal melting profiles of triple helical DNA, poly(dA)•2poly(dT), in the absence or in the presence of spermine or the copolymer. In the absence of spermine or the copolymer at physiological ionic strength, the triple helical DNA melts at 37°C (the transition observed at lower temperature). While the T_m of the triplex-helical DNA in the presence of spermine increased to 60°C, it increased to 87°C in the presence of the copolymer, thus demonstrating stronger stabilization effect of the copolymer.

Despite the strong stabilizing effect of the copolymer, the reversible association of ss DNAs to form triple-helical DNA was apparently observed in the cooling process. A kinetic study using a surface plasmon apparatus revealed that the copoly-

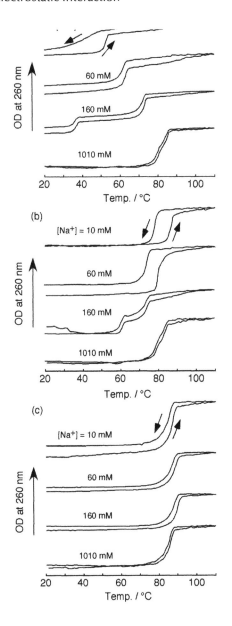

FIGURE 4.9 Salt dependencies of thermal melting and reassociation profiles of poly(dA)•2poly(dT) triple-helical DNA in the absence (a) or the presence (b) of 100 µM spermine or polylysine-*graft*-dextran copolymer (c) at polymer/DNA charge ratio of 2. (From Maruyama, A. et al., *Colloids Surf. B*, 16, 273, 1999, with permission.)

mer accelerates association of DNAs to form a hybrid.[36] In Figure 4.9, spermine at lower ionic strength caused hysteresis of the transition whereas the copolymer did not induce hysteresis. Spermine is known to condense DNA into globular conformation at low salt concentration. This spermine/DNA interaction may hinder the association of DNAs. In contrast to spermine, the ability of the copolymer to maintain DNA in a native structure may permit hybrid formation without hysteresis.

The copolymer was also demonstrated to considerably accelerate the strand exchange reaction between ds DNA and its complementary ss DNA, while stabilizing the ds DNA.[37] It is interesting that the copolymer promotes the strand exchange reaction in which dissociation of parent ds DNA must be involved. These observations with the copolymer imply that the rationale design of polyion complexes is a successful strategy to manipulate nucleic acid hybridization.

4.7 CONCLUSION

Electrostatic interactions play pivotal roles in assembling and recognition of biomolecules such as proteins and nucleotides. In general, van der Waals interactions are used for precise folding and recognition in living systems, whereas polyionic properties are employed for regulation of the interaction. In DNA-binding proteins, while ionic interactions are mainly employed for nonspecific binding to DNA, and other interactions accomplish accurate molecular recognition of base sequences. The nonspecific ionic interactions, however, play the significant role of recruiting the protein to DNA, thereby increasing the overall association rate by increasing the local concentrations of the proteins.

It remains difficult to construct biomaterials that undergo precise folding and assembling, like proteins, using van der Waals interactions. On the other hand, the stability and stoichiometry seen in polyion complexes permit us to design well-defined self-assembling biomaterials. One of these biomaterials may serve as a polycationic vector for gene therapy (see Chapter 12). Self-assembling of polyions is also employed for fabrication of multilayered membranes (see Chapter 5). The fundamental knowledge accumulated from these studies has greatly facilitated progress of supramolecular biomaterials.

REFERENCES

1. Voet, D.J., Voet, G., *Biochemistry*, 2nd ed., John Wiley & Sons, New York, Chap. 7, 1995.
2. Wada, A., The alpha-helix as an electric macro-dipole, *Adv. Biophys.*, 1, 1976.
3. Saenger, W., *Principles of Nucleic Acid Structure*, Springer-Verlag, Heidelberg, Chap. 18, 1983.
4. Hol, W.G.J., van Duijnen, P.T., and Berebdsen, H.C., The α-helix dipole and the properties of proteins, *Nature*, 273, 443, 1978.
5. Manning, G.S., Limiting laws and counterion condensation in polyelectrolyte solutions. I. Colligative properties, *J. Chem. Phys.*, 51, 924, 1969.
6. Manning, G.S., On the application of polyelectrolyte "limiting laws" to the helical-coil transition of DNA. VI. The numerical value of the axial phosphate spacing for the coil form, *Biopolymers*, 11, 937, 1972.
7. Anderson, C.F. and Record, M.T., Jr., Polyelectrolyte theories and their applications to DNA, *Annu. Rev. Phys. Chem.*, 33, 191, 1982.
8. Anderson, C.F. and Record, M.T., Jr., Ion distributions around DNA and cylindrical polyions: theoretical descriptions and physical implications, *Annu. Rev. Biophys. Chem.*, 19, 423, 1990.

9. Record, M.T., Jr., Effects of Na⁺ and Mg⁺⁺ ions on the helix-coil transition of DNA, *Biopolymers*, 14, 2137, 1975.

10. Record, M.T., Jr., Anderson, C.F., and Lohman, T.M., Thermodynamic analysis of ion effects on the binding and conformational equilibria of proteins and nucleic acids: the roles of ion association or release, screening, and ion effects on water activity, *Q. Rev. Biophys.*, 11, 103, 1978.

11. Nielsen, P.E. et al., Sequence-selective recognition of DNA by strand displacement with a thymine-substituted polyamide, *Science*, 254, 1497, 1991.

12. Betts, L. et al., A nucleic acid triple helix formed by a peptide nucleic acid-DNA complex, *Science*, 270, 1838, 1995.

13. Tomac, S. et al., Ionic effects on the stability and conformation of peptide nucleic acid complexes, *J. Amer. Chem. Soc.*, 118, 5544, 1997.

14. Bond, J.P., Anderson, C.F., and Record, M.T., Jr., Conformational transitions of duplex and triplex nucleic acid helices: Thermodynamic analysis of effects of salt concentration on stability using preferential interaction coefficient, *Biophys. J.*, 67, 825, 1994.

15. Booij, H.L. and Bungenberg-deJong, H.G., *Biocolloids and their Interaction*, Springer, Vienna, 1956.

16. Michaels, A.S., Polyelectrolyte complexes, *Ind. Eng. Chem.*, 57, 32, 1965.

17. Fuoss, R.M. and Sadek, H., Mutual interaction of ployelectrolyes, *Science*, 110, 554, 1949.

18. Michaels, A.S. and Miekka, G.L.R.G., Polycation–polyanion complexes. Preparation and properties of poly-(vinylbenzyltrimethylammonium) poly-(styrenesulfonate), *J. Phys. Chem.*, 65, 1765, 1961.

19. Tsuchida, E., Osada, Y., and Sanada, K., Interaction of poly(styrene sulfonate) with polycations carrying charges in the chain backbone, *J. Polym. Sci.*, 10, 3397, 1972.

20. Kabanov, V.A. and Zezin, A.B., A new class of complex water-soluble polyelectrolytes, *Macromol. Chem., Suppl.*, 6, 259, 1984.

21. Kabanov, A.V. and Kabanov, V.A., DNA complexes with polycations for the delivery of genetic material into cells, *Bioconjugate Chem.*, 6, 7, 1995.

22. Lohman, T.M., Haseth, P.L., and Record, M.T., Jr., Pentalysine–deoxynucleic acid interactions: a model for the general effects of ion concentrations on the interactions of proteins with nucleic acids, *Biochemistry*, 19, 3522, 1980.

23. Mascotti, D.P. and Lohman, T.M., Thermodynamic extent of counterion release upon binding oligolysines to single-stranded nucleic acids, *Proc. Natl. Acad. Sci. U.S.A.*, 87, 3142, 1990.

24. Mascotti, D.P. and Lohman, T.M., Thermodynamics of oligoarginines binding to RNA and DNA, *Biochemistry*, 36, 7272 , 1997.

25. Record, M.T., Jr., Lohman, T.M., and Haseth, P. L., Ion effects on ligand-nucleic acid interactions, *J. Mol. Biol.*, 107, 145, 1976.

26. Mascotti, D.P. and Lohman, T.M., Thermodynamics of charged oligopeptide–heparin interactions, *Biochemistry*, 34, 2908, 1995.

27. Tsuboi, M. and Matsuo, K., Interaction of poly-L-lysine and nucleic acids, *J. Mol. Biol.*, 15, 256, 1966.

28. Hampel, K.J., Crosson, P., and Lee, J.S., Polyamines favor DNA triplex formation at neutral pH, *Biochemistry*, 30, 4455, 1991.

29. Thomas, T. and Thomas, T.J., Selectivity of polyamines in triplex DNA stabilization, *Biochemistry*, 32, 14068, 1993.

30. Musso, M. and van Dyke, M.W., Polyamine effects on purine–purine–pyrimidine triple helix formation by phophodiester and phosphorothioate oligodeoxyribonucleotides, *Nucleic Acid Res.*, 23, 2320, 1995.

31. Maruyama, A. et al., Comb-type polycations effectively stabilize DNA triplex, *Bioconjugate Chem.*, 8, 3, 1997.

32. Maruyama, A. et al., Characterization of interpolyelectrolyte complexes between double-stranded DNA and polylysine comb-type copolymers having hydrophilic side chains, *Bioconjugate Chem.*, 9, 292, 1998.

33. Ferdous, A. et al., Poly(L-lysine) graft dextran copolymer: Amazing effect on triplex stabilization under physiological relevant conditions (*in vitro*), *Nucleic Acid Res.*, 26, 3949, 1998.

34. Ferdous, A. et al., Comb-type copolymer: stabilization of triplex DNA and possible application in antigene strategy, *J. Pharm. Sci.*, 87, 1400, 1998.

35. Maruyama, A. et al., Polycation comb-type copolymer reduces counterion condensation effect to stabilize DNA duplex and triplex formation, *Colloids Surf. B.*, 16, 273, 1999.

36. Torigoe, H. et al., Poly(L-lysine)-graft-dextran copolymer promotes pyrimidine motif triplex DNA formation at physiological pH. Thermodynamic and kinetic studies, *J. Biol. Chem.*, 274, 6161, 1999.

37. Kim, W.J. et al., Comb-type cationic copolymer expediates DNA strand exchange while stabilizing DNA duplex, *Eur. Chem. J.*, 7, 176, 2001.

5 Physical Adsorption for Supramolecular Design

Takeshi Serizawa

CONTENTS

5.1 INTRODUCTION

Adsorption of molecules onto material surfaces is a fundamental process in supramolecular design for biological applications. When certain solid materials are immersed in solutions containing synthetic polymers or biopolymers, the polymers spontaneously adsorb onto the material surfaces as a result of concentration-dependent interactions. Two types of physical and chemical adsorption have been defined. The first is governed by van der Waals interactions such as London forces, dipole–dipole interactions, and so on, between the polymers and the material surfaces, without any orbital overlapping. The second involves the formation of chemical bonds or overlapping of molecular orbitals by electrostatic, hydrogen bond, or charge-transfer interactions. The classification of physical or chemical adsorption is difficult in most cases of polymer adsorptions, because various functional groups exist in polymers and on material surfaces. Some researchers in biology utilize terms such as "specific" and "nonspecific" adsorption to describe these biomolecular interactions. Specific adsorption usually includes adsorption based on multiple structurally regulated interactions, such as antibody to antigen, adsorption of sugar-binding proteins (lectins) to corresponding sugars, or other specific-bindings between biomolecules. Nonspecific adsorption includes adsorption of other molecules to various material surfaces without any specific interactions. The present section describes the basis of physical adsorption of various molecules. Although nonspecific adsorption is not strictly defined as physical adsorption, it is included here.

0-8493-0965-4/02/$0.00+$1.50
© 2002 by CRC Press LLC

83

Adsorption of biomolecules is the initial step when materials make contact in biological environments. Proteins, for example, adsorb onto the surfaces of various materials that have potential applications in biomedical fields. The quantities, species, and conformational changes of biomolecules adsorbed induce various significant bioactivities. Cells will adhere onto a material surface onto which cell-adhering proteins have been adsorbed. Certain material surfaces adsorb plasma proteins and platelets, and can induce the sequential events leading to coagulation. The native structure of some proteins is denatured by adsorption. Characteristics of materials are sometimes determined by the characteristics of the surfaces contacting the biomolecules. Accordingly, it is important to analyze phenomena associated with the adsorption of biomolecules to material surfaces by using suitable methodologies. In other words, selective adsorption of certain biomolecules onto material surfaces sometimes can induce specific bioactivities. There are great advantages to the preparation of materials that utilize nonprotein adsorption, in order to obtain bioinert material surfaces. This can be achieved by specific design of the chemical structures of the materials and/or by surface modification of materials with suitable chemical species.

It is important to chemically and physically analyze adsorption of polymers including biomolecules onto certain materials in order to study supramolecular design for biological applications. The amounts of biomolecules adsorbed are usually much smaller than adsorption of other materials. The thicknesses of the adsorbed layers are also small — typically less than 100 nm. It is difficult to analyze amounts or adsorption processes. Novel techniques suitable for analysis of small adsorption amounts have been developed in recent years, although conventional analysis is still useful. The apparatus for such techniques is commercially available and relatively easy to operate. This section describes current methodologies for analyzing adsorption.

In order to design "intelligent" materials for biological applications, a basic analysis of the physical adsorption capabilities of various molecules including supermolecules is significant. This chapter discusses a basic strategy for physical adsorption from the viewpoint of biological applications. The adsorption of proteins, surfactants, and linear polymers is discussed. These processes are schematically represented in Figure 5.1. There are variations in the manner of adsorption, dependent on the species of adsorbate. The theoretical aspects of these processes are not discussed. Further details regarding theory may be obtained from other reference books.[1-3]

5.2 ADSORPTION ISOTHERMS

Adsorption isotherms and isobars are commonly utilized to describe the physical adsorption of molecules to material surfaces. The former are profiles of equilibrium adsorption amounts measured against the concentration or vapor pressure of an adsorbate at a constant temperature. The latter are plotted against temperature at a constant pressure. These profiles are helpful in the characterization of certain

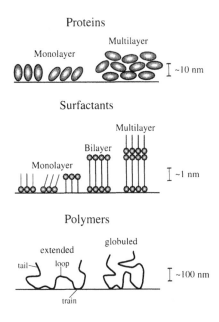

Proteins

Monolayer

Multilayer

$\sim$10 nm

Surfactants

Monolayer

Bilayer

Multilayer

$\sim$1 nm

Polymers

extended

globuled

tail

loop

train

$\sim$100 nm

FIGURE 5.1 Adsorption schemes of biorelated molecules.

adsorption processes. Various significant parameters (e.g., adsorption/desorption constants) that define the adsorption process can be also obtained from a physical analysis of these profiles. With respect to biological applications, adsorption isotherms are readily available because biological supermolecules tend to be denatured by changes in temperature. This in turn affects the adsorption isobars by causing changes in these highly ordered structures. It is easier to change the concentration or pressure of the adsorbates and maintain a constant temperature. Some of the various adsorption isotherms are described below.

The simplest isotherm is derived from Langmuir adsorption. This has been applied to monolayer adsorption of certain molecules onto material surfaces. Two assumptions are inherent in this isotherm. One is equivalent adsorption of adsorbates at each adsorption site, indicating that the adsorption mechanism is essentially the same at any point in time and at a specific concentration (or relative pressure). Another is that no interaction between adsorbates occurs after their adsorption, even if they exist in close proximity on the surface of the adsorbent. Langmuir isotherms are often observed in the physical adsorption of biomolecules from their aqueous solutions. In this case, the above assumptions might not be strictly satisfied, because biomolecules (e.g., proteins) can be denatured by adsorption and may subsequently interact with each other via secondary interactions. In addition, Langmuir isotherms are usually typical of a chemical adsorption onto surfaces, which is reasonable, given the inherent assumptions. However, fitting to a Langmuir isotherm still necessitates a discussion of the physical adsorption of biomolecules and requires the estimation of an adsorption constant.

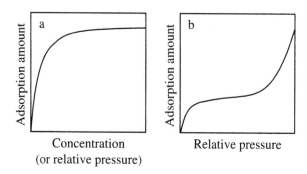

FIGURE 5.2 Langmuir (a) and BET (b) isotherms.

The Langmuir isotherm (Figure 5.2a) for physical adsorption from a solution of a certain adsorbate is expressed using the Langmuir equation as follows:

$$\frac{m}{m_{max}} = \frac{KC}{1 + KC} \tag{1}$$

where m is the amount of adsorbate adsorbed, m_{max} is the maximum adsorption amount, K is the apparent adsorption constant, and C is the concentration of adsorbate. When adsorption occurs in the gas phase, C is changed to a relative pressure value. The left side of the equation (1) is sometimes expressed as follows:

$$\theta = \frac{m}{m_{max}} \tag{2}$$

K indicates the ratio between the adsorption (k_a) and desorption (k_d) rate constants as follows:

$$K = \frac{k_a}{k_d} \tag{3}$$

K can be compared with the value estimated from the rate constants that are estimated by the time dependence of the adsorption amount. Equation (1) is transformed as follows:

$$\frac{C}{m} = \frac{C}{m_{max}} + \frac{1}{K \cdot m_{max}} \tag{4}$$

This equation indicates that m_{max} and K are calculated from the slope and intercept, respectively, of a linear plot of C/m against C. In other words, a linear relationship is necessary in order to apply Langmuir adsorption. When concentrations and adsorption data are given, they are fitted to Equation (4). K is independent of m_{max}. Even if m_{max} is very small, K can be very large. These variables must be considered independently in adsorption analyses. Other experiential isotherms are used to describe monolayer adsorption (Temkin isotherm, Freundlich isotherm, and so on), which correct the assumptions of the Langmuir equation. These can similarly be applied, depending on the species of adsorbate.

The Langmuir equation ignores multilayer adsorption on surfaces. Use of the Brunauer–Emmett–Teller (BET) isotherm (Figure 5.2b) for multilayer adsorption is well known. This isotherm is characterized by strong interactions in adsorption of the first monolayer and subsequent weak interactions (as for liquefaction heating) for multilayer adsorption. The adsorption amount increases infinitely with increasing vapor pressure. This isotherm is normally applicable to adsorption of small molecules (also supermolecules) on adsorbents in the gas phase. When the adsorption of certain molecules shows a BET-like isotherm, the data can be fitted to the following equation:

$$\frac{m}{m_{mono}} = \frac{cz}{(1-z)\{1-(1-c)z\}}$$

(5)

where m is the amount of adsorbates adsorbed, m_{mono} is the amount of monolayer adsorption, and c is a constant. The z can be expressed as follows:

$$z = \frac{P}{P_{sat}}$$

(6)

where P is the vapor pressure and P_{sat} is saturated vapor pressure. Equation (5) is transformed as follows:

$$\frac{z}{(1-z)m} = \frac{c-1}{c \cdot m_{mono}}z + \frac{1}{c \cdot m_{mono}}$$

(7)

This equation indicates that m_{mono} and c can be calculated from the slope of a linear plot of the left term against z. A linear relationship is necessary to apply BET adsorption. Certain biomolecules (e.g., proteins) sometimes show multilayer adsorption from solutions. The surfaces of monolayers of proteins might behave as adsorbents due to denaturing after adsorption. In this case, adsorption data might also be fitted to the BET equation. The constant c suggests a degree of multilayer adsorption and is normally around 20 to 500 as shown in Figure 5.2b. A larger c means a difficulty with multilayer adsorption. In order to determine the surface areas of supramolecular assemblies such as porous particles and their adsorbed surfaces, BET analysis using an inactive gas such as nitrogen or argon as the adsorbate is useful. In cases involving multilayer adsorption, the Frenkel-Halsey-Hill isotherm can be applied in certain cases.

5.3 HEAT OF ADSORPTION

Adsorption heat is essential for physical adsorption as well as adsorption isotherms. Adsorption normally involves an exothermic phenomenon. The heat produced is the heat of adsorption. Although adsorption results in an entropy decrease due to restriction of molecular motion of adsorbates, this is compensated for by enthalpy derived from adsorbate-adsorbent and adsorbate–adsorbate interactions. Heat of adsorption can be directly measured by calorimeters using isothermal or adiabatic systems. In the isothermal system in gas phases, heat of adsorption (q) is calculated by the Clapeyron-Clausius equation as follows:

$$q = -R\left[\frac{\partial lnP}{\partial(1/T)}\right]_P \tag{8}$$

where R is the gas constant, P is the vapor pressure, and T is the temperature. In solutions, careful measurements using calorimeters are necessary for accurate analysis of heat of adsorption.

5.4 METHODOLOGIES

5.4.1 STATIC ANALYSIS

Physical adsorption is analyzed by various static techniques (Figure 5.3). The most primitive method for measuring the physical adsorption of certain molecules onto material surfaces is a direct weighing of the molecules adsorbed or the molecules remaining in solution after adequate incubation time by using a microbalance. However, weighing is usually difficult because the adsorption amount is quite small relative to the weight of the adsorbent. The use of colloidal particles as adsorbents may potentially increase the relative adsorption amounts due to their larger surface areas. Most techniques have limitations.

When adsorbates absorb UV/Vis light or emit fluorescence, the detection of small amounts in supernatants becomes easier, although application of this method requires that adsorbates have large molar absorptivity.[4] In the case of adsorption of biomolecules such as proteins, various reagents that have chromophores that react

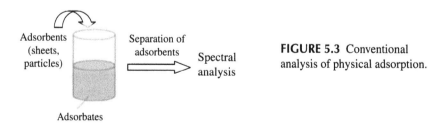

Adsorbents (sheets, particles)   Separation of adsorbents   Spectral analysis

Adsorbates

FIGURE 5.3 Conventional analysis of physical adsorption.

with them, are available. IR and CD spectra are also useful in the detection of bio-molecules. However, denaturing of adsorbed biomolecules makes detection difficult because of changes in peak areas.

5.4.2 DYNAMIC ANALYSIS

Dynamic analyses of physical adsorption are required to calculate rate constants for adsorption and desorption and obtain adsorption isotherms. Dynamic analysis is difficult using the conventional methodologies described above. Two recently developed techniques are applicable to dynamic analysis of physical adsorption as follows.

A quartz crystal microbalance (QCM) (Figure 5.4) can be used to quantitatively detect the mass of adsorbate on its electrodes. When certain molecules are adsorbed onto a QCM, the resonant frequency is decreased in proportion to the mass of adsorbate. The relationship between the frequency decrease (ΔF) and the mass (Δm) is described as follows:[5]

$$-\Delta F = \frac{2F_0^2}{A\sqrt{\rho_q \mu_q}} \times \Delta m \qquad (9)$$

where F_o is the parent frequency of the QCM, A is the electrode area, ρ_q is the density of the quartz (2.65 g/cm^3), and μ_q is the shear modulus (2.95 × 10^{11} dyne/cm^2). Equation (9) indicates that the sensitivity of the QCM is dependent on the parent frequency. QCMs with parent frequencies around 5 to 27 MHz are commercially available. When a 27-MHz QCM is utilized, monolayer adsorptions of small molecules (molecular weights below 100 and several angstroms in size) can be analyzed *in situ*. An adsorption amount of less than 50 ng/cm^2 can be monitored by the sensitive QCM method. The monolayer adsorption of acetic acid onto self-assembled monolayers prepared on a 27-MHz QCM has been demonstrated.[6] Even when a QCM with a

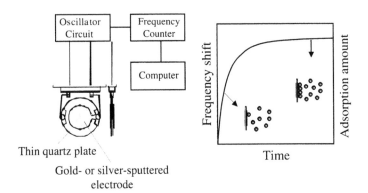

FIGURE 5.4 QCM analysis.

small resonant frequency is utilized, submicrograms per square centimeter of adsorbate can be monitored. A QCM can be utilized in both gas phases and solutions. Equation (9) however, is most reliable when adsorption experiments are performed in gas phases, because the viscosity of the media in solutions affects the frequency change. In gas phases, the mass of the solvents is never detected as a frequency shift, and the effect of the viscosity of the adsorbent on the frequency can be ignored. In order to analyze adsorption in solutions, adequate calibration or theoretical treatment is necessary for accuracy. The frequency is also affected by the elasticity of the adsorbate. In an ideal analysis, adsorbates should be hard materials. In fact, various molecules including biomolecules, can be detected.[7,8] The use of other materials as adsorbents for the analysis of physical or chemical adsorption can modify the electrode of the QCM.

Surface plasmon resonance (SPR), which is the resonance between the evanescent and surface plasmon waves (Figure 5.5), can also be used to monitor *in situ* adsorption processes.[9-11] When certain molecules are adsorbed onto the surface of a gold-sputtered prism, the resonance angle shifts ($\Delta\Theta$), depending on the refractive index (n) and thickness (d) of the adsorbate as follows:

$$\Delta\theta = f(n,d) \tag{10}$$

The sensitivity of this method is similar to that of the 27-MHz QCM.[12,13] The mass of adsorbates can be estimated by using calibration curves. *In situ* analysis of the change in resonance angle allows a dynamic analysis of adsorption processes. Other materials can be used as adsorbents for the analysis of physical adsorption to modify the gold surface.

5.5 RECENT ADVANCES IN PHYSICAL ADSORPTION FOR SUPRAMOLECULAR DESIGN

Scanning probe microscopy (SPM) techniques (Figure 5.6) such as atomic force microscopy (AFM)[14] and scanning tunnel microscopy (STM)[15] are useful tools for the

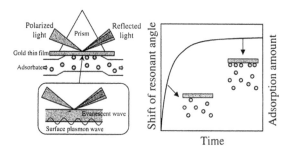

FIGURE 5.5 SPR analysis.

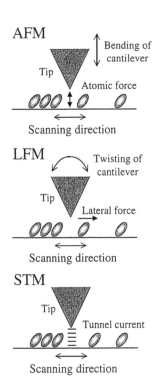

AFM

Bending of
cantilever

Tip

Atomic force

Scanning direction

LFM

Twisting of
cantilever

Tip

Lateral force

Scanning direction

STM

Tip

Tunnel current

Scanning direction

FIGURE 5.6 SPM analysis.

static analysis of physical adsorption. AFM can relay images of the surface topologies of certain materials by using a cantilever at the molecular level. Adsorption onto a surface is recognized by an increase in height of several nanometers. Two modes are available for analysis: the noncontact mode and the contact mode. The noncontact mode seems to be better than the contact mode for work with boimolecules. AFM images reveal differences in height more accurately than lateral resolution, due to curvature of the cantilever. This means that AFM sometimes overestimates real two-dimensional nano-ordered sizes.

It is difficult to apply AFM to monolayer adsorptions with very small differences in heights (less than 1 Å). In this case, lateral force microscopy (LFM), which creates two-dimensional images of the lateral forces at surfaces, might be applicable. Adhesion forces can be analyzed using AFM apparatus, in which corresponding molecules are conjugated onto both a substrate and a cantilever.[16] STM, which creates two-dimensional images of differences in tunnel currents, can also be applied to the analysis of physical adsorption when absorbates are conductive. Laser and x-ray reflection (ellipsometry and small-angle x-ray diffraction (SANX), respectively) can be utilized for detection of the mean thicknesses of adsorbed layers. As both analyses are strongly influenced by adsorption density on surfaces, careful treatment of the data is necessary.

Layer-by-layer (LbL) assembly is a potentially significant new technique that uses physical (nonspecific) adsorption of certain polymers in the preparation of polyelectrolyte multilayers (Figure 5.7). Decher et al.[17] found that a stepwise immersion of substrates into aqueous solutions of oppositely charged polymers created layered ultrathin polymer films with controllable thicknesses in nanometer levels. In each step, the adsorbed polymer is rendered insoluble by nonspecific polyion complex formation on the substrate, resulting in a stable ultrathin film. LbL assembly involves the simple alternate immersion of a substrate into oppositely charged polymer solutions, followed by sequential physical adsorption. LbL assemblies have been applied to water-soluble linear-charged polymers, viruses, proteins, colloids, dyes, metal oxides, and amphiphiles. Charge-transfer and hydrogen-bonding interactions between certain polymers are utilized to facilitate ultrathin film deposition. The concept of LbL assembly suggests that certain polymers can be assembled on a substrate by stabilization after adsorption due to polymeric interactions. LbL assembly of stereoregular poly(methyl methacrylate)s (PMMAs) is an important system that utilizes physical adsorption of polymers.[18] Isotactic (it) and syndiotactic (st) PMMAs form stereocomplexes with double-stranded helical structures in polar organic solvents. LbL assembly from both solutions using a QCM substrate revealed that the stereocomplex was formed at the adsorption step of st-PMMA after the physical adsorption of the it-PMMA step on the assembly surface.

Physical adsorption is a useful measurement when certain materials are immersed in solutions containing certain molecules. The mechanism of physical adsorption is sometimes difficult to analyze. However, several techniques that involve physical adsorption appear to have great potential in supramolecular design.

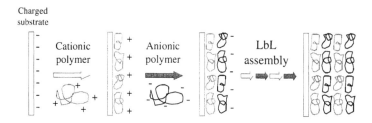

FIGURE 5.7 LbL assembly.

REFERENCES

1. Bruch, L.W., Cole, M.W., and Zaremba, E., *Physical Adsorption: Forces and Phenomena*, Oxford University Press, Oxford, 1997.
2. Fleer, G.J. et al., *Polymers at Interfaces*, Chapman & Hall, London, 1993.
3. Dash, J.G., *Films on Solid Surfaces: The Physics and Chemistry of Physical Adsorption*, Academic Press, New York, 1975.
4. Aston, J.R. et al., *Adsorption at the Gas–Solid and Liquid–Solid Interface*, Rouquerol, J. and Sing, K.S., Eds., Elsevier, Amsterdam, 1983.
5. Sauerbrey, G., Quartz oscillators for weighing thin layers and for microweighing, *Z. Phys.*, 155, 206, 1959.
6. Matsuura, K., Ebara, Y., and Okahata, Y., Gas phase selective adsorption on functional monolayers immobilized on a highly sensitive quartz-crystal microbalance, *Langmuir*, 12, 1023, 1996.
7. Hook, F. et al., The dissipative QCM technique: interfacial phenomena and sensor applications for proteins, biomembranes, living cells and polymers, in *Proc. Jt. Meet. Eur. Freq. Time Forum IEEE Int. Control Symp.*, Vol. 2, Institute of Electronics Engineering, New York, 1999, 966.
8. White, R.M., Acoustic sensors for physical, chemical and biochemical applications, in *Proc. IEEE Int. Freq. Control Symp.*, Institute of Electrical and Electronics Engineers, New York, 1998, 587.
9. Brockman, J.M., Nelson, B.P., and Corn, R.M., Surface plasmon resonance imaging measurements of ultrathin organic films, *Annu. Rev. Phys. Chem.*, 51, 41, 2000.
10. Otsuni, E., Yan, L., and Whitesides, G.M., The interaction of proteins and cells with self-assembled monolayers of alkanethiolates on gold and silver, *Colloids Surf., B*, 15, 3, 1999.
11. Hanken, D.G. et al., Surface plasmon resonance measurements of ultrathin organic films at electrode surfaces, *Electroanal. Chem.*, 20, 141, 1998.
12. Kaiser, T. et al., Biotinylated steroid derivatives as ligands for biospecific interaction analysis with monoclonal antibodies using immunosensor devices, *Anal. Biochem.*, 282, 173, 2000.
13. Okahata, Y. et al., Kinetic measurements of DNA hybridization on an oligonucleotide-immobilized 27-MHz quartz crystal microbalance, *Anal. Chem.*, 70, 1288, 1998.
14. Takahara, A. et al., *In situ* atomic force microscopic observation of albumin adsorption onto phase-separated organosilane monolayer surface, *J. Biomater. Sci. Polymer Edn*, 11, 111, 2000.
15. You, H.X. et al., Physical adsorption of immunoglobulin G on gold studied by scanning tunneling microscopy, *Int. J. Biol. Macromol.*, 16, 87, 1994.
16. Ludwig, M. et al., AFM, a tool for single-molecules experiments, *Appl. Phys. A: Mater. Sci. Process*, A68, 173, 1999.
17. Decher, G., Fuzzy nanoassemblies: toward layered polymeric multicomposites, *Science*, 277, 1232, 1997.
18. Serizawa, T. et al., Stepwise stereocomplex assembly of stereoregular poly(methyl methacrylate)s on a substrate, *J. Am. Chem. Soc.*, 122, 1891, 2000.

6 Gels and Interpenetrating Polymer Networks

Takashi Miyata

CONTENTS

0-8493-0965-4/02/$0.00+$1.50
© 2002 by CRC Press LLC

6.1 INTRODUCTION

Gels are cross-linked networks of polymers or the networks swollen with liquids. They are insoluble in any solvents.[1] Gels are classified as hydrogels swollen in aqueous solvents, organogels swollen in organic solvents, and xerogels without solvents. Gels swollen in solvents have unique properties in that they show both liquid-like and solid-like behavior. Such swollen gels are interesting from the viewpoint of fundamental science and because they have various applications due to their unique properties. The term "gel" often means a gel swollen in solvents and does not include xerogels. Most gels used for biological applications are hydrogels swollen in water or physiological solutions, so this chapter focuses on hydrogels.

Hydrogels (abbreviated as *gels* hereafter) are hydrophilic polymer networks swollen in aqueous solutions (Figure 6.1). The polymeric chains are covalently or noncovalently cross-linked together. Some noncovalently cross-linked natural polymer gels such as agar and jelly are well known. Most biological systems are based on

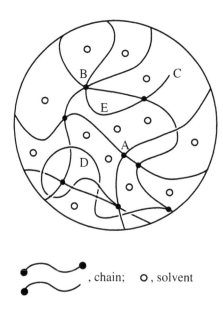

, chain;   o , solvent

FIGURE 6.1 Structure of a gel swollen in an aqueous solution: (A) tetrafunctional cross-links; (B) multifunctional cross-links; (C) chain end; (D) entanglements; and (E) loops.

natural polymer gels consisting of proteins, saccharides, etc. Covalently cross-linked synthetic gels are useful in the biochemical and biomedical fields because water-swollen gels are very similar to natural tissues and often exhibit good biocompatibility due to their high water content.[2-4] These qualities imply the potential of gels as the next generation of functional materials. The abilities of gels are strongly dependent upon their physical and chemical structures. For example, the cross-linking structures enable the gels to retain their shapes and to keep solvents within their networks. The characteristics of constituent polymer chains in gels govern their swelling behavior, e.g., gels consisting of hydrophilic polymer chains are swollen in water but gels of hydrophobic chains are shrunken. Consequently, many potential applications of gels are determined by their structural designs from the viewpoint of the cross-linking structures and constituent polymer chains.

Ideally, a gel is a single polymer molecule in which all the monomer units are connected. Therefore, we can observe the behavior of a single polymer molecule as swelling behavior of gels on a macroscopic scale. Polymer chains in gels behave cooperatively because all chains are connected to each other. The covalent or noncovalent bonds as cross-links in gels play important roles in fabricating gel structures and acting as functional materials. Such gel systems are very similar to the supramolecular systems in which covalent or noncovalent bonds are used to fabricate suprastructured molecules with smart functions although molecular architectures in most gels are not designed as precisely as supermolecules. Furthermore, the biological molecules and systems that represent the goals of supramolecular chemistry are almost based on gels having both liquid- and solid-like properties. This suggests potential contributions of gels to supramolecular chemistry in a broad sense.

Various unique features of gels have attracted considerable attention in fundamental and practical science fields. In particular, the discovery of volume phase transition of gels led to the establishment of gel science,[1,5,6] which is essentially associated with understanding the structures and functions of biomolecules such as proteins and saccharides. The volume phase transition of gels provides the tools for creating intelligent materials that simultaneously serve such functions as sensing a signal (sensor), judging its magnitude (processor), and altering its function in direct response (effector).[5,6] Stimuli-responsive behaviors including volume phase transition of gels can be applied to construct intelligent devices for sensors, drug delivery systems, separation, actuators and so on, which can control their functions in response to environmental stimuli such as changes in pH, temperature, and ionic strength, etc.[3-10]

Many researchers have focused on interpenetrating polymer networks (IPNs) having well organized structures compared to conventional gels. In general, IPNs are defined as combinations of two or more polymers in network form, at least one of which is synthesized and/or cross-linked in the immediate presence of the others.[11-13] Similarly to simple polymer blends, a polymer or network of an IPN is not covalently bonded to the other polymer networks. However, IPNs do not dissolve in solvents as their constituent polymers are physically and strongly entangled with the other polymer networks. Thus, IPNs are distinguished from simple polymer blends. IPNs, in which three-dimensional polymer networks are entangled in the other networks, are

(a) IPN   (b) semi-IPN

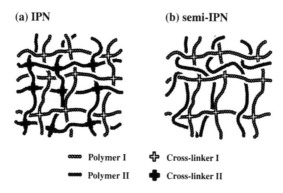

ᴑᴑᴑᴑ Polymer I   ⊹ Cross-linker I

▬▬▬ Polymer II   ✚ Cross-linker II

FIGURE 6.2 Structures of IPN (a) and semi-IPN (b).

simply called IPNs; whereas IPNs whose linear polymers are entangled are named semi-IPNs (Figure 6.2). The original concept of the IPNs suggested having a homogeneous structure based on miscible polymer blends. In practice, however, most IPNs do not interpenetrate perfectly on a molecular scale due to immiscible composition, and often exhibit phase separation. On the whole, IPNs have better mechanical properties than polymer blends since IPNs have more entanglements than polymer blends. In addition, IPNs may be regarded as interlocked polymers, similarly to polyrotaxane and polycatenane (see Chapter 7). The unique network structures of IPNs attract much attention because of their functions and performance factors such as mechanical properties. Interlocked structures in some IPN gels play important roles in exhibiting stimuli-responsive behavior. Thus, since IPNs have well organized structures compared to conventional gels, they may be more relevant to supramolecular chemistry.

This chapter focuses on polymer gels and IPNs for biological and biomedical applications, and describes their fundamentals and strategies for gel synthesis and characterization. Biological and biomedical applications of gels and IPNs are described in detail in other chapters. (Chapter 9 addresses stimuli-responsive gels, Chapter 10 addresses modulated drug delivery systems, and Chapter 16 addresses the biological interactions between gel surfaces and biomolecules.)

6.2 THERMODYNAMICS AND KINETICS

6.2.1 Volume Phase Transition

The volume of a gel swollen in a solvent is strongly dependent upon its constituent polymer chains and cross-linking structures. For example, gels with ionized groups swell strongly in water and gels with high cross-linking density exhibit low swelling ratios. Furthermore, some gels are found to undergo drastic changes in volume in response to environmental changes such as solvent composition, temperature, pH, etc. Reversible and discontinuous volume changes of gels are envisaged as primary phase transitions, that is, volume phase transitions.[1,14-23] Tanaka et al.[14,15] discovered the volume phase transitions of gels experimentally. Their theoretical studies revealed that the volume phase transition should be universally observed in all gels, similarly to volume changes of low molecular weight molecules from liquid states to gas states. The swollen and collapsed phases of gels correspond to the gas and liquid states, respectively. Such volume phase transition of gels can be understood using a mean field theory on the basis of Flory–Huggins thermodynamics for polymers.[14,15,20,24]

The contributions of mixing, elasticity, and ions to the Gibbs free energy of an ionic gel swollen in a solvent (Figure 6.3) are given by:

$$\Delta G_{mixing} = kT[n\ln(1-\phi)+\chi n\phi] \tag{1}$$

$$\Delta G_{elastic=} \frac{3vkT}{2}(\alpha^2 -1-\ln\alpha) \tag{2}$$

$$\Delta G_{ion} = -vfkT\ln\left(\frac{V_0\alpha^3}{nv_1}\right) \tag{3}$$

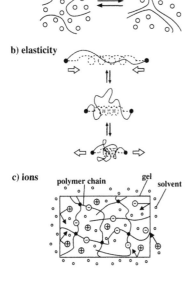

a) mixing

polymer solvent

b) elasticity

c) ions

polymer chain gel solvent

FIGURE 6.3 Free energy contributions of mixing (a), elasticity (b), and ions (c) for the state of a gel swollen in a solvent.

where ΔG_{mixing}, $\Delta G_{elastic}$, and ΔG_{ion} are Gibbs free energy contributions of mixing, elasticity, and ions, n is the number of solvent molecules in the gel, ϕ is the volume fraction of the polymer network, χ is the polymer–solvent interaction parameter, v is the total number of chains in the gel, α is the linear swelling ratio, V_0 is the volume of the gel when its network has a random walk configuration, v_l is the molar volume of the solvent, k is the Boltzmann constant, T is the absolute temperature, and f is the number of counter ions per chain. It should be kept in mind that a chain in the gel is defined as a portion of the structure extending from a cross-linkage to the next one occurring along the given primary molecule (see Figure 6.1). Therefore, total Gibbs free energy of the ionic gel in the solvent becomes:

$$\Delta G = \Delta G_{mixing} + \Delta G_{elastic} + \Delta G_{ion} = kT[n\ln(1-\phi) + \chi n\phi] + \frac{3vkT}{2}(\alpha^2 - 1 - \ln\alpha) - vfkT\ln\left(\frac{V_0\alpha^3}{nv_l}\right)$$

(4)

The Gibbs free energy of the gel is related to the osmotic pressure Π of gels by Equation (5).

$$\Pi = -\frac{N}{v_1}\left(\frac{\partial\Delta G}{\partial n_1}\right)_{T.P}$$

(5)

Therefore, the osmotic pressure of the gel is given by:

$$\Pi = \Pi_{mixing} + \Pi_{elastic} + \Pi_{ion}$$

$$= \frac{NkT}{v_1}[\phi + \ln(1-\phi) + \chi\phi^2] + vkT\left[\frac{\phi}{2\phi_0} - \left(\frac{\phi}{\phi_0}\right)^{1/3}\right] + vfkT\left(\frac{\phi}{\phi_0}\right)$$

(6)

where Π_{mixing}, $\Pi_{elastic}$, and Π_{ion} are the osmotic pressure contributions of mixing, elasticity, and Donnan-type potential, respectively, ϕ_0 is the volume fraction of polymer when the gel network has a random walk configuration, and n is the number of constituent chains per unit volume at $\phi = \phi_0$. As the osmotic pressure of the gel in equilibrium with a surrounding solvent should be zero ($\Pi = 0$), the equilibrium state of the gel can be expressed as:

$$\tau = 1 - 2\chi = \frac{vv_1}{N\phi^2}\left[(2f+1)\left(\frac{\phi}{\phi_0}\right) - 2\left(\frac{\phi}{\phi_0}\right)^{1/3}\right] + 1 + \frac{2}{\phi} + \frac{2\ln(1-\phi)}{\phi^2}$$

(7)

where the parameter τ is called the reduced temperature, which changes with solvent composition and temperature.

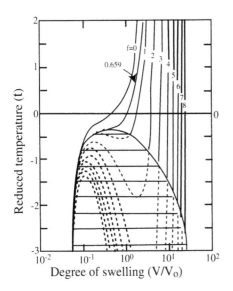

FIGURE 6.4 Theoretical relationship between the reduced temperature τ and equilibrium swelling ratio V/V_0 of gels. An increase of f means an increase in the degree of ionization of the gel network. (From Dusek, K., *Responsive Gels, Volume Transitions, I,* Advances in Polymer Science, Vol. 109, Springer, Berlin, 1993, with permission.)

Equation (7) is fundamental for representing the volume phase transitions of gels. Equation (7) means that τ is a function of f and a volume fraction of the polymer. Thus, the relationship between the reduced temperature and the equilibrium swelling ratio for gels with various degrees of ionization can be plotted, based on Equation (7) (Figure 6.4).[5,15] Figure 6.4 demonstrates the presence of an unstable Maxwell's loop for gels with a high degree of ionization, similarly to that for van der Waals fluid. As shown in Figure 6.4, therefore, Equation (7) predicts that the gels with the high degree of ionization exhibit discontinuous volume phase transition.

Figure 6.5 shows the experimental volume phase transition of positively and negatively ionized poly(acrylamide) (PAAm) gels in acetone/water mixtures.[16] The positively and negatively ionized PAAm gels were prepared by copolymerization of acrylamide and a cross-linker with (methacrylamidopropyl)trimethylammonium chloride (MAPTAC) having cationic groups and sodium acrylate having an anionic group, respectively. The ionized PAAm gels with low contents of the ionized groups underwent continuous volume changes as a function of acetone concentration, but the gels with high contents of the ionized groups exhibited discontinuous volume changes. These results indicate that the ionization of gels plays an important role in their discontinuous volume phase transition. Thus, the experimental results support the theoretical results based on Flory–Huggins thermodynamics.

Discontinuous volume phase transition of the ionic gels can be described qualitatively and simply as follows: In an ionic gel in a solvent, the repulsion of ionic groups and osmotic pressure by counterions cause swelling of the gel, and the attraction based on polymer–polymer interactions becomes the force to collapse gels. The balance of their forces determines two stable states of gels — the swollen state and the collapsed state. When each force is very strong, the balance is easily lost. Losing the balance gives rise to volume phase transition of gels from one state to

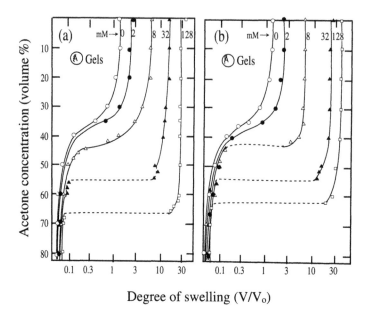

Acetone concentration (volume %)

Degree of swelling (V/V₀)

FIGURE 6.5 Effect of the acetone concentration on the swelling ratio of (a) positively and (b) negatively ionized poly(acrylamide) gels. The positively and negatively ionized gels were prepared by copolymerization of acrylamide and a cross-linker with (methacrylamidopropyl)trimethylammonium chloride (MAPTAC) and sodium acrylate, respectively. The concentration of MAPTAC and sodium acrylate in the gels ranges from 0 to 128 mM. (From Hirokawa, Y., Tanaka, T., and Sato, E., *Macromolecules*, 18, 272, 1985, with permission.)

another state. The volume phase transition of gels is universally similar to that from water to vapor. Tanaka et al. reported various types of volume phase transitions of gels as a function of solvent composition,[14-16,18,19,21] pH,[15] temperature[14,18,20] electric field,[17] light,[22] specific molecules,[23] and so on. The relationship between fundamental interactions of polymer chains and volume phase transitions of gels is described in detail in Section 6.3.

6.2.2 KINETICS OF SWELLING

This section describes a theory for the kinetics of the swelling of a gel in a solvent. Tanaka et al.[25,26] derived a theoretical formula for the equation of motion for a gel. When the gel is transferred into a large volume of the solvent, the gel network begins to expand by absorbing the solvent. The diameter of the gel changes from a_0 to a. Tanaka's theory used the displacement vector, $u(r, t)$, which denotes the displacement of a point on the network from its final equilibrium location after the gel is swollen (Figure 6.6). The equation of the network motion in the solvent is given by:

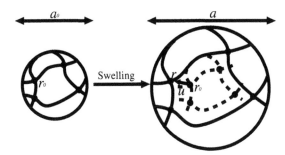

FIGURE 6.6 Swelling change of a gel. The diameter of the gel changes from a_0 to a, then a point r_0 on the network moves to a point r; u represents the displacement vector.

$$\rho \frac{\partial^2 u}{\partial t^2} = \nabla \cdot \tilde{\sigma} - f \frac{\partial u}{\partial t}$$

(8)

where ρ is the mass density of the gel, $\tilde{\sigma}$ is the stress tensor, and f is the friction coefficient between the network and the solvent. The left-hand side of Equation (8) represents the acceleration term of the equation of the motion, and the first and second terms of the right-hand side mean the elastic and the friction terms between the network and solvent, respectively. The component σ_{ij} of the stress tensor and the component u_{ij} of the strain tensor are defined as:

$$\sigma_{ij} = K \nabla \cdot u \delta_{ij} + 2\mu \left(u_{ij} - \frac{1}{3} \nabla \cdot u \delta_{ij} \right)$$

(9)

$$u_{ij} = \frac{1}{2} \left(\frac{\partial u_i}{\partial x_j} + \frac{\partial u_j}{\partial x_i} \right)$$

(10)

where K and μ are the bulk and shear moduli, respectively; δ_{ij} and u_i are the unit tensor and the i-th component of u, respectively. In the case of the diffusion of the gel network, since the acceleration term of the left-hand side of Equation (8) is much smaller than the terms of the right-hand side, it is negligible. By using Equations (8) and (9), therefore, Equation (8) can be rewritten as:

$$\frac{\partial u}{\partial t} = \left(\frac{K + \mu/3}{f}\right)\nabla(\nabla \cdot u) + \left(\frac{\mu}{f}\right)\nabla^2 u \tag{11}$$

Equation (11) is the diffusion equation of a gel and provides the diffusion coefficient as follows:

$$D = \frac{K + 4\mu/3}{f} \tag{12}$$

As the polymer chains in a gel are connected through covalent bonds, electrostatic interactions, hydrogen bonds, etc., all segments in the network move collectively. Therefore, the diffusion coefficient of segments in a gel means the collective diffusion coefficient D, which is much lower than the self-diffusion coefficient of the solvent molecules. Equation (11) is fundamental for discussing kinetics of a gel. The friction coefficient f and the shear modulus μ can be measured by dynamic light scattering.

6.2.2.1 Spherical Gels[25,27]

In the case of a spherical gel, as the displacement vector u is spherically symmetric, Equation (11) can be rewritten as:

$$\frac{\partial u}{\partial t} = D_0 \frac{\partial}{\partial r}\left\{\frac{1}{r^2}\left[\frac{\partial}{\partial r}(r^2 u)\right]\right\} \tag{13}$$

When the radius of a spherical gel changes from initial a_0 to final radius a of an equilibrium state, the kinetics of the gel with zero shear modulus is given by:

$$\Delta a(t) = u(a,t) = \frac{6\Delta a_0}{\pi^2}\sum_{n=1}^{\infty} n^{-2}\exp\left(-\frac{n^2 t}{\tau}\right) \tag{14}$$

$$\tau = \frac{a^2}{\pi^2 D_0} \tag{15}$$

where $\Delta a(t)$ is the radius change of the gel at time t, Δa_0 is the total change of the radius, i.e., $\Delta a_0 = a - a_0$, and τ is the relaxation time for swelling. Equations (14) and (15) enable us to determine the relaxation time τ and the collective diffusion coefficient D_0. Furthermore, Equation (15) indicates that τ is proportional to the square of the gel radius and the inverse of the collective diffusion coefficient. Figure 6.7 shows τ for the swelling of spherical poly(acrylamide) gels as a function of a^2.[25] The rela-

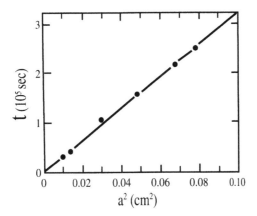

FIGURE 6.7 Relaxation time τ for swelling of spherical poly(acrylamide) gels as a function of the square of the final radius a. (From Tanaka, T. and Fillmore, D.J., *J. Chem. Phys.*, 70, 1214, 1979, with permission.)

tionship between τ and a^2 is found to be linear in agreement with the theoretical prediction of Equation (15). Thus, Equation (15) suggests that designing gel size is of great importance in biomedical applications of swelling or shrinking of gels.

6.2.2.2   Cylindrical Gels and Disk Gels[26]

During swelling of asymmetric gels, the shear modulus μ in Equation (11) is not negligible since the nonisotropic deformation of the gel induces a shear energy. Therefore, the kinetics for a spherical gel is insufficient to describe the swelling and shrinking processes for asymmetric gels because of the existence of the shear modulus of their network. The total energy of a gel is comprised of a bulk energy and a shear energy. The former is related to the volume change, and the latter can be instantly minimized by readjusting the shape of the gel. The shear energy of a gel is represented as:

$$F_{sh} = \mu \int \left[\left(u_{xx} - \frac{T}{3} \right)^2 + \left(u_{yy} - \frac{T}{3} \right)^2 + \left(u_{zz} - \frac{T}{3} \right)^2 \right] dV \qquad (16)$$

where $T = (u_{xx} + u_{yy} + u_{zz})$ is the trace of the strain tensor u_{ij}. The shear energy of a gel is always minimized during a swelling and shrinking process, and the change of total shear energy should be zero:

$$\delta F_{sh} = 0 \qquad (17)$$

The kinetics of the swelling and shrinking for asymmetric gels should be discussed on the basis of both Equations (11) and (17). Tanaka et al. considered an infinitesimally small swelling process as a combination of two consecutive small processes: a pure diffusion process described by equation (11) and a shear relaxation process described by Equation (17). The details of the method are described in Tanaka's paper.[26] This section focuses on only important results concerning the swelling of asymmetric gels such as long cylindrical gels and large disk gels.

The apparent collective diffusion coefficient D_e for asymmetric gels is smaller than the collective diffusion coefficient D_0 for spherical gels due to the reduction effect of the shear process. The relationships between D_0 and D_e for cylindrical gels and large disk gels at their boundaries (their surfaces; $r = a$) are summarized as follows:

$$D_e(a,t) = \frac{2}{3}D_0 \quad \text{(cylindrical gels)} \tag{18}$$

$$D_e(a,t) = \frac{1}{3}D_0 \quad \text{(disk gels)} \tag{19}$$

Figure 6.8 shows the effective collective diffusion coefficient normalized by the collective diffusion coefficient of spherical gels as a function of radial position.[26] It becomes clear from these results that the swelling rate of the disk gel is governed by the thickness. Consequently, the kinetics for swelling and shrinking of gels is strongly dependent upon gel size and shape. In the applications of stimuli-responsive gels, the gel size and shape should be designed for constructing gel systems with fast responses.

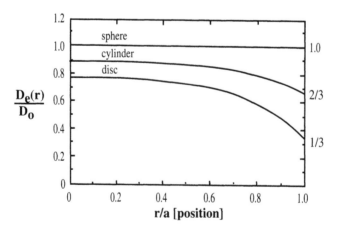

FIGURE 6.8 Position dependence of the effective collective diffusion coefficient normalized by the collective diffusion coefficient of spherical gels, $D_0 = (K + 4\mu/3)/f$. At the boundary, the values for sphere, cylinder, and disk are 1, 2/3, and 1/3, respectively. (From Li, Y. and Tanaka, T., *J. Chem. Phys.*, 92, 1365, 1990, with permission.)

6.2.3 DIFFUSION IN GELS

6.2.3.1 Fick's Law

Diffusion of solvents and solutes in gels is an important factor to determine gel functions such as stimuli responsiveness and drug delivery. This section focuses on diffusion of solvents and small solutes in gels on the basis of Fick's law. The basic equation for diffusion in isotropic media is Fick's first law as follows:

$$J = -D \left(\frac{\partial C}{\partial x} \right) \tag{20}$$

where J is the flux, i.e., the rate of transfer of mass Q per unit cross-sectional area A, C is the concentration of diffusing substance, x is the space coordinate measured normal to the section, and D is the diffusion coefficient. By considering the mass balance of a volume element in which diffusion takes place, the rate of the concentration change is given by:

$$\frac{\partial C}{\partial t} = D \left(\frac{\partial^2 C}{\partial x^2} \right) \tag{21}$$

where Equation (21) is obtained under the condition that D is constant. The condition of constant D is valid in the absence of structural inhomogeneity or anisotropy. Equation (21) is well known as Fick's second law of fundamental differential equation of diffusion.

6.2.3.2 Time Lag[28,29]

In the case of diffusion of penetrant passing through a gel film, Equation (21) can be solved under the specified boundary conditions. The conditions are as follows: the film is initially completely free of the penetrant; the penetrant is first admitted to one side of the film and is continually removed from the other side (the low concentration side; $C_2 = 0$); the amount Q_t of the penetrant passing through the film in time t is given by:

$$Q_1 = \frac{DC_1}{l} \left(t - \frac{l^2}{6D} \right) - \frac{2lC_1}{\pi^2} \sum_{n=1}^{\infty} \frac{(-1)^n}{n^2} \exp\left(\frac{-Dn^2\pi^2 t}{l^2} \right) \tag{22}$$

where l is the film thickness and C_1 is the concentration at the upstream side.

When the steady state is achieved at a large t, the exponential terms of Equation (22) become negligibly small. Then Equation (22) becomes:

$$Q_1 = \frac{DC_1}{l} \left(t - \frac{l^2}{6D} \right) \tag{23}$$

Equation (23) suggests that a plot of t vs. Q_l yields a straight line. The intercept L on the t axis, which is called time lag, is given by:

$$L = \frac{l^2}{6D} \tag{24}$$

Consequently, D can be determined from Equation (24) by measuring time lag L. Tokita[30] determined the diffusion coefficient of the probe molecule in a gel film from time lag (Figure 6.9) and revealed that it agreed rather well with the diffusion coefficient determined from electrophoretic mobility of the molecule in the gel film.

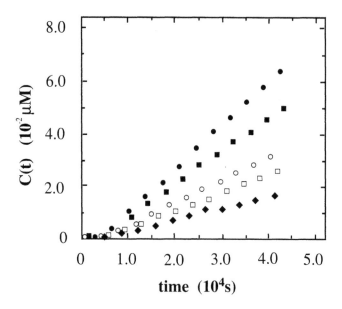

FIGURE 6.9 Elution time course of the probe molecule through a gel film. The initial concentration of the probe molecule in the upstream side: ◆, 4.1 mM; □, 6.1 mM; ○, 8.1 mM; ■, 12.1 mM; ●, 16.2 mM. (From Tokita, M., *Jpn. J. Appl. Phys.*, 34, 2418, 1995, with permission.)

6.2.3.3   Sorption and Desorption Kinetics[28,29,31]

The sorption method is popular in determination of diffusion coefficients since the uptake of the penetrant can be easily monitored by weighing and other appropriate techniques. The solution of the diffusion equation for sorption of penetrant into a gel film with constant D is given by:

$$\frac{M_t}{M_\infty} = 1 - \frac{8}{\pi^2}\sum_{m=0}^{\infty}\frac{1}{(2m+1)^2}\exp\left(\frac{-D(2m+1)^2\pi^2t}{l^2}\right) \qquad (25)$$

where M_t is the total amount of penetrant adsorbed into the film at time t, M_∞ is the equilibrium sorption, and l is the film thickness. Also, with suitable interpretation of M_t and M_∞, Equation (25) describes desorption from the same film. For long times, Equation (25) is approximated by:

$$\frac{M_t}{M_\infty} = 1 - \frac{8}{\pi^2}\exp\left(\frac{-\pi^2 Dt}{l^2}\right) \qquad (26)$$

The approximation for a short time becomes:

$$\frac{M_t}{M_\infty} = \frac{4}{l}\left(\frac{Dt}{\pi}\right)^{1/2} \qquad (27)$$

Equation (27) indicates that a plot of $t^{1/2}$ vs. M_t/M_∞ is initially linear. Therefore, the diffusion coefficient can be determined from the initial slope of the plot.

6.2.3.4 Anomalous Diffusion

The diffusion of penetrant in some polymers cannot be described adequately by Fick's law of a concentration-dependent form (Case I), especially when the penetrant causes extensive swelling of the polymers. This is designated anomalous diffusion, and Case II diffusion and Super-Case II diffusion are known as non-Fickian behaviors.[28,29] Since the boundary between swollen region and glassy core changes as a function of time during swelling of gels in solvents, the diffusions of solvents and/or solutes in gels are almost based on anomalous diffusion.

In general, the total amount M_t of the penetrant sorbed into a polymer at time t is given by:

$$M_t = kt^n \qquad (28)$$

where k and n are constant. If Case I diffusion (Fickian) occurs, $n = 1/2$ (Equation (27), while for Case II diffusion, $n = 1$.[32] Therefore, index n determined from a plot of t vs. M_t provides information about diffusion mechanisms of solvents or solutes in gels.

6.2.3.5 Free Volume Theory

Free volume theory is based on the fact that a polymer has a substantial portion of void space or unoccupied volume. The theory is used for the description of gas permeation through polymer membranes. The free volume theory can be applied to the diffusion of solutes in water-swollen gels.[33,34] In the case of water-soluble solutes, it may be assumed that the effective free volume available for solute permeation is essentially the free volume of water, and that the solutes are not permeated through the polymer matrix. If the interaction between the polymer and the solute is negligible, the solute diffusion in the water-swollen gel can be written as:

$$\frac{D_{2,13}}{D_{2,1}} = \varphi(q_2)\exp\left[-B\left(\frac{q_2}{V_{f,1}}\right)\left(\frac{1}{H}-1\right)\right]$$

(29)

where the suffixes 1, 2, 3, and 13 designate water, solute, polymer, and water-swollen gel, respectively, q_2 is a cross-sectional area of the solute, $\varphi(q_2)$ is the volume fraction of medium filled up by pores equal to or larger than q_2, B is a proportionality factor, $V_{f,1}$ is the free volume of pure water that is available for the permeation of solutes in the water, H is the water content of the gel.

Yasuda et al.[33] measured the diffusion coefficient of sodium chloride in various gel membranes as a function of hydration. A straight line of the plot of $1/H$ vs. D_2 shown in Figure 6.10 demonstrates that Equation (29) is a valid description of the solute diffusion in water-swollen gels.

6.2.3.6   Scaling Theory[35]

A probe molecule fluctuates thermally in time and space when dissolved in a simple fluid. The diffusion coefficient D_0 of the probe molecule is given by the Stokes–Einstein relationship[36] as follows:

$$D_0 = \frac{kT}{6\pi\eta R}$$

(30)

where k is Boltzmann's constant, T is the absolute temperature, η is the viscosity of the fluid, and R is the hydrodynamic radius of the probe molecule.

On the other hand, the diffusion of a probe molecule in a gel is inhibited by the presence of polymer networks, since they behave as fixed obstacles due to the much smaller collective diffusion coefficient of the gel than that of the probe molecules. When the interaction between the polymer networks and the probe molecules is negligible, the diffusion of the probe molecules is governed only by the mesh size of the network and the sizes of the probe molecules. Based on the scaling theory,[37] the diffusion coefficient D of the probe molecules in gel is represented as:

$$\frac{D}{D_0} = f\left(\frac{R}{\xi}\right)$$

(31)

where D_0 is the diffusion coefficient of the probe molecule in the simple fluid, R is the size of the probe molecule, ξ is the correlation length of the network, and $f(x)$ is

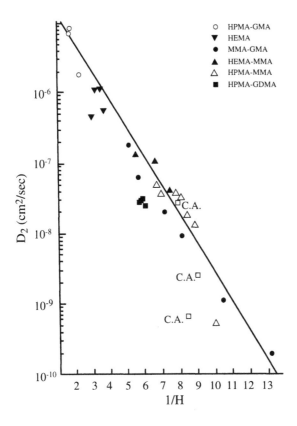

FIGURE 6.10 Diffusion coefficient of NaCl in various membranes as a function of reciprocal hydration. (From Yasuda, H., Lamae, C.E., and Ikenberry, L.D., *Makromol. Chem.*, 118, 19, 1968, with permission.)

the scaling function. R/ξ is the ratio of characteristic lengths of the probe molecule and networks. R and ξ have a power law relationship for the molecular weight M of the probe molecule and the predetermined concentration ϕ of monomer in the pregel solution. Since the scaling function of the diffusion coefficient is expected to be $f(x)$ = exp($-x$) according to hydrodynamic theory,[38] the diffusion coefficient of the probe molecule in the gel is given by:

$$\frac{D}{D_0} = \exp(-M^{1/3}\phi^{3/4}) \tag{32}$$

Theoretical results obtained on the basis of Equation (32) were in good agreement with the experimental results using a pulsed field gradient NMR technique (Figure 6.11).[35]

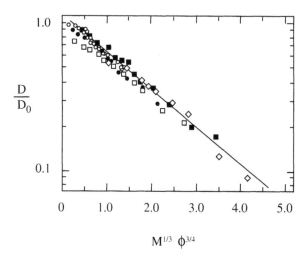

FIGURE 6.11 Relationship between the normalized diffusion coefficients D/D_0 of the probe molecules in the gel and the scaling variable $M^{1/2}\phi^{3/4}$. ○ water; ●, ethanol; □, glycerin; ■, poly(ethyleneglycol), and ◇, sucrose. (From Tokita, M. et al., *Phys. Rev. E*, 53, 1823, 1996, with permission.)

6.3   FUNDAMENTAL INTERACTIONS IN GELS

Volume phase transition of gels is a unique feature that provides many opportunities to use this feature to develop intelligent materials in biological and biomedical fields. The thermodynamics of volume phase transition are described in Section 6.2.1. The balance of the repulsion and attraction forces of polymer chains in gels plays an important role in volume phase transition. For example, when the repulsion between polymer chains is more dominant than the attraction, the gel swells. The strong attraction between polymer chains causes shrinking of the gel. Such repulsion and attraction between polymer chains are mainly generated by four fundamental molecular interactions: van der Waals interaction, hydrophobic interaction, hydrogen bonding, and electrostatic interaction. The volume phase transition of gels visualizes fundamental molecular interactions operating polymer chains. Fundamental researches on volume phase transition of gels contributes significantly to our understanding of superstructures and functions of biological molecules and systems based on a variety of interactions. In the following section, four fundamental interactions from the viewpoint of volume phase transition of gels (Figure 6.12) are described.[39]

6.3.1   VAN DER WAALS INTERACTION

The fundamentally weak van der Waals interaction that results from the attraction between dipoles induced by fluctuation of electron in neutral molecules. Volume phase transition of hydrophilic gels in a mixed solvent is basically caused by van der Waals interaction (Figure 6.12 a). For example, ionized poly(acrylamide) (PAAm)

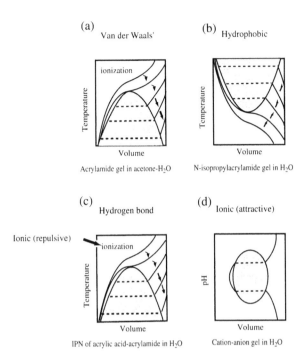

FIGURE 6.12 Volume phase transitions of gels induced by four fundamental interactions; (a) van der Waals interaction, (b) hydrophobic interaction, (c) hydrogen bonding, and (d) electrostatic interaction. (From Ilman, F., Tanaka, T., and Kokufuta, E., *Nature*, 349, 400, 1991, with permission.)

gels undergo discontinuous volume phase transition in an acetone–water mixture (Figure 6.5).[15,16] PAAm is very soluble in pure water since its amide groups have strong interactions with water molecules. In the PAAm gels, the strong interaction between the amide groups and water molecules causes the swelling of the gels and van der Waals interaction between PAAm chains is the attraction that collapses the gels. In the ionized PAAm gels in the acetone–water mixture, however, the presence of acetone results in decreasing interactions between the amide groups and water molecules because acetone as a nonpolar solvent plays an important role in decreasing the dielectric constant of the solvent. In ionized PAAm gels in an acetone–water mixture, the van der Waals interaction between PAAm chains is the most important interaction governing the state of the gels since the van der Waals interaction becomes more predominant than the interaction between the amide groups and water molecules. Thus the ionized PAAm gels collapse in the acetone–water mixture, based on the van der Waals interaction. The ionization of the PAAm gels gives rise to discontinuous volume phase transition in the acetone–water mixture. In the case of an acetone–water mixture with a fixed acetone concentration, ionized PAAm gels shrink at low temperatures and swell at high temperatures because the van der Waals interaction becomes weaker with rising temperature, i.e., a negative function of temperature.

6.3.2 Hydrophobic Interaction

Some poly(alkylacrylamide) gels are well-known to undergo volume phase transition in water by varying the temperature.[18,20,40] Unlike the positively temperature-dependent swelling change of hydrolyzed PAAm gels in an acetone–water mixture described in Section 6.3.1, a poly(N-isopropylacrylamide) (PNIPAAm) gel in water collapses with rising temperature. The negative swelling change of the PNIPAAm gel implies that the volume phase transition is based on a molecular interaction that becomes stronger with temperature, i.e., hydrophobic interaction (Figure 6.12b). Water molecules around hydrophobic polymer chains form ordered structures similar to the ice structure. The formation of ordered structures of water molecules lowers both enthalpy and entropy of the system and is an exothermic process. Therefore, the hydrophobic polymer chains prefer to interact with each other at higher temperatures to prevent the formation of the ordered structures of water molecules. This is the hydrophobic interaction acting on the hydrophobic polymer chains (see Chapter 2). As the hydrophobic interaction becomes stronger with rising temperature due to entropic contributions, the PNIPAAm gel undergoes volume phase transition in water from a swollen state at low temperatures to a collapsed state at high temperatures. Molecular design to control hydrophobic interaction is important in synthesizing the gels that undergo volume phase transition.

6.3.3 Hydrogen Bonding

Hydrogen bonding plays important roles in fabricating the structures of biological molecules and systems. For example, DNA composed of nucleotides forms double or triple strands with its complementary base pairs by hydrogen bonding. Details of hydrogen bonding are described in Chapter 3. It should be kept in mind that the hydrogen bond has a directional preference. This means that polymer architectures such as sequences and shapes strongly affect the formation of hydrogen bonds. In biological molecules and systems, the directional preference of the hydrogen bond enables them to fabricate their superstructures. Hydrogen bonding between polymer chains sometimes exhibits a cooperative activity called the "zipper" effect. Volume changes driven by hydrogen bonding were observed for IPN gels consisting of poly(acrylic acid) (PAAc) and PAAm.[39,41-43] The pioneer studies by Okano et al.[41-43] demonstrated that the PAAc/PAAm IPN gel without ionized groups undergoes a continuous volume change from a collapsed state to a swollen state via rising temperature. The positively temperature-dependent swelling changes are due to the weakening of the hydrogen bond with rising temperature, i.e., a negative function of temperature. In addition, slight ionization of the PAAc/PAAm IPN gel induced the discontinuous volume phase transition in response to temperature in pure water (Figure 6.12c).[39] However, the PAAc/PAAm gels without IPN structures exhibited no discontinuous volume phase transition. This leads us to the conclusion that cooperative hydrogen bonding by "zipper" effect gives rise to positively temperature-dependent volume changes.

6.3.4 ELECTROSTATIC INTERACTION

Electrostatic interaction is a long range order interaction that is the strongest in four fundamental molecular interactions. The interaction between negative and positive charges induces the attraction, and the interaction between similar charges gives rise to the repulsion. Thus positively or negatively charged groups in gels strongly dominate their swelling behavior. For example, gels with ionizable groups swell by ionization of the groups because the osmotic pressure increases due to counterions localized near the ionized groups. The repulsion by similar charges on the polymer chains also causes strong swelling of the gels. On the other hand, the attraction between negative and positive charges induces discontinuous volume phase transition in polyampholyte gels (Figure 6.12d). The polyampholyte gels consisting of acrylamide sodium acrylate and methacrylamidopropyltrimethylammonium chloride (MAPTAC) swell at acidic and basic pH, but shrink at neutral pH.[44] In polyampholyte gels, positively charged groups have attractive interactions with negatively charged groups over long ranges, but the similarly charged groups repel each other over short ranges. At neutral pH, therefore, the polyampholyte gels shrink by attraction since each ionizable group has negative or positive charges. Positive charges at acidic pH or negative charges at basic pH result in drastic swelling of the polyampholyte gels by their repulsion. The presence of several phases (multiple phases) was found between the fully swollen and collapsed phases (Figure 6.13).[45] The multiple phases of the gels are attributable to complicated balances of repulsion and attraction on the basis of electrostatic interactions between positive and negative charges. The multiple phases of the gels may be associated with the superstructured folding of proteins.

To summarize, van der Waals interaction and hydrogen bonding cause volume phase transition that causes gels to swell at high temperatures and shrink at low temperatures since their interactions have negative temperature dependences. On the other hand, hydrophobic interaction enables gels to collapse at high temperatures due to their positive temperature dependence. In volume phase transition based on these three interactions, the ionization of polymer chains plays important roles in discontinuous volume phase transition. In addition, electrostatic interaction gives rise to swelling or shrinking due to repulsion or attraction which depends on the combination of positive and negative charges. One or more of these four fundamental interactions determine specific phases of a gel. Therefore, a gel is at a stable phase while maintaining the balance of the interactions, and undergoes unique volume phase transition when the balance is lost. Four fundamental interactions are essential factors that determine the swelling behaviors of gels, such as volume phase transition. Knowledge gained from volume phase transition induced by fundamental interactions provides a basis for synthesis of stimuli-responsive gels and provides more insight into superstructures of biomolecules and folding of proteins.

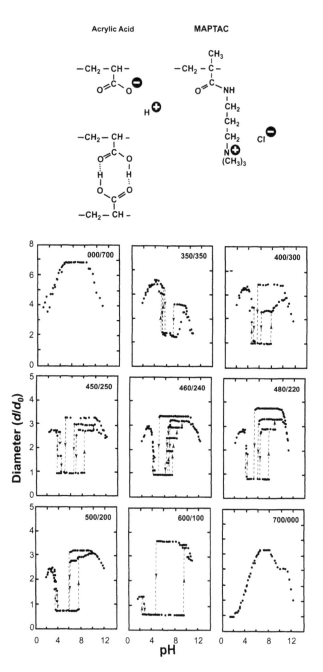

FIGURE 6.13 Equilibrium swelling ratios of copolymer gels consisting of acrylic acid and MAPTAC in water, as a function of pH, at 25°C. Acrylic acid and MAPTAC ratios are indicated in the figures. (From Annaka, M. and Tanaka, T., *Nature*, 355, 430, 1992, with permission.)

6.4 SYNTHESIS OF GELS AND IPNs

6.4.1 COVALENTLY CROSS-LINKED GELS

6.4.1.1 Polymerization

Covalently cross-linked gels can be synthesized by radical copolymerization of vinyl monomers with divinyl compounds or by condensation polymerization of monomers with functional groups (Figure 6.14a). Radical polymerization is one of the most popular methods of synthesizing gels. Radical polymerizations are classified into bulk, solution, suspension, emulsion, plasma, and photo polymerizations. Bulk and solution radical polymerizations are often used for gel preparation. In most cases of bulk and solution polymerizations, vinyl and/or (meth)acryl monomers are copolymerized with divinyl or di(meth)acryl monomers as cross-linkers by various initiators.

Acrylamide, N-isopropylacrylamide, (meth)acrylic acid, 2-hydroxyethyl methacrylate, N-vinyl-2-pyrrolidone, and other hydrophilic monomers are the main monomers for synthesizing gels for biological and biomedical applications. Ethylene glycol dimethacrylate and N,N'–methylene bisacrylamide are widely used as cross-linkers of covalently cross-linked gels. Their chemical structures are shown in Figure 6.15.

Azobisisobutyronitrile (AIBN), benzoyl peroxide (BPO), and ammonium persulfate (APS) are common initiators of radical polymerization. As the addition of a reducing agent accelerates radical formation from peroxide, the redox initiators such as hydrogen peroxide/reducing agent enable us to polymerize monomers at low temperatures. Metal ions in reduced states such as Fe^{2+} or Cu^+ are commonly used as reducing agents. In solution polymerization, solvents affect the polymerization, which dominates the structures and properties of the resultant gels. For example, using a poor solvent for the resultant polymers sometimes gives rise to precipitation without

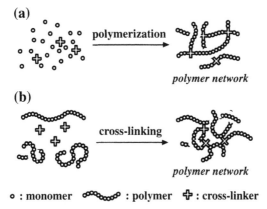

FIGURE 6.14 Methods to synthesize covalently cross-linked gels: (a) polymerization; (b) cross-linking of polymers.

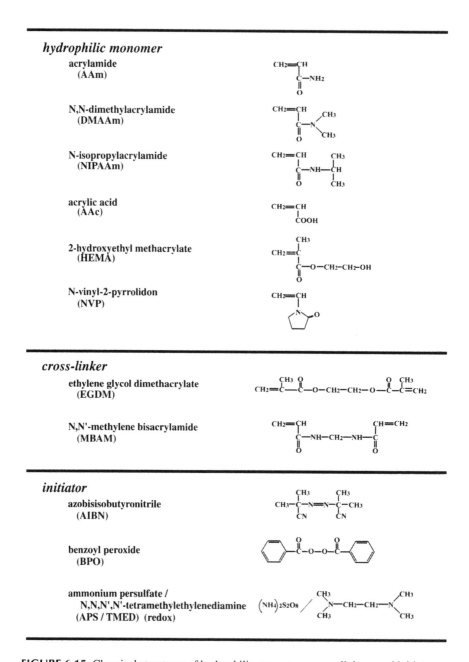

FIGURE 6.15 Chemical structures of hydrophilic monomers, cross-linkers, and initiators.

forming swollen gels. Therefore, the solvent for solution polymerization should be carefully selected to ensure homogeneously swollen gels. Most gels prepared by radical polymerization have heterogeneous network structures due to differences in reactivity between cross-linkers and hydrophilic monomers and between two vinyl groups of cross-linkers. Suspension and emulsion polymerizations are effective to prepare gel particles;[46-48] whereas plasma and photo polymerizations are useful to form gel layers on films or membranes by graft copolymerizations.[49,50]

Condensation polymerization requries monomers with polyfunctional groups to form three-dimensional networks. Condensation polymerization of monomers with bifunctional groups produces linear polymers; the presence of monomers with three or more groups results in the formation of three-dimensional networks. For example, condensation polymerization of ethylene glycol and adipic acid leads to a linear polyester, but condensation polymerization of glycerol and adipic acid produces a three-dimensional polyester network. Since the resultant three-dimensional network has high cross-linking density, the gel hardly swells in a solvent. The kind of monomer with polyfunctional groups and main monomers should be carefully chosen for preparing soft gels for biological and biomedical applications.

6.4.1.2 Cross-Linking of Polymers

One method to synthesize gels is direct cross-linking of linear or branched polymers using a small amount of a cross-linking agent (Figure 6.14b). In most cases, the cross-linking reaction is performed in a solution containing hydrophilic polymers; aqueous solutions are usually used in synthesizing gels as biomaterials. Polymers with hydroxyl groups such as poly(vinyl alcohol) (PVA) and cellulose can be cross-linked with aldehydes, dicarbonic acids, bisepoxides, diisocyanates, etc. Diol and diamine are cross-linking agents for polymers with isocyanate groups. Polymers with amino groups form gels by cross-linking with aldehydes. On the whole, cross-linking of hydrophilic polymers with functional groups provides more homogeneous gels than polymerization using cross-linking monomers. However, since the cross-linking reaction does not proceed perfectly, the resultant network often has some defects such as unreacted polymer chains, entanglements and loops.

Linear or branched polymers can be cross-linked by γ-ray irradiation and electron beam irradiation in aqueous solutions. For example, γ-ray irradiation for an aqueous solution of poly(vinyl methyl ether) (PVME) produces a PVME gel with a porous structure that is formed by phase separation through heating under the irradiation.[51,52] The fine porous structures of the PVME gel cause a quick response during shrinking in response to temperature changes. Cross-linking by radioactive rays has some advantages: (1) it does not need initiator; (2) it can be carried out at a low temperature; (3) relatively homogeneous gels can be obtained due to good reproducibility of radioactive rays; (4) cross-linking structures of the resultant gels can be controlled by irradiation dose, time, temperature, polymer concentration, solvent, etc. However, since cross-linking reaction by radioactive rays is strongly dependent upon the kind of polymer and some polymers do not produce homogeneous gels, one should pay attention to cross-linking conditions.

6.4.2 NonCovalently Cross-Linked Gels

6.4.2.1 Cross-Linking by Hydrogen Bonds

Agars of natural polymers are known to form gels by cooling to 30°C after melting at more than 90°C. The gelation by cooling is attributed to the association of double helices induced by hydrogen bonding between hydroxyl groups of saccharides (Figure 6.16a).[53] An aqueous gelatin solution is gelated by cooling to a temperature of less than 25°C due to the association of a triple helix formed by hydrogen bonding between N–H and C=O groups in polypeptides. The aqueous solutions of their natural polymers undergo reversible sol–gel phase transitions in response to temperature changes on the basis of the association and dissociation of the helix structure by hydrogen bonding. These classical phenomena suggest that gels can be prepared by cross-linking through hydrogen bonding. Hydrogen bonding has been used to prepare natural polymer gels and synthetic polymer gels. Repetitive freezing and thawing of an aqueous PVA solution produces a PVA gel with a strong three-dimensional network structure.[54-56] The gel is formed by the cooperative hydrogen bonding among hydroxyl groups. The mechanical strength of the PVA gel can be improved by increasing the number of freezing/thawing cycles, which encourages the formation of hydrogen bonds as cross-links. Cross-linking by hydrogen bonding has an important

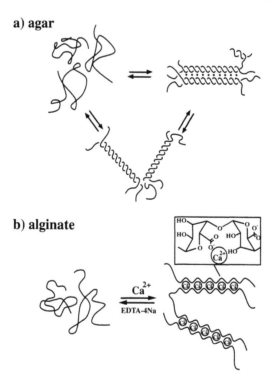

FIGURE 6.16 Examples of noncovalently cross-linked gels: gelation of (a) agar and (b) alginate.

advantage in preparing gels used in biomedical fields; the cross-linking agents, most of which are harmful to the human body, are unnecessary in gel preparation. This is one reason why the PVA gel is a promising biomaterial.

6.4.2.2 Cross-Linking by Ionic Bonds and Coordinate Bonds

Alginates are linear polysaccharides containing β-D-mannuronic acid and α-L-gu-luronic acid residues. Alginate gels can be prepared by adding a solution of sodium alginate into an aqueous solution of divalent cross-linking agents such as Ca^{2+}, Sr^{2+} and Ba^{2+}. The gelation is mainly achieved by the exchange of sodium ions from the guluronic acids with divalent cations and by the stacking of these guluronic groups to form the characteristic egg-box structure (Figure 6.16b).[57,58] The divalent cations bind to the α-L-guluronic acid blocks in a highly cooperative manner. Each alginate chain can be dimerized to form cross-links with many other chains, and as a result gel networks rather than insoluble precipitates are formed. Unique bioconjugate gels were recently synthesized by assembling water-soluble synthetic polymers and a well-defined coiled-coil protein through complexation between metal-chelating li-gands and metals.[59,60]

6.4.3 IPNs[11-13]

6.4.3.1 Sequential Method

This method initially requires preparation of polymer network I. The resulting net-work I is swollen by monomers, cross-linker, and activator. Polymer network II is then synthesized in the first polymer network I *in situ* (Figure 6.17a). An example of the sequential method is as follows. A network of poly(ethyl acrylate) (PEA) is ini-tially prepared by the photopolymerization of ethyl acrylate and tetraethyleneglycol dimethacrylate (TEGDM) as a cross-linker, with benzoin as a photosensitizer. After the resulting PEA network is swollen in the styrene monomer containing TEGDM and benzoin, another photopolymerization is performed to form the second poly(styrene) (PS) network. Thus, PEA/PS IPNs can be prepared by the sequential method.[61] In general, swelling of the polymer network I by monomer II, cross-linker, and activator governs the morphologies and properties of the resulting IPNs since the swelling influences entanglements between polymer networks I and II. This means that morphology of the resulting IPNs can be controlled by structural designs of poly-mer network I. When a linear polymer is used in place of polymer network I, the semi-IPN in which a linear polymer is entrapped in the second polymer network II is obtained.

6.4.3.2 Simultaneous Method

Monomers and/or prepolymers are simultaneously mixed with cross-linkers and ac-tivators to form both networks. The simultaneous polymerizations are carried out by noninterfering reactions (Figure 6.17b). The simultaneous method requires choosing

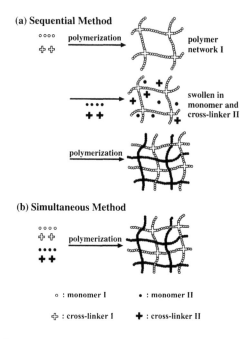

FIGURE 6.17 Basic synthesis methods for IPNs: (a) sequential IPNs; (b) simultaneous IPNs.

a different reaction mechanism for each monomer to form polymer networks I and II. In general, a combination of radical polymerization and condensation polymerization can minimize the interference of each reaction. For example, a mixture of butyl acrylate and an epoxy compound can be simultaneously polymerized by application of light and heat to yield a simultaneous IPN.[62] During simultaneous polymerizations, the gelation of polymer I and polymer II and phase separation take place. Their order, depending on the combination of the monomers, dominates the morphologies and properties of the resulting IPNs. If one polymerization provides cross-linked networks and the other provides linear polymers, the simultaneous polymerizations result in formation of a semi-IPN.

6.5 STRUCTURES AND CHARACTERIZATIONS OF GELS AND IPNs

6.5.1 Swelling Ratio

The swelling of gels is the most important property, and the degree of swelling must be evaluated quantitatively. In general, the degree of swelling is typically expressed as the equilibrium volume swelling ratio or the equilibrium weight swelling ratio. The equilibrium volume swelling ratio q is defined as the volume V of the equilibrium swollen gel divided by the volume v_2 of the same gel before swelling as follows:

$$q = \frac{V}{\upsilon_2} \qquad (33)$$

Similarly, the equilibrium weight swelling ratio is the corresponding ratio of the weights of the two gel states. The water content (%H_2O) is also an indicator to estimate the degree of swelling. The water content is typically defined as:

$$\%H_2O = \frac{w_s - w_d}{w_s} \qquad (34)$$

where w_s and w_d are the weights of the swollen gel and dried gel, respectively. Highly swollen gels show the swelling ratio from 10 to 1000, depending on their chemical and physical structures. Then the highly swollen gels retain solvents of more than 90%.

6.5.2 CROSS-LINKING DENSITY

Cross-linking density of gels governs their physical properties. Therefore, determination of cross-linking density is the most important aspect in characterization of gels. Most researchers use two methods to determine cross-linking density of gels — the determination from the swelling ratio using the Flory-Rehner equation and the determination from the elastic modulus. The fundamental theory in their methods can be used on the assumption that the microscopic relative average positions of cross-linking points must change in proportion to the changes in macroscopic dimensions of the gels. It should be kept in mind that their methods provide only average values for the cross-linking density of the gels, and most gels have heterogeneously cross-linking structures such as irregularly, loosely, and imperfectly cross-linked networks. However, the cross-linking density determined by their methods leads to a better understanding of the structures and functions of gels.

6.5.2.1 Cross-Linking Density from Swelling Ratio[24,63]

The state of a nonionic gel swollen in a solvent was discussed by Flory and Rehner.[24,63] The swelling equilibrium equation is comprised of mixing and elastic terms as follows:

$$-\left[\ln(1-\upsilon_2)+\upsilon_2+\chi\upsilon_2^2\right] = v_1(v_e/V_0)(\upsilon_2^{1/3}-\upsilon_2/2) \qquad (35)$$

where υ_2 is the equilibrium polymer volume fraction, χ is the Flory polymer–solvent interaction parameter, v_1 is the molar volume of the solvent, v_e is the effective number of chains in the network, and V_0 is the volume of the relaxed network before swelling. For the definitions of chains in the network, see section 6.2.1 and Figure 6.1. Therefore, v_e/V_0 corresponds to the cross-linking density of the gel. By neglecting the higher terms in the series expansion of the left-hand member of Equation 35, the equation can be solved for $v_2 = 1/q$ with the following result:

$$q^{5/3} \cong (V_0 / v_e)(1/2 - \chi)/v_1 \tag{36}$$

where q is the equilibrium volume swelling ratio. Therefore, if χ is known, the cross-linking density of the gel can be easily determined by swelling measurements, using Equation (36). If χ is unknown, it must be predetermined by other methods. It should be noted that the cross-linking density determined by this method is strongly affected by heterogeneity of the gel structure. The average molecular weight M_c between cross-links can be obtained by:

$$v_e = (V / \bar{\upsilon} M_c)(1 - 2M_c / M) \tag{37}$$

where, V is the total volume and $\bar{\upsilon}$ is the specific volume of the polymer. The factor $(1 - 2M_c/M)$ is the correction for network imperfections resulting from chain ends. Therefore, for a perfect network ($M = \infty$), the factor $(1 - 2M_c/M)$ reduces to unity.

In the case of ionic gels, the terms for osmotic pressure arising from the difference in the mobile ion concentration must be added to Equation (36) as follows:

$$q^{5/3} \cong \left[\left(i / 2v_u C_s^{1/2} \right)^2 + (1/2 - \chi)/v_1 \right] / (v_e / V_0) \tag{38}$$

where i is the number of electronic charges per polymer unit in a polyelectrolyte, v_u is the molar volume of a structural unit, and C_s is the ionic strength. The determination of the cross-linking density of ionic gels from their swelling ratio is more complicated than the procedure for nonionic gels, because of the need to know χ and also i.

6.5.2.2 Cross-Linking Density from Elastic Modulus[24,64,65]

The cross-linking density of gels is an important factor in governing their elasticity. Let us assume that a cross-linked network formed at volume V_0 is isotropically swollen in a solvent to volume V. When the cross-linked network swollen in the solvent acts as an elastomer, the configurational entropy change ΔS relative to the initial state is given on the assumption of an affine transformation as follows:

$$\Delta S = -\left(\frac{kv_e}{2\upsilon_2^{2/3}} \right) \left(\alpha^2 + \frac{2}{\alpha} - 3 + \ln\upsilon_2 \right) \tag{39}$$

where k is Boltzmann's constant, α is deformation of a network structure by elonga-
tion ($\alpha = L/L_0$), υ_2 is the volume fraction of polymer, and v_e is the effective number
of chains in the network.

The elastic retractive force (f) for an ideal rubber is given by:

$$f = -\left(\frac{T}{L_0}\right)\left(\frac{\partial S}{\partial \alpha}\right)_{T,V} \qquad (40)$$

From Equations (39) and (40), the tension τ expressed as retractive force per unit
of initial cross-sectional area of the swollen unstretched gel is given by:

$$\tau = \left(\frac{RT\upsilon_e}{V\upsilon_2^{2/3}}\right)\left(\alpha - \frac{1}{\alpha^2}\right) = \left(\frac{RTv_e}{V_0}\upsilon_2^{1/3}\right)\left(\alpha - \frac{1}{\alpha^2}\right) \qquad (41)$$

where v_e is given in moles. Equation (41) corresponds to the relationship between the
stress (τ) and the strain ($\alpha - 1/\alpha^2$) for the gel. The factor $RTv_e\upsilon_2^{1/3}/V_0$ represents the
elastic modulus of the gel. Consequently, since the plot of τ vs. ($\alpha - 1/\alpha^2$) gives us
the elastic modulus from the slope, the cross-linking density (v_e/V_0) of the gel can be
determined by using Equation (41). The elastic modulus can be measured easily by
a variety of methods, and provides knowledge of cross-linking structures more directly than the swelling ratio. For example, the cross-linking structures of gels with
phosphate groups[66] or bioconjugates gels containing lectin[67] were investigated by
measuring compressive modulus. Thus, determinations of the cross-linking density
of a gel from its elastic modulus might be easier and more accurate than those from
swelling ratios, since the determination from swelling ratios require the Flory polymer–solvent interaction parameter and the number of electronic charges, and the
elastic modulus reflects network structures directly.

6.5.3 MICROSCOPIC STRUCTURES

Microscopic structures such as spatial inhomogeneity are not only attractive objects
from the scientific standpoints but also important factors that should be designed to
control properties of gels. Several techniques such as light scattering, small-angle neutron scattering (SANS), and small-angle X-ray scattering (SAXS) allow us to better
understand the microscopic structures of gels. Thermal motions of polymer molecules
in a solution cause space and time fluctuations of polymer concentration. Most scattering techniques detect such fluctuations of polymer concentration. However, the investigations of gel structures by scattering techniques have some difficulties because
of their connected polymer chains. Light scattering has been used for investigating the
structural inhomogeneities of gels. The friction coefficient f and the shear modulus μ
(see Section 6.2.2) can be measured by dynamic light scattering. The investigation of
microscopic structures and determination of kinetic parameter of gels by light

scattering have been described.[68-74] This section focuses on studies on spatial inhomogeneity of gels by using SANS.

SANS has some advantages in investigating the homogeneitie of gels — variety of labeling techniques, high contrast between hydrogen and deuterium, and strong transmission power. By using SANS, therefore, many researchers have investigated microscopic structures of gels, focusing on cross-links[75,76] Microscopic structures of gels can be characterized by the correlation length ξ of the polymer chains, which indicates "blob" size (mesh size) composed of polymer chains entangled with each other. In the case of semi-dilute polymer solutions, the elastic scattered intensity $I_L(q)$ is expressed as a function of the transfer wave vector q by the Ornstein–Zernike (OZ) equation:

$$I_L(q) = \frac{I_L(0)}{1+\xi^2 q^2} \tag{42}$$

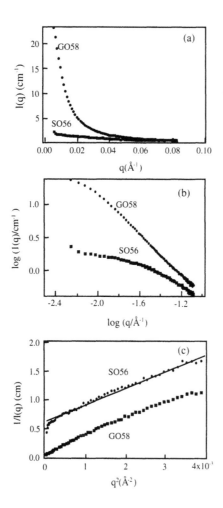

FIGURE 6.18 Small-angle neutron scattering intensity profiles for the PNIPAAm gel (G083) and the PNIPAAm solution (S056): (a) linear plot; (b) log–log plot; and (c) Ornstein–Zernike plot. The straight line in (c) indicates the fit with Equation (42). (From Shibayama, M., Tanaka, T., and Han, C.C., *J. Chem. Phys.*, 97, 6829, 1992, with permission.)

The correlation length ξ indicates the range of the spatial correlation of concentration fluctuation in the polymer solution. However, the concentration fluctuations in gels are perturbed due to the presence of cross-links, and do not obey Equation (42). Hechet et al.[77] divided the scattering intensity function into the solution-like and solid-like contributions. The solution-like contribution is expressed by Equation (42). Horkay et al.[78,79] used the form of $\exp[-\Xi^S q^S]$ as a scattering function for the regions in which the mobility of polymer chains is restricted by the cross-links, and provided an appropriate scattering intensity function for gels as follows:

$$I(q) = I_G(0)\exp(-\Xi^s q^s) + \frac{I_L(0)}{1+\xi^2 q^2} \tag{43}$$

where Ξ is the mean size of the solid-like nonuniformity. The first and second terms of the right-hand side represent solid-like and solution-like contributions, respectively. Shibayama et al.[80] exchanged the solid-like contribution in Equation (43) with the "Guinier" function by using the radius of gyration of the polymer rich (or poor) domains ($R_g = 3^{1/2}\Xi$) as follows:

$$I(q) = I_G(0)\exp\left(\frac{-R_g^2 q^2}{3}\right) + \frac{I_L(0)}{1+\xi^2 q^2} \tag{44}$$

Based on Equations (42) and (44), the scattering intensity functions for PNIPAAm solutions and PNIPAAm gels in D_2O were compared in SANS experiments. Figure 6.18c demonstrates that the application of Equation (42) for polymer solutions is valid. It is noteworthy that the PNIPAAm gels exhibit a strong scattering at low q region due to their heterogeneity (Figure 6.18b). Curve fittings for the scattering intensity as a function of q in the PNIPAAm solutions and gels provided the correlation lengths ξ of 21.3 Å and 45.3 Å, respectively. From the discussion about the correlation length ξ of polymer solutions and gels, it was clear that the introduction of cross-links caused a change in the solvent quality from a good solvent to a θ solvent. In addition, the curve fitting for gels revealed that a static inhomogeneity of characteristic size $R_g = 146$ Å was superimposed (Figure 6.19).

6.5.4 MORPHOLOGY OF IPNs

Most multicomponent polymers consisting of immiscible polymers have macro- or microphase separations with various morphologies. Since IPNs are multicomponent polymer networks in which two or more polymers are interlocked in a three-dimensional structure, phase separation takes place in IPNs of combinations of immiscible polymers.[11-13] Morphology of IPNs is an important factor to dominate the material properties strongly. It can be controlled by chemical compatibility of the polymers, interfacial tension, cross-linking density, polymerization method, IPN composition, etc.

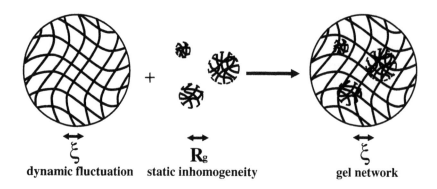

dynamic fluctuation   static inhomogeneity   gel network

FIGURE 6.19 Schematic diagram for the concentration fluctuations in gels.

Microscopy is a useful tool for observing the morphologies of IPNs directly. Observation of coarse structures at a magnification range about 1000 times is possible with optical microscopy. Transmission electron microscopy (TEM) enables us to study morphological details at magnifications of 100,000 times. In TEM observations, most samples must be stained by OsO_4[81] or RuO_4.[82] TEM image contrast caused by staining reveals the morphologies of IPNs. Many researchers have investigated the effects of some factors on the morphologies of IPNs using TEM. For example, Huelck et al.[83,84] observed the morphologies of sequential IPNs of poly(ethyl acrylate) (PEA: polymer I) and poly(methyl methacrylate) (PMMA: polymer II), or of PEA (polymer I) and poly(styrene) (PS: polymer II). The PEA/PMMA IPNs, whose components are isomeric and nearly compatible, have fine structures with dispersed phase domains less than 100 Å in size (Figure 6.20a). In the PEA/PS of the much less compatible combination, however, a cellular structure of about 1000 Å in size was found (Figure 6.20b). Thus, IPNs for higher compatibility systems have morphologies with a smaller domain size than those for lower compatibility systems. Furthermore, some TEM observations revealed that increasing cross-linking density in polymer network I clearly decreases the domain size of polymer II and that variation of cross-linking density in the polymer network II has little effect on IPN morphology.[85,86]

Many studies on sequential IPNs led to the following generalizations about their morphologies: (1) polymer I tends to form a continuous phase for all compositions; (2) IPNs containing polymer II at high concentrations tend to have dual phase continuity; (3) domain sizes of IPNs change from about 100 nm for highly immiscible polymer combinations to about 10 nm for microheterogeneous combinations; (4) increasing cross-linking density results in decreasing domain size. It is noteworthy that the morphology of IPNs can be controlled by the cross-links as well as the compatibility between polymer I and polymer II.

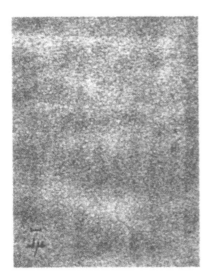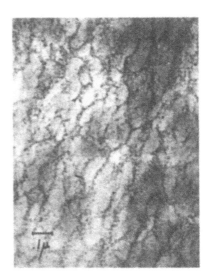

FIGURE 6.20 Transmission electron micrographs of sequential IPNs of (a) PEA/PMMA (72.2/27.8) and (b) PEA/PSt (48.8/51.2). (From Huelck, V., Thomas, D.A., and Sperling, L.H., *Macromolecules*, 5, 340, 1972, with permission.)

On the other hand, the control of the morphology of simultaneous IPNs might be more difficult than those of sequential IPNs, since both networks are formed at the same time in the simultaneous IPNs. Frish et al.[87] explored the effect of mutual solubility on the morphology of polyurethane (PU)-based simultaneous IPNs. The PU/PMMA combination provides a closer match in solubility parameters than the PU/PSt combination. As a result, the PU/PMMA IPNs exhibited significantly greater molecular mixing than the PU/PSt IPNs.

6.6 UNIQUE PROPERTIES AND BIOLOGICAL APPLICATIONS OF GELS AND IPNs

Gels exhibit both liquid-like and solid-like behaviors. Such behaviors are closely associated with their unique properties such as water adsorption, biocompatibility, separation characteristics, stimuli-responsiveness, etc. The important point is that physical properties of water-swollen gels are similar to those of living bodies. Gels have great potential in a variety of biomedical and pharmaceutical applications. In particular, they are promising candidates as biomaterials due to their high water content and special surface properties. Gels have some advantages as biological and biomedical materials:

(1) They can adsorb and retain a large amount of water.
(2) Their soft nature minimizes mechanical and frictional irritation to surrounding tissue.

(3) Their zero or very low interfacial free energy in surrounding biological fluids and tissue minimizes the physicochemical driving forces for protein adsorption and cell adhesion.

(4) They allow and control the permeation and diffusion of low molecular weight solutes such as drugs.

(5) They respond to environmental changes and induce their own structural changes.

The ability to absorb and retain water enables us to use gels as super-water absorbents in products such as disposable diapers. In general, polyelectrolyte gels can absorb over 100 times more weight of water than the weight of the polymer network. The polyelectrolyte gels are used in disposable diapers because they retain large amounts of water.

The second and third advantages are concerned with the biocompatibility of gels in biomedical and pharmaceutical applications. Contact lenses are the most outstanding examples of successful biomedical application of gels. Unique surface properties of a few gels prevent biological responses such as toxic and foreign-body reactions.[4,88-90] Chapter 16 focuses on the biocompatibility of biomaterials from the viewpoint of their protein adsorption and anticoagulation. Commercially available hemodialysis membranes are considered water-swollen gels due to their potentially high water-swollen states. Thus, membranes for artificial kidneys, artificial liver, artificial pancreas, and plasmapheresis are based on the properties cited in items (3) and (4).[4,91] A variety of gel drug delivery systems and smart biomaterials have been developed, using the properties described in items (4) and (5).[2,10,92,93] The stimuli-responsive behavior described in item (5) indicates that gels simultaneously fulfill sensor, processor, and effector functions. In particular, volume phase transition of gels by environmental changes enables a biological signal to be transduced and amplified. Modulated drug delivery using stimuli-responsive gels appears promising as described in Chapters 9 and 10. In addition, the interlocked structures of IPN gels have some utility in the development of stimuli-responsive gels for use in the biological and biomedical fields. For example, IPN gels consisting of PAAc and PAAm exhibit positively temperature-dependent swelling changes through the "zipper" effect of cooperative hydrogen bonding.[41-43] IPN or semi-IPN structures were introduced into temperature-responsive gels to improve their responsiveness and mechanical strength.[94-97] The interlocked structures of biodegradable gelatin–dextran IPN gels enable dual-stimuli-responsive degradation by enzymes due to physical chain entanglements between chemically different polymer networks.[98-100] The semi-IPN structures of stimuli-responsive gels that have antigen–antibody bindings play an important role in reversibility of their antigen-responsive swelling changes.[101,102] Stimuli-responsive gels with IPN structures and the drug delivery systems using such gels are described in Chapters 9 and 10. The studies on IPN-structured gels reveal the significance of IPNs in developing novel biological and biomedical gels. The important properties of gels suggest many potential applications in biological and biomedical fields. Some fine reviews dealing with various aspects of biological applications of gels appear in other chapters of this book.

6.7 OUTLOOK

Gels are very classical materials that have become increasingly important because of their potential applications in a variety of biomedical fields. Gels represent the next generation of materials suitable for biological and biomedical applications. Their unique behaviors such as volume phase transition and cooperative diffusion are closely associated with structures and functions of biological molecules and systems, i.e., the essence of life. The structures of most synthetic gels have not been well defined yet. However, the IPN form of gel has an interlocked structure that enhances its performance and functions, similarly to catenane and rotaxane in supramolecular chemistry. A few researchers are trying to introduce supramolecular structures such as proteins and polyrotaxane into gels.[23,59,60,67,101-105] Their studies reveal that designing gel architectures represents a breakthrough for developing novel materials. Thus, studies of gels fall within the discipline of supramolecular chemistry. Supramolecular chemistry targets the well-organized structures and intelligent functions of biological molecules and systems. The goals of most studies on gels agree with those of supramolecular chemistry although the approaches might be different. The fundamentals described in this chapter will surely lead to a better understanding of the structures and functions of gels and also to promising strategies to develop novel gels.

REFERENCES

1. Tanaka, T., Gels, *Sci. Am.*, 244, 123, 1981.
2. Peppas, N.A., *Hydrogels in Medicine and Pharmacy*, CRC Press, Boca Raton, FL, 1987.
3. DeRossi, D., Kajiwara, K., Osada, Y., and Yamauchi, A., *Polymer Gels, Fundamentals and Biomedical Applications*, Plenum Press, New York, 1991.
4. Tsuruta, T. et al., *Biomedical Applications of Polymeric Materials,* CRC Press, Boca Raton, FL, 1993.
5. Dusek, K., *Responsive Gels, Volume Transitions I*, Advances in Polymer Science, Vol. 109, Springer, Berlin, 1993.
6. Dusek, K., *Responsive Gels, Volume Transitions II*, Advances in Polymer Science, Vol. 110, Springer, Berlin, 1993.
7. Osada, Y. and Ross-Murphy, S.B., Intelligent gels, *Sci. Am.*, 268, 82, 1993.
8. Hoffman, A.S., "Intelligent" polymers in medicine and biotechnology, *Macromol. Symp.*, 98, 645, 1995.
9. Hoffman, A.S., Application of thermally reversible polymers and hydrogels in therapeutics and diagnostics, *J. Controlled Release,* 6, 297, 1987.
10. Okano, T., *Biorelated Polymers and Gels*, Academic Press, Boston, 1998.
11. Sperling, L.H., *Interpenetrating Polymer Networks and Related Materials*, Plenum, New York, 1981.
12. Sperling, L.H., Interpenetrating polymer networks: an overview, in *Interpenetrating Polymer Networks*, Klempner, D. et al., Eds., American Chemical Society, Washington, 1994.
13. Sperling, L.H., *Polymeric Multicomponent Materials,* John Wiley & Sons, New York, 1997.

14. Tanaka, T., Collapse of gels and the critical endpoint, *Phys. Rev. Lett.*, 40, 820, 1978.

15. Tanaka, T. et al., Phase transition in ionic gels, *Phys. Rev. Lett.*, 45, 1636, 1980.

16. Hirokawa, Y., Tanaka, T., and Sato, E., Phase transition of positively ionized gels, *Macromolecules*, 18, 2782, 1985.

17. Tanaka, T. et al., Collapse of gels in an electric field, *Science*, 218, 467, 1982.

18. Hirokawa, Y. and Tanaka, T., Volume phase transition in a nonionic gel, *J. Chem. Phys.*, 81, 6379, 1984.

19. Amiya, T. and Tanaka, T., Phase transitions in cross-linked gels of natural polymers, *Macromolecules*, 20, 1162, 1987.

20. Hirotsu, S., Hirokawa, Y., and Tanaka, T., Volume-phase transitions of ionized N-iso-propylacrylamide gels, *J. Chem. Phys.*, 87, 1392, 1987.

21. Amiya, T. et al., Reentrant phase transition of N-isopropylacrylamide gels in mixed solvents, *J. Chem. Phys.*, 86, 2375, 1987.

22. Suzuki, A. and Tanaka, T., Phase transition in polymer gels induced by visible light, *Nature*, 346, 345, 1990.

23. Kokufuta, E., Zhang, Y.-Q., and Tanaka, T., Saccharide-sensitive phase transition of a lectin-loaded gel, *Nature*, 351, 302, 1991.

24. Flory, P. J., *Principles of Polymer Chemistry*, Cornell University Press, Ithaca, NY, 1953.

25. Tanaka, T. and Filmore, D. J., Kinetics of swelling of gels, *J. Chem. Phys.*, 70, 1214, 1979.

26. Li, Y. and Tanaka, T., Kinetics of swelling and shrinking of gels, *J. Chem. Phys.*, 92, 1365, 1990.

27. Sato-Matsuo, E. and Tanaka, T., Kinetics of discontinuous volume-phase transition of gels, *J. Chem. Phys.*, 89, 1695, 1988.

28. Crank, J. and Park, G.S., *Diffusion in Polymers*, Academic Press, New York, 1968.

29. Crank, J., *The Mathematics of Diffusion*, Clarendon Press, Oxford, 1975.

30. Tokita, M., Time-lag method and transport properties of gel, *Jpn. J. Appl. Phys.*, 34, 2418, 1995.

31. Kaneko, Y., Sakai, K., and Okano, T., Temperature-responsive hydrogels as intelligent materials, in *Biorelated Polymers and Gels*, Okano, T., Ed., Academic Press, Boston, 1998, 29.

32. Alfrey, T., Gurnee, E.F., and Lloyd, W.O., Diffusion in glassy polymers, *J. Polym. Sci., Part C*, 12, 249, 1966.

33. Yasuda, H., Lamaze, C.E., and Ikenberry, L.D., Permeability of solutes through hy-drated polymer membranes. Part I. Diffusion of sodium chloride, *Makromol. Chem.*, 118, 19, 1968.

34. Yasuda, H. et al., Permeability of solutes through hydrated polymer membranes. Part III. Theoretical background for the selectivity of dialysis membranes, *Makromol. Chem.*, 126, 177, 1969.

35. Tokita, M. et al., Probe diffusion in gels, *Phys. Rev. E*, 53, 1823, 1996.

36. Einstein, A., *Investigations on the Theory of Brownian Movement*, Dover, New York, 1956.

37. de Gennes, P.G., *Scaling Concept in Polymer Physics*, Cornell University Press, Ithaca, NY, 1979.

38. Cukier, R.I., Diffusion of Brownian spheres in semidilute polymer solutions, *Macromolecules*, 17, 252, 1984.

39. Ilman, F., Tanaka, T., and Kokufuta, E., Volume transition in a gel driven by hydrogen bonding, *Nature*, 349, 400, 1991.

40. Inomata, H., Goto, S., and Saito, S., Phase transition of N-substituted acrylamide gels, *Macromolecules*, 23, 4887, 1990.

41. Katono, H. et al., Thermo-responsive swelling and drug release switching of inter-penetrating polymer networks composed of poly(acrylamide-co-butyl methacrylate) and poly(acrylic acid), *J. Controlled Release*, 16, 215, 1991.

42. Katono, H. et al., Drug release OFF behavior and deswelling kinetics of thermo-responsive IPNs composed of poly(acrylamide-co-butyl methacrylate) and poly(acrylic acid), *Polym. J.*, 23, 1179, 1991.

43. Aoki, T. et al., Temperature-responsive interpenetrating polymer networks constructed with poly(acrylic acid) and poly(N,N-dimethylacrylamide), *Macromolecules*, 27, 947, 1994.

44. Katayama, S., Myoga, A., and Akahori, Y., Swelling behavior of amphoteric gel and the volume phase transition, *J. Phys. Chem.*, 96, 4698, 1992.

45. Annaka, M. and Tanaka, T., Multiple phases of polymer gels, *Nature*, 355, 430, 1992.

46. Makino, K. et al., Surface structure of latex particles covered with temperature-sensitive hydrogel layers, *J. Colloid Interface Sci.*, 166, 251, 1994.

47. Nakazawa, Y. et al., Preparation and structural characteristics of stimuli-responsive hydrogels microsphere, *Angew. Makromol. Chem.*, 240, 187, 1996.

48. Okubo, M., Ahmad, H., and Komura, M., Preparation of temperature-sensitive polymer particles having different lower critical solution temperatures, *Colloid Polym. Sci.*, 274, 1188, 1996.

49. Iwata, H. and Matsuda, T., Preparation and properties of novel environment-sensitive membranes prepared by graft polymerization onto a porous membrane, *J. Membrane Sci.*, 38, 185, 1988.

50. Yamaguchi, T. et al., Development of a fast response molecular recognition ion gating membrane, *J. Am. Chem. Soc.*, 121, 4078, 1999

51. Hirasa, O. et al., Thermoresponsive polymer hydrogel, in *Polymer Gels*, DeRossi, D., et al., Eds., Plenum Press, New York, 1991, 247.

52. Hirasa, O. et al., Preparation and mechanical properties of thermo-responsive fibrous hydrogels made from poly(vinyl methyl ether)s, *Kobunshi Ronbunshu*, 46, 661, 1989 (in Japanese).

53. Clark, A.H. and Ross-Murphy, S.B., Structural and mechanical properties of biopolymer gels, *Adv. Polym. Sci., 83, 57, 1987.*

54. Hassan, C.M., Stewart, J.E., and Peppas, N.A., Diffusional characteristics of freeze/thawed poly(vinyl alcohol) hydrogels: applications to protein controlled release from multilaminate devices, *Eur. J. Pharm. Biopharm.*, 49, 161, 2000.

55. Mongia, N.K., Anseth, K.S., and Peppas, N. A., Mucoadhesive poly(vinyl alcohol) hydrogels produced by freezing/thawing processes: applications in the development of wound healing systems, *J. Biomater. Sci. Polym. Ed.*, 7, 1055, 1996.

56. Hassan, C.M. and Peppas, N.A., Structure and applications of poly(vinyl alcohol) hydrogels produced by conventional crosslinking or freezing/thawing methods, *Adv. Polym. Sci.*, 153, 37, 2000.

57. Rees, D.A. and Welsh, E.J., Secondary and tertiary structure of polysaccharides in solution and gels, *Angew. Chem. Int. Ed. Engl.*, 16, 214, 1977.

58. Ree, D.A., Polysaccharide shapes and their interactions — some recent advances, *Pure Appl. Chem.*, 53, 1, 1981.

59. Wang, C., Stewart, R.J., and Kopecek, J., Hybrid hydrogels assembled from synthetic polymers and coiled-coil protein domains, *Nature*, 397, 417, 1999.

60. Chen, L., Kopecek, J., and Stewart, R.J., Responsive hybrid hydrogels with volume transitions modulated by a titin immunoglobulin module, *Bioconjugate Chem.*, 11, 734, 2000.

61. Sperling, L.H. and Friedman, D.W., Synthesis and mechanical behavior of interpenetrating polymer networks. Poly(ethyl acrylate) and polystyrene, *J. Polym. Sci. A-2*, 7, 425, 1969.

62. Touhsanent, R.E., Thomas, A., and Sperling, L. H., Epoxy/acrylic simultaneous interpenetrating networks, *J. Polym. Sci. C*, 46, 175, 1974.

63. Flory, P.J. and Rehner, R., Jr., Statistical mechanics of crosslinked polymer networks. I. Rubberlike elasticity, *J. Chem. Phys.*, 11, 52, 1943.

64. Treloar, L.R.G., *The Physics of Rubber Elasticity*, Clarendon Press, Oxford, 1958.

65. Mark, J.E., The use of model polymer networks to elucidate molecular aspects of rubberlike elasticity, *Adv. Polym. Sci.*, 44, 1, 1982.

66. Miyata, T. et al., Stimuli-sensitivities of hydrogels containing phosphate groups, *Macromol. Chem. Phys.*, 195, 1111, 1994.

67. Miyata, T. et al., Preparation of poly(2-glucosyloxyethyl methacrylate)-concanavalin A complex hydrogel and its glucose-sensitivity, *Macromol. Chem. Phys.*, 197, 1135, 1996.

68. Tanaka, T., Hocker, L.O., and Benedek, G.B., Spectrum of light scattered from a viscoelastic gel, *J. Chem. Phys.*, 59, 5151, 1973.

69. Munch, J.P. and Candau, S., Spectrum of light scattered from viscoelastic gels, *J. Polym. Sci., Polym. Phys. Ed.*, 14, 1097, 1976.

70. Oikawa, H. and Murakami, K., Dynamic light scattering of swollen rubber vulcanizates and the swelling mechanism, *Macromolecules*, 24, 1117, 1991.

71. Oikawa, H. and Nakanishi, H., A light scattering study on gelatin gels chemically crosslinked in solution, *Polymer*, 34, 3358, 1993.

72. Koike, A. et al., Dynamic light scattering and dynamic viscoelasticity of PVA in aqueous borax solutions, *Macromolecules*, 28, 2339, 1995.

73. Burchard, W., Kajiwara, K., and Neger, D., Static and dynamic scattering behavior of regularly branched chains: a model of soft-sphere microgels, *J. Polym. Sci., Polym. Phys. Ed.*, 20, 157, 1982.

74. Asnagli, D. et al., Large-scale microsegregation in polyacrylamide gels (Spinodal gels), *J. Chem. Phys.*, 102, 9736, 1995.

75. Candau, S., Bastide, J., and Delsanti, M., Structural, elastic, and dynamic properties of swollen polymer networks, *Adv. Polym. Sci.*, 44, 27, 1982.

76. Kajiwara, K. et al., Characterization of gel structure by means of SAXS and SANS, in *Polymer Gels, Fundamentals and Biomedical Applications*, DeRossi, D., et al., Eds., Plenum Press, New York, 1991, 3.

77. Hecht, A.-M., Duplessix, R., and Geissler, E., Structural inhomogeneities in the range 2.5–2500 Å in polyacrylamide gels, *Macromolecules*, 18, 2167, 1985.

78. Mallam, S. et al., Microscopic and macroscopic thermodynamic observations in swollen poly(dimethylsiloxane) networks, *Macromolecules*, 24, 543, 1991.

79. Horkay, F. et al., Macroscopic and microscopic thermodynamic observations in swollen poly(vinyl acetate) networks, *Macromolecules*, 24, 2896, 1991.

80. Shibayama, M., Tanaka, T., and Han, C.C., Small angle neutron scattering study on poly(N-isopropyl acrylamide) gels near their volume-phase transition temperature, *J. Chem. Phys.*, 97, 6829, 1992.

81. Andrews, E.H. and Stubbs, J.M., A new freezing head for the ultramicrotomy of rubbers, *J. Roy. Microscop. Soc.*, 82, 221, 1964.

82. Trent, J.S., Scheinbeim, J. I., and Couchman, P. R., Ruthenium tetraoxide staining of polymers for electron microscopy, *Macromolecules*, 16, 589, 1983.

83. Huelck, V., Thomas, D.A., and Sperling, L.H., Interpenetrating polymer networks of poly(ethyl acrylate) and poly(styrene-co-methyl methacrylate). I. Morphology via electron microscopy, *Macromolecules*, 5, 340, 1972

84. Huelck, V., Thomas, D.A., and Sperling, L.H., Interpenetrating polymer networks of poly(ethyl acrylate) and poly(styrene-co-methyl methacrylate). II. Physical and mechanical behavior, *Macromolecules*, 5, 348, 1972

85. Sperling, L.H., *Recent Advances in Polymer Blends, Grafts, and Blocks,* Plenum Press, New York, 1974.

86. Donatelli, A.A., Sperling, L.H., and Thomas, D.A., A semiempirical derivation of phase domain size in interpenetrating polymer networks, *J. Appl. Polym. Sci.*, 21, 1189, 1977.

87. Kim, S.C. et al., Polyurethane interpenetrating polymer networks. I. Synthesis and morphology of polyurethane-poly(methyl methacrylate) interpenetrating polymer networks, *Macromolecules*, 9, 258, 1976.

88. Ikada, Y., Interfacial biocompatibility, in *Polymers of Biological and Biomedical Significance,* Shalaby, S.W. et al., Eds., American Chemical Society, Washington, 540., 37, 1994.

89. Merrill, E.W., Pekala, R.W., and Mahmud, N.A., Hydrogels for blood contact, in *Hydrogels in Medicine and Pharmacy,* Vol. III, Peppas, N. A., Ed., CRC Press, Boca Raton, FL, 1987.

90. Klee, D. and Höcker, H., Polymers for biomedical applications: improvement of the interface compatibility, *Adv. Polym. Sci.*, 149, 1, 2000.

91. Paul, J.P. et al., *Biomaterials in Artificial Organs*, Macmillan, London, 1984.

92. Piskin, E. and Hoffman, A.S., *Polymeric Biomaterials*, Martinus Nijhoff, Dordrecht, The Netherlands, 1986.

93. Langer, R., Drug delivery and targeting, *Nature*, 392, 5, 1998.

94. Bae, Y.H., Okano, T., and Kim, S.W., A new thermo-sensitive hydrogel: interpenetrating polymer networks from N-acryloylpyrrolidine and poly(oxyethylene), *Makromol. Chem., Rapid Commun.*, 9, 185, 1988.

95. Mukae, K. et al., A new thermosensitive hydrogel — poly(ethylene oxide-dimethyl siloxane-ethylene oxide)/poly(N-isopropyl acrylamide) interpenetrating polymer networks. 1. Synthesis and characterization, *Polym. J.*, 22, 206, 1990.

96. Bae, Y.H. and Kim, S.W., Hydrogel delivery systems based on polymer blend, block — copolymers or interpenetrating networks, *Adv. Drug Delivery Rev.*, 11, 109, 1993.

97. Gutowska, A. et al., Thermosensitive interpenetrating polymer networks — synthesis, characterization, and macromolecular release, *Macromolecules*, 27, 4167, 1994.

98. Yamamoto, N., Kurisawa, M., and Yui, N., Double-stimuli-responsive degradable hydrogels: interpenetrating polymer networks consisting of gelatin and dextran with different phase separation, *Macromol. Rapid Commun.*, 17, 313, 1996.

99. Kurisawa, M., Terano, M., and Yui, N., Double-stimuli-responsive degradation of hydrogels consisting of oligopeptide-terminated poly(ethylene glycol) and dextran with and interpenetrating polymer network, *J. Biomater. Sci. Polym. Edn.*, 8, 691, 1997.

100. Kurisawa, M. and Yui, N., Dual-stimuli-responsive drug release from interpenetrating polymer network-structured hydrogels of gelatin and dextran, *J. Controlled Release,* 54, 191, 1998.

101. Miyata, T., Asami, N., and Uragami, T., Preparation of an antigen-sensitive hydrogel using antigen-antibody bindings, *Macromolecules*, 32, 2082, 1999.

102. Miyata, T., Asami, N., and Uragami, T., A reversibly antigen-responsive hydrogel, *Nature,* 399, 766, 1999.

103. Obaidat, A.A. and Park, K., Characterization of glucose dependent gel-sol phase transition of the polymeric glucose-concanavalin A hydrogel system, *Pharm. Res.,* 13, 989, 1996.

104. Obaidat, A.A. and Park, K., Characterization of protein release through glucose-sensitive hydrogel membranes, *Biomaterials,* 18, 801, 1997.

105. Ichi, T. et al., Controllable erosion time and profile in poly(ethylene glycol) hydrogels by supramolecular structure of hydrolysable polyrotaxane, *Biomacromolecules,* 1, 204, 2001.

7 Interlocked Molecules

Nobuhiko Yui and Taichi Ikeda

CONTENTS

7.1 INTRODUCTION

In 1957, Pedersen reported the synthesis of crown ether,[1] a cyclic oligoether that can selectively form an inclusion complex with a cationic ion in relation to its ring size.[2] Since the discovery of crown ether, many cyclic molecules have been studied, for instance, cyclodextrin,[3] cyclophane,[4] and calixarene.[5] These studies contributed to the establishment of the new field of host–guest chemistry. Host-guest chemistry has now become an important part of a more general concept known as supramolecular chemistry.[6]

These studies led to the preparation of interlocked molecules, e.g., rotaxanes (polyrotaxane) and catenanes (polycatenane). "Rotaxane" is derived from the Latin words for wheel (*rota*) and axle (*axis*). A cyclic molecule is threaded on a linear compound capped with bulky blocking groups (Figure 7.1a). [*n*]-Rotaxane consists of *n* – 1 cyclic molecules. In general, a rotaxane consisting of many cyclic molecules is called a polyrotaxane (Figure 7.1b). The inclusion complex without bulky end groups is known as pseudorotaxane (pseudopolyrotaxane). "Catenane" is derived from the Latin word for chain (*catena*). Two cyclic molecules in the catenane molecule are mechanically entangled with each other (Figure 7.1c). [*n*]-Catenane consists of *n* interlocked cyclic molecules. A polymeric chain cross-linked by a catenane structure is a polycatenane (Figure 7.1d).

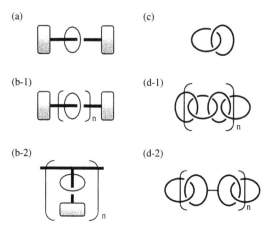

FIGURE 7.1 Examples of interlocked molecules. (a) [2]-rotaxane; (b-1) polyrotaxane; (b-2) side-chain polyrotaxane; (c) [2]-catenane; (d-1) and (d-2) polycatenane.

Although the idea of interlocked molecules has a long history, early studies did not provide any clear evidence for interlocked structures, mainly due to the lack of powerful synthetic and analytical methods that are now available. Highly resolved NMR and x-ray crystallography techniques reveal the three-dimensional structures of interlocked molecules. The progress in host–guest chemistry enables us to produce high yields of interlocked molecules. Detailed information on interlocked molecules is available from many excellent books and reviews.[7-13]

Interlocked molecules are attractive for their unique topological, mechanical, and physicochemical properties. For instance, the interlocked cyclic compound in a rotaxane can slide or rotate against the axis, and this discovery led to fabrication of the nanoscale equipment. For another example, it takes more time to hydrolyze a pseudopolyrotaxane consisting of polyester in comparison to hydrolysis of the polyester without cyclic compounds because the cyclic compounds hinder the hydrolysis of the included polyester. These fascinating features of interlocked molecules stimulated us to design supramolecular biomaterials. It is impossible to discuss all of the studies on interlocked molecules in this chapter. Therefore, we will introduce preparation methods, functions, and principles involved in characterization of interlocked molecules. These topics should stimulate interest in supramolecular designs for biological applications.

7.2 STRATEGY TO PREPARE INTERLOCKED MOLECULES

Interlocked molecules were prepared by means of directed or statistical methods in early studies. In the directed methods, the precursor of the interlocked molecule, in which interlocked components are linked by a covalent bond, is built up by organic synthesis. Finally, the interlocked molecule can be obtained by the cleavage of the

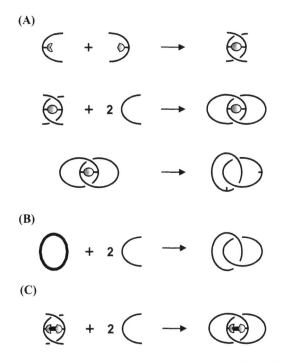

FIGURE 7.2 Strategy to prepare interlocked molecules: (A) directed method; (B) statistical method; (C) template-directed method.

covalent bond between the components (Figure 7.2a). In the statistical method, the components are statistically interlocked in the solution containing large amounts of constituents (Figure 7.2b). Since no attractive interaction exists between the components, the yield of the product is quite low. In recent studies, the interlocked molecules were prepared by the template-directed method. An attractive interaction among the components assisted the formation of interlocked structure (Figure 7.2c).

This method drastically improves the yield of interlocked molecules. Inclusion complexation by cyclic molecules, e.g., cyclodextrin, crown ether, and cyclophane, affords the precursor of the interlocked molecule (Figure 7.3). The dimensions of cyclodextrin and crown ether are summarized in Tables 7.1 and 7.2. The dimensions of the cyclic host molecule are on the order of 10^{-9} to 10^{-10} m. Therefore, the dimensions of the interlocked molecules are 10^{-8}–10^{-9} m.

7.3 TEMPLATE-DIRECTED PREPARATION OF ROTAXANES AND CATENANES

Various kinds of rotaxanes and catenanes have been reported in last three decades. In this subsection, they are classified into five categories based on their templates

TABLE 7.1

Dimension of Cyclodextrin[3]

n		Cavity diameter (Å)	Height of torus (Å)
6	α-CD	4.7–5.3	7.9 ± 0.1
7	β-CD	6.0–6.5	7.9 ± 0.1
8	γ-CD	7.5–8.3	7.9 ± 0.1

TABLE 7.2

Dimensions of Crown Ether

n		Diameter (Å)
1	12C4	1.2–1.5
2	15C5	1.7–2.2
3	18C6	2.6–3.2
4	21C7	3.4–4.3

Source: From Vögtle, F., *Supramolecular Chemistry*, John Wiley & Sons, 38, 1991. With permission.

(cyclodextrin, crown ether, cyclophane, hydrogen bond between amide bonds, and transition metal templates).

Cyclodextrin (CD) is a useful host molecule for preparing interlocked molecules.[14] CD is a cyclic oligomer of α-D-glucose linked by α-1,4-glycoside bonds (Figure 7.3a). The most familiar members are α-, β-, and γ-CDs consisting of six, seven, and eight glucose units, respectively. CD has a hollow truncated cone-like structure, and the environment inside the cavity of CD is hydrophobic and cationic due to C^3H, C^5H, and C^6H hydrogen. CD can form inclusion complexes with various types of compounds, and the property of inclusion complexation has been well studied. The equilibrium constant for the most stable inclusion complexation pair, i.e., β–CD and adamantane derivatives, is in the order of 10^5 M^{-1}.[15] Several kinds of interactions and factors participate in inclusion complexation: van der Waals interaction, hydrophobic effect, electrostatic interaction, desolvation of the guest molecule, etc.[16] The aliphatic and aromatic derivatives have been used as backbones to prepare CD-template interlocked molecules due to their strong interactions with CD. Figure 7.4 shows an example of a cyclodextrin template rotaxane.[17]

NMR measurements are helpful for characterizing supramolecular structures. Aromatic guest molecules often affect the chemical shift of protons and carbons inside the CD cavity (C^3H and C^5H) due to anisotropic shielding of the aromatic ring.

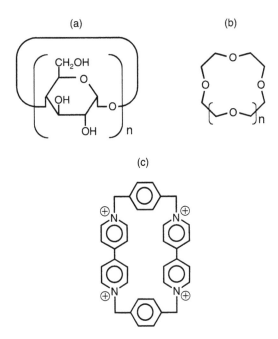

FIGURE 7.3 Cyclic molecules for preparing interlocked molecules: (a) cyclodextrin; (b) crown ether; (c) cyclophane (cyclobis(paraquat-*p*-phenylene)).

In some systems, a chemical shift change of protons and carbons assigned to guest molecules is also observed. For instance, the NMR peak assigned to the aliphatic protons shifts to a lower field by inclusion complexation with CD.[18] Nuclear Overhauser effect (NOE) measurement enables us to perform conformational analysis of the CD inclusion complex. Induced circular dichroism (ICD) also affords information on the orientation of guest molecules in the CD cavity. Nakashima et al. analyzed the change in the location of α-CD in response to the light irradiation by means of NOE and ICD measurements (Figure 7.5).[19] In the case of *trans* azobenzene, azobenzene moiety was captured in the cavity of α-CD from ICD spectra. On the other hand, the result of NOE measurement indicated that α-CD exists at the methylene spacer in the case of *cis* azobenzene.

Crown ether and its derivatives serve as ionophores for cations, i.e.,they have strong affinities with alkali and alkaline earth cations (Figure 7.3b).[1,2] Dibenzo[24]crown-8 (DB24C8) forms a stable inclusion complex with secondary dialkylammonium salt derivatives in CHCl₃ ($K_a = 10^4\ M^{-1}$).[20] Therefore, the preparation of rotaxanes consisting of DB24C8 and secondary dialkylammonium salt derivatives have been studied extensively.[21-25] The main driving force is considered to be electrostatic interaction and hydrogen bond. Figure 6 shows the x-ray structure of the rotaxane based on the crown ether template.[24] As shown in Figure 7.6, four hydrogen bonds stabilize the inclusion complex. In this system, the preparation condition has been improved. Takata et al. reported the preparation of an interlocked molecule in 89% yield by using tributylphosphine (excellent catalyst for acylation) (Figure 7.7).[25]

It was found that π-electron-deficient cyclophane, cyclobis(paraquat-p-pheny-lene) (Figure 7.3c) forms a stable inclusion complex with a π-electron-rich guest compound, 1,4-bis(2,2,2-(hydroxyethoxy(ethoxy)))benzene apolar solvent (K_a = 2200 M^{-1}).[26] Based on the crystal structure, three driving forces for inclusion com-plexation are proposed: π-π overlap of the π-electron-rich hydroquinone rings and the π-electron-deficient bipyridinium units, edge-to-face interactions of the p-xylyl spacers in the cyclophane with two of the hydroquinone ring hydrogen atoms, and

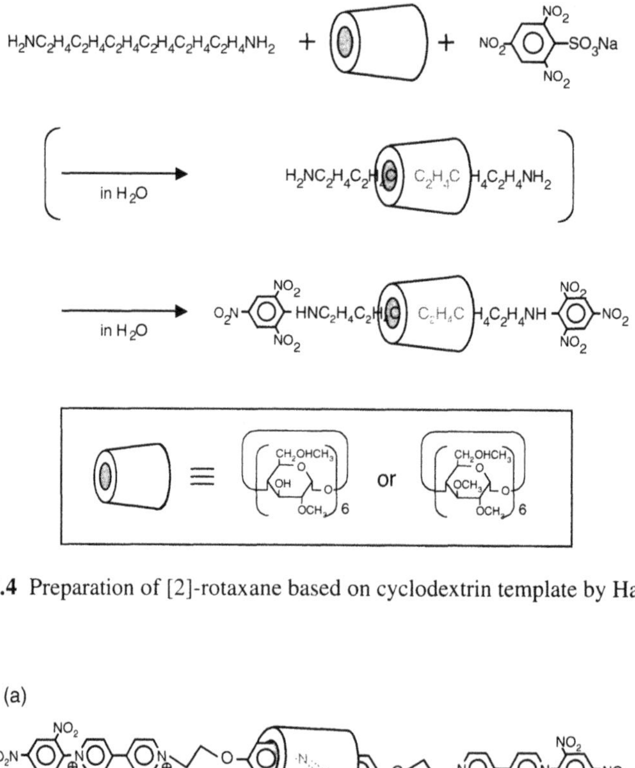

FIGURE 7.4 Preparation of [2]-rotaxane based on cyclodextrin template by Harada et al.[17]

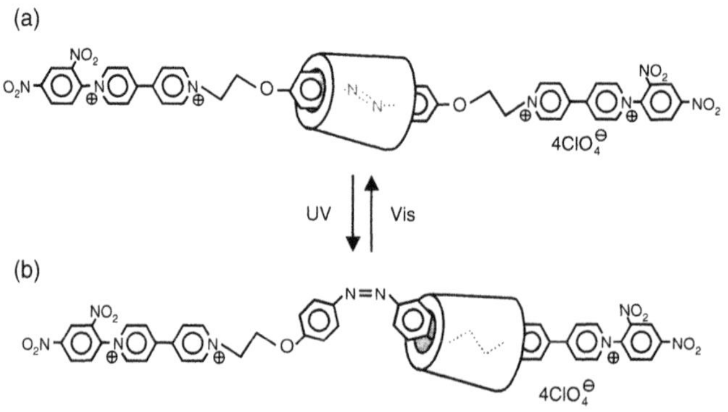

(a)

(b)

FIGURE 7.5 Light-driven molecular shuttle by Nakashima et al.[19] (a) *trans* isomer; (b) *cis* isomer.

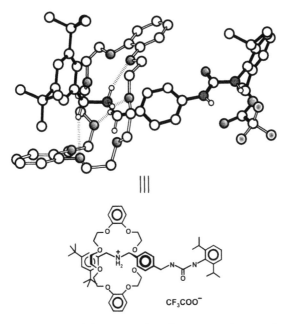

FIGURE 7.6 X-ray structure of [2]-rotaxane based on crown ether template. (From Cantrill, S. J. et al., *Chem. Eur. J.*, 6, 2274, 2000. With permission.)

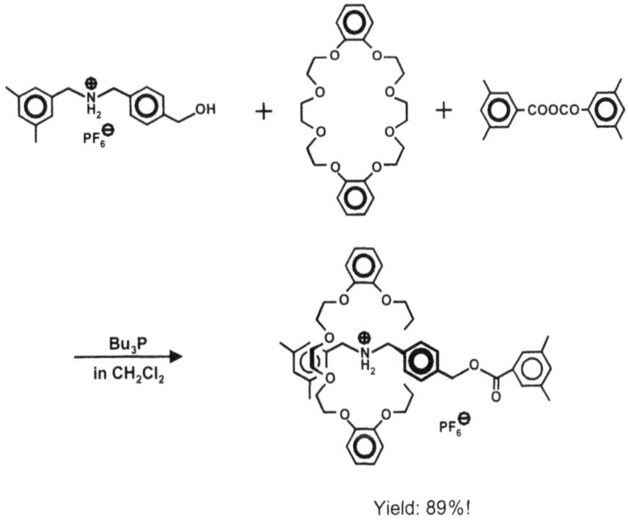

Yield: 89%!

FIGURE 7.7 High-yield preparation of [2]-rotaxane based on crown ether template by Takata et al.[25]

hydrogen bonds (Figure 7.8).[26] Stoddart and his coworkers extensively studied the interlocked molecules by using this template.[27] They demonstrated control of the location of a cyclic component against acyclic (rotaxane) or another cyclic component (catenane) (see section 7.7).[28] These studies utilized novel nanotechnology devices.[29]

Hunter serendipitously found [2]-catenane formation.[30] Figure 7.9 shows the x-ray structure of the interlocked molecule based on hydrogen bonding between amide bonds.[31] Six hydrogen bonds between the amide bonds play an important role in stabilizing the precursor of [2]-rotaxane. $\pi-\pi$ interaction also assists the self-assembly. Based on Hunter's prototype, Leigh et al. reported synthesis of [2]-catenane from *iso*-phthaloyl chloride and 1,4-bis(aminomethyl)benzene (Figure 7.10).[32] One can easily obtain interlocked molecules from inexpensive commercial sources. Leigh et al. reported various rotaxane and catenane derivatives by using this protocol and analyzed the molecular motions in the interlocked molecules.[33-36]

In early studies of the template-directed method, the transition metal coordination template was useful for preparing catenane (Figure 7.11).[37] Sauvage and his coworkers worked on the preparation and characterization of transition metal template rotaxanes and catenanes.[38] The most fascinating feature of the transition-metal coordination templates is that they represent switchable interaction sites by electrochemical interconversion between oxidation states of different coordination geometries. Bipyridine (bipy) has been the most useful ligand for transition metal complexation. The association constant of Cu^{2+}(bipy) reaches the order of 10^9.[39,40]

Transition metal complex is also used to interlock the supramolecular structure. In the first cyclodextrin-template rotaxane, cobalt complex was used for end-capping.[41] Fujita et al. found that the catenane structure was easily obtained from a mixture of pyridine derivatives and paradium complex (Figure 7.12).[42]

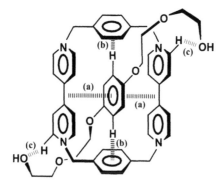

FIGURE 7.8 Structure and interaction of pseudorotaxane consisting of cyclobis(paraquat-*p*-phenylene) and a hydroquinone derivative; (a) $\pi-\pi$ interaction; (b) edge-to-face interactions (T-type interaction); (c) hydrogen bond.[29]

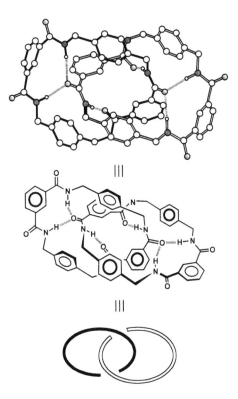

FIGURE 7.9 X-ray structure of [2]-catenane based on hydrogen bonds between amide bonds. (From Deleuze, M.S. et al., *J. Am. Chem. Soc.*, 121, 2364, 1999. With permission.)

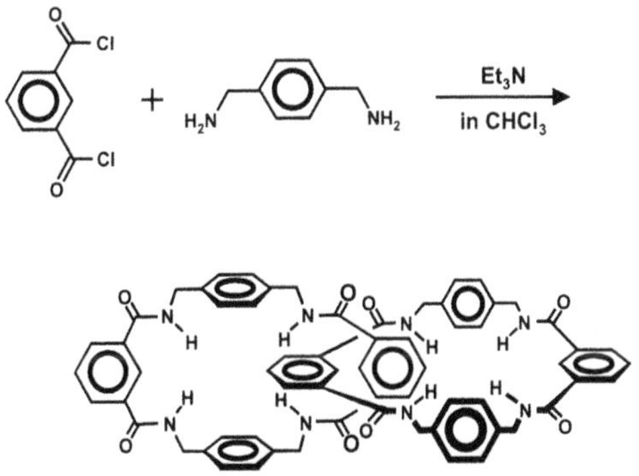

FIGURE 7.10 Preparation of [2]-catenane based on hydrogen bonds between amide bonds by Leigh et al.[33]

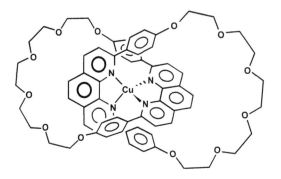

FIGURE 7.11 [2]-Catenane based on transition metal template by Sauvage et al.[37]

(A)

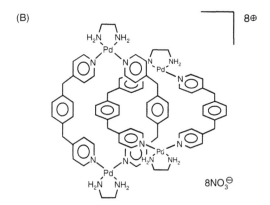

FIGURE 7.12 (A) [2]-Rotaxane by Ogino.[41] (B) [2]-Catenane by Fujita et al.[42]

(B)

8⊕

8NO₃⊖

7.4 PREPARATION OF CYCLODEXTRIN-TEMPLATE POLYROTAXANES

The preparation of pseudopolyrotaxanes and polyrotaxanes has been demonstrated by many research groups.[7-12] The same templates described in the previous subsection are used for the preparation of pseudopolyrotaxanes, i.e., cyclodextrin, crown ether, cyclophane, hydrogen bond between amide bonds, and transition metal templates.

This subsection focuses on the preparation of cyclodextrin-template (pseudo)polyrotaxanes[14] because the cyclodextrin-template polyrotaxanes have much potential for functional devices by means of the modification of their own many hydroxyl groups. Table 7.3 summarizes cyclodextrin template pseudopolyrotaxanes.

In 1976, Ogata et al. prepared pseudopolyrotaxanes consisting of β-cyclodextrins by polycondensation reaction of diamines and dichlorides in the presence of β-cyclodextrins.[43] This method is categorized as template-directed, since β-CD forms an inclusion complex with lipophilic monomers by means of hydrophobic interaction. Based on this prototype, several kinds of pseudopolyrotaxanes have been prepared by polymerization in the presence of cyclodextrins.[44-47]

Wenz et al. prepared pseudopolyrotaxanes consisting of α-CD and poly(iminooligomethylene)s.[48-50] The pseudopolyrotaxanes they prepared were water soluble in acidic conditions. Hydrophobic interaction between cyclodextrin and a methylene spacer is considered to play an important role in inclusion complexation. Wenz introduced bulky stoppers on the polymer chains to prepare the polyrotaxane.[48]

Harada et al. discovered a new type of pseudopolyrotaxane formation by cyclodextrins and polymers.[51-55] When poly(ethylene glycol) (PEG) solution is added to α-CD saturated solution, the mixture solution becomes turbid within a few minutes and one can easily obtain pseudopolyrotaxane as the precipitate (Figure 7.13a). β-CD does not form pseudopolyrotaxane with PEG, but does so with poly(propylene glycol) (PPG). It is clear that cyclodextrin recognizes the cross-sectional dimension of the polymer. Although the driving force of this system is not clear, hydrogen bonds between hydroxyl groups on adjacent CDs are considered to play a critical role in inclusion complexation. Some biodegradable polymers, e.g. polyesters,[56,57] poly(ε-caprolactone),[58] and poly(ε-lysine)[59] also form inclusion complexes with α-CD. Some inorganic[60] and conductive polymers[61] also form inclusion complexes with CDs.

Based on these findings, Harada et al. prepared a polyrotaxane consisting of PEG and α-CD by the end capping with dinitrofluorobenzene[62,63] (Figure 7.13b). They successfully prepared a tubular conjugate of "molecular tube" by cross-linking hydroxyl groups of adjacent α-CDs in the polyrotaxane[64] (Figure 7.13c). Such template synthesis is a smart approach to constructing new nanostructures.

7.5 PREPARATION OF POLYCATENANES

Polycatenanes such as structure d-1 in Figure 7.1 have not yet been prepared, although an oligomeric catenane chain was prepared by the stepwise approach.[65] Some polymeric products linked by [2]catenane structures, namely poly[2]catenanes, were prepared by polymerization of bifunctional [2]catenanes (d-2 in Figure 7.1). The preparations of bifunctional [2]catenanes were demonstrated by means of the hydrogen bonds between amide bonds,[66] the transition metal coordination template,[67] and the cyclophane template.[68,69] The mechanically interlocked polymer may be more flexible than the conventional polymer linked by the covalent bond.

TABLE 7.3

Cyclodextrin-Template Pseudopolyrotaxane

Polymer, Oligomer	Cyclic component	Reference
$\{NH(CH_2)_6NHCO\text{-}C_6H_4\text{-}CO\}_n$	β-CD	43
$\{NH(CH_2)_6NHCO\text{-}C_6H_4(CO)\}_n$	β-CD	43
$\{NHCH_2\text{-}C_6H_4\text{-}CH_2NHCO\text{-}C_6H_4\text{-}CO\}_n$	β-CD	43
$\{NHCH_2\text{-}C_6H_4(CH_2NHCO\text{-}C_6H_4\text{-}CO)\}_n$	β-CD	43
$\{CC_2CH_2\}_n$	β-CD	44
$\{NH(CH_2)_{10}CO\}_n$	β-CD	45
$\{N\cap N(CH_2)_{10}CO\}_n$	α-CD	45
$\{N(CH_3)\cap N(CH_3)(CH_2)_{10}CO\}_n$	α-CD	45
$\{NH(CH_2)_{10}NHCO(CH_2)_8CO\}_n$	α-CD	45
$\{(CH_2)_{11}\text{-}N\text{-}C_6H_4\text{-}C_6H_4\text{-}N\text{-}(CH_2)_{11}O\}_n$	α-CD	46
$\{O(CH_2)_6O\text{-}C_6H_4\text{-}O(CH_2)_6OCONH\text{-}C_6H_4\text{-}CH_2\text{-}C_6H_4\text{-}NHCO\}_n$	α-CD β-CD	47
$\{NH_2(CH_2)_3NH_2(CH_2)_{10}\}_n$	α-CD	48
$\{NH_2(CH_2)_{11}\}_n$	α-CD	48
$\{NH_2(CH_2)_6NH_2(CH_2)_{10}\}_n$	α-CD	49
$\{NH_2(CH_2)_6NH_2(CH_2)_{12}\}_n$	α-CD	49

TABLE 7.3 (CONTINUED)

Polymer, Oligomer	Cyclic component	Reference
$\left[N(CH_3)_2(CH_2)_{10} \right]_n$	α-CD	49
$\left[N\bigcirc\!\!-\!\!\bigcirc N\!-\!(CH_2)_{10} \right]_n$	α-CD	50
$\left[CH_2CH_2O \right]_n$	α-CD, γ-CD	51,52,53
$\left[CH(CH_3)CH_2O \right]_n$	β-CD, γ-CD	53,54
$\left[CH_2CH(OCH_3) \right]_n$	γ-CD	53
$\left[CH_2CH_2 \right]_n$	α-CD	55
$\left[CH_2CH(CH_3)CH_2CH_2 \right]_n$	β-CD, γ-CD	55
$\left[CH_2C(CH_3)_2 \right]_n$	β-CD, γ-CD	55
$\left[CO(CH_2)_4COO(CH_2)_2O \right]_n$	α-CD, γ-CD	56
$\left[CO(CH_2)_4COO(CH_2)_3O \right]_n$	α-CD, γ-CD	56
$\left[CO(CH_2)_4COO(CH_2)_4O \right]_n$	α-CD, γ-CD	56
$\left[CO(CH_2)_8OCO(C_2H_4O)_{20} \right]_n$	α-CD, β-CD	57
$\left[CO(CH_2)_5O \right]_n$	α-CD	58
$\left[COCH(NH_2)(CH_2)_5NH \right]_n$	α-CD	59
$\left[Si(CH_3)_2O \right]_n$	β-CD, γ-CD	60
$\left[\bigcirc\!-\!N_H \right]_n$	β-CD	61

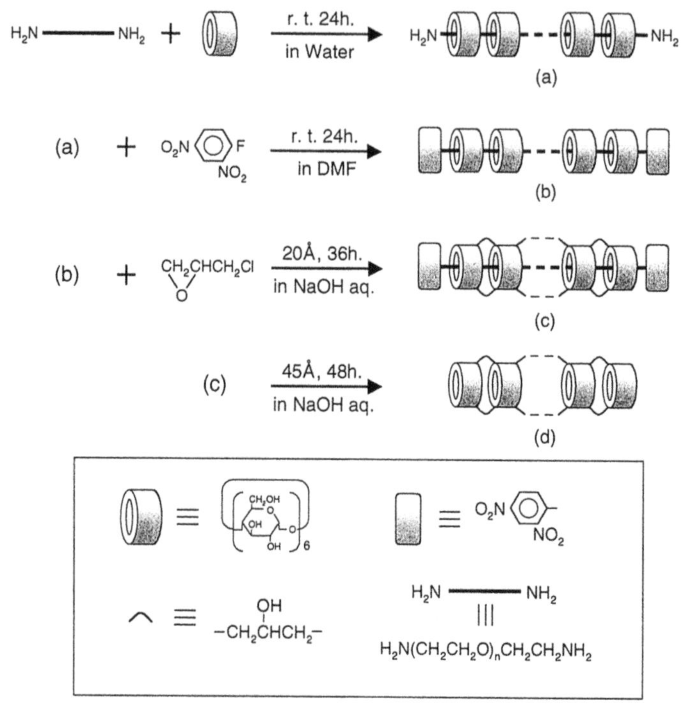

FIGURE 7.13 Preparation of (a) pseudopolyrotaxane, (b) polyrotaxane and (c) cyclodextrin-based molecular tube by Harada et al.[63,64]

7.6 SUPRAMOLECULAR POLYMERS AND NETWORKS

Supramolecular polymers and networks are polymeric products and networks cross-linked by supramolecular structures, respectively. The formation of supramolecular polymers and networks by the association of complementary components via hydrogen bonding in the liquid crystalline state has been well studied.[70] In principle, various kinds of supramolecular assemblies can be created through self-organization (Figure 7.14). In a similar manner, supramolecular assemblies are prepared through the inclusion complex of CD[71] or a cyclodextrin-based molecular tube.[72,73]

Daisy chain polypseudorotaxanes are prepared by a self-complementary monomer that consists of host and guest components. The stiffness of the monomer compound is important in order to prevent the formation of an intramolecular inclusion complex and a cyclic daisy chain. Tabushi et al. confirmed the daisy chain structure of mono-*tert*-butylsulfonyl-substituted β-cyclodextrin in solid state by x-ray crystallographic study.[74] Gibson et al. synthesized a self-complementary monomer consisting of crown ether and paraquat components (Figure 7.15).[75] The chemical shift of ^{1}H NMR suggested that a noncovalently bounded polymer with 50 monomer units should be formed in high-concentration solution. Harada et al. confirmed that

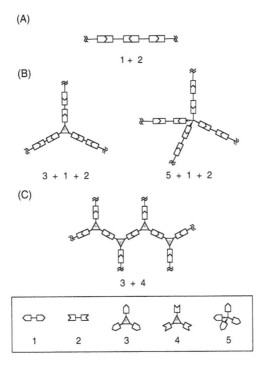

(A)

1 + 2

(B)

3 + 1 + 2   5 + 1 + 2

(C)

3 + 4

1   2   3   4   5

FIGURE 7.14 Supramolecular assemblies: (A) linear polymeric supermolecules; (B) two- and three-dimensional supramolecular networks; (C) self-assembled dendrimer and related species. (From Lehn, J.-M., *Makromol. Chem., Macromol. Symp.*, 69, 1, 1993. With permission.)

6-cynnamoyl β-cyclodextrin forms a cyclic daisy chain.[76] Furthermore, they successfully prepared a cyclic tri[2]-rotaxane (daisy chain necklace) by attaching a bulky stopper (Figure 7.16).

Yui et al. prepared a polyrotaxane hydrogel cross-linked by poly(ethylene glycol) between cyclic molecules in the polyrotaxane (Figure 7.17).[77] The polyrotaxane had hydrolyzable bulky end-groups. It was confirmed that the polyrotaxane dissociates in a few days by the hydrolysis of the end-groups. However, it takes several months to degrade the polyrotaxane hydrogel. The degradation time can be controlled by the amount and the length of the cross-linker. The details are discussed in Chapter 9.

7.7 FUNCTIONAL INTERLOCKED MOLECULES

The interlocked molecules are characterized by sliding or rotation of the cyclic component against an acyclic molecule (rotaxane) or another cyclic molecule (catenane). The representative of functional interlocked molecules is a molecular shuttle in which a cyclic component moves back and forth between two identical stations in

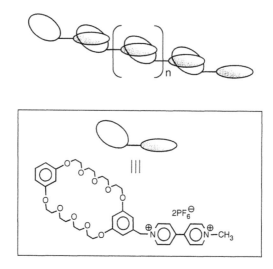

FIGURE 7.15 Linear daisy chain by Gibson et al.[75]

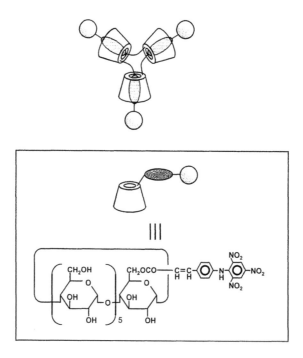

FIGURE 7.16 Cyclic daisy chain. Daisy chain necklace by Harada et al.[76] (From Hoshino, T. et al., *J. Am. Chem. Soc.*, 122, 9876, 2000. With permission.)

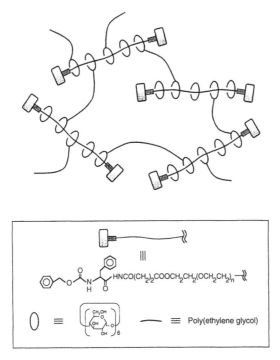

FIGURE 7.17 Poly(ethylene glycol) hydrogel cross-linked by hydrolyzable polyrotaxane by Yui et al.[77]

another acyclic or cyclic component. Stoddart et al. first reported a molecular shuttle by using a cyclophane template (Figure 7.18).[78] Two hydroquinol rings that correspond to the stations in the axial compound, interact with cyclobis (paraquat-p-phenylene). The locations of cyclic molecules exchange between the two stations thermodynamically. The exchange rate depends on the experimental temperature. Stoddart's group improved the design of the molecular shuttle by aiming at the switch devices in the nanoscale.[28]

Some research groups proposed a controllable molecular shuttle in response to pH,[79-81] solvent,[82] light,[19,83] and oxidization–reduction reaction.[84-87] Sauvage et al. prepared a rotaxane dimer of "molecular muscle" that can contract and stretch in response to chelate species.[88] As shown in Figure 7.19, the doubly threaded compound can bind simultaneously two metal centers in a four-coordinate or a five-coordinate geometry. The four-coordinate situation corresponds to an expanded state, whereas the five-coordinate situation leads to a contracted state.

Regulation of the location of cyclic molecules in polyrotaxane was also examined. Yui et al. prepared a polyrotaxane consisting of β-CD and PEG-b-PPG-b-PEG triblock copolymer (Figure 7.20).[89] The number of β-CDs locating on the PPG segment increased with temperature based on ICD and NMR measurements. This is

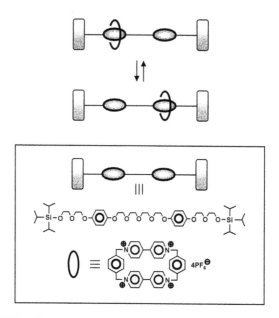

FIGURE 7.18 Molecular shuttle by Stoddart et al.[78]

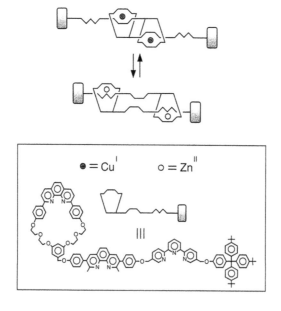

FIGURE 7.19 Molecular muscle by Sauvage et al.[88] (From Jimenez, M.C. et al., *Angew. Chem. Int. Ed.*, 39, 3284, 2000. With permission.)

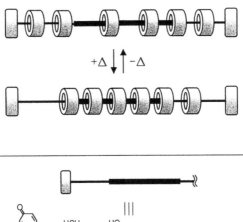

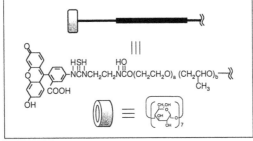

FIGURE 7.20 Thermally induced localization of β-cyclodextrins in a polyrotaxane consisting of β-cyclodextrins and poly(ethylene glycol)–poly(propylene glycol) triblock copolymer by Yui et al.[89]

attributed to the enhanced hydrophobic interaction between the β-CD cavity and the PPG segment.

Another characteristic feature of interlocked molecules is the mechanically interlocked structure, i.e., the components can dissociate by the removal of the bulky end-groups. Yui et al. prepared polyrotaxanes with enzymatically degradable bulky end-groups with the intent of developing a drug delivery system (Figure 6.21).[90-93] When the peptide bonds between the polymer backbone and terminal groups are cleaved by an enzyme, drug-immobilized α–cyclodextrins are released as the result of the dissociation of the supramolecular structure.

Although polymeric chains exhibit their random coil conformations in solution, the flexibility of polymeric chains is strongly limited by inclusion complexation with cyclic compounds. As a result, anisotropy in the shape of polyrotaxanes observed by light scattering measurement has been considered one of their structural characteristics.[91]

7.8 THERMODYNAMICS

In this subsection, thermodynamic analysis is briefly introduced. In the system in which inclusion complexation accompanies a physical property change, one can estimate the equilibrium constant from the physical property change in relation to the

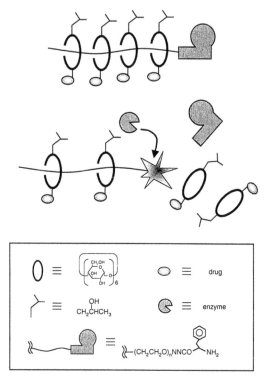

FIGURE 7.21 Biodegradable polyrotaxane for drug delivery system by Yui et al.[90-93]

concentration of the host molecule.[94] In the simplest case, in which host and guest form a 1:1 complex (Equation 1), the equilibrium constant is often evaluated by the following equations:

$$[\text{Host}] + [\text{Guest}] \rightleftharpoons [\text{Complex}] \tag{1}$$

$$\frac{[\text{Host}]_t [\text{Guest}]_t}{\Delta x} = \frac{1}{cK_a} + \frac{[\text{Host}]_t}{c} \tag{2}$$

$$\Delta x = A_G - A_{obs} \quad \text{for absorption spectroscopy}$$

$$\Delta x = F_G - F_{obs} \quad \text{for fluorescence spectroscopy}$$

$$\Delta x = \delta_G - \delta_{obs} \quad \text{for NMR}$$

where $[Host]_t$, $[Guest]_t$ represents the total molar concentrations of host and guest molecules, respectively, K_a is the association constant (= $[Complex]/[Host][Guest]$), c is a constant value, A_G, F_G and δ_G are the absorbance, fluorescence intensity, and chemical shift assigned to the guest molecule in the absence of the host molecule, respectively, and A_{obs}, F_{obs} and δ_{obs} represent the observed values of absorbance, fluorescence intensity, and chemical shift in the presence of the host molecule,

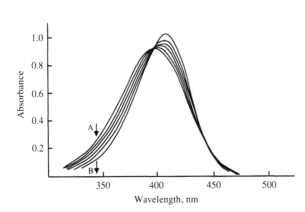

FIGURE 7.22 Spectra of p-nitrophenol anion at varying α-cyclodextrin concentrations. Solvent: phosphate buffer. pH: 11.0 (I = 0.5). Temperature: 20°C. The cyclodextrin concentrations are 0.0, 2.5 × 10^{-4}, 5.0 × 10^{-4}, 1.0 × 10^{-3}, 5.0 × 10^{-3}, and 1.0 × $10^{-2} M$ from A to B. The concentration of p-nitrophenol is 5.0 × $10^{-5} M$. (From Cramer, F. et al., *J. Am. Chem. Soc.*, 89, 14, 1967, with permission.)

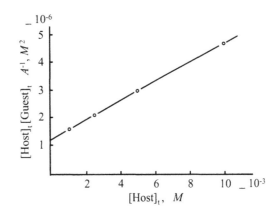

FIGURE 7.23 Determination of the equilibrium constant of p-nitrophenol–α-cyclodextrin complex according to Benesi–Hildebrand plot. (From Cramer, F. et al., *J. Am. Chem. Soc.*, 89, 14, 1967, with permission.)

respectively. [Host]$_t$ should be high enough to ignore the concentration change of the host molecule by inclusion complexation ([Host] = [Host]$_t$). In other words, [Host]$_t$ should be much higher than the total concentration of guest molecule ([Host]$_t$ >> [Guest]$_t$). Cramer et al. estimated the association constant for the inclusion complexation between 4-nitrophenol and α-CD from absorption spectra (Figures 7.22 and 7.23).

Isothermal titration calorimetry (ITC) has been extensively applied for thermodynamic analysis of inclusion complexation in recent years. This is because ITC allows simultaneous determination of both free energy (ΔG) and enthalpy changes (ΔH) at a given temperature and precise determination of heat capacity changes from measurements at different temperatures.[95] From titration curves, one can estimate ΔH and K$_a$. From these parameters, ΔG and entropy change (ΔS) were calculated as follows:

$$\Delta G = -RT \ln K_a \tag{3}$$

$$\Delta G = \Delta H - T\Delta S \tag{4}$$

Yui et al. analyzed thermodynamics for inclusion complexation between an α-cyclodextrin-based molecular tube and sodium alkyl sulfonate by means of ITC (Figure 7.24).[96] Thermodynamic parameters suggest that van der Waals interaction and hydrophobic effect play important roles in inclusion complexation.

The thermodynamic parameters of cyclodextrins[16] and crown ether[97] have been reviewed.

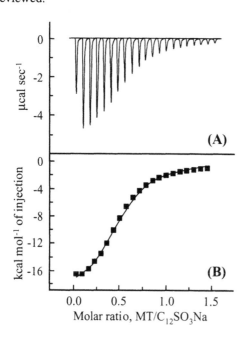

FIGURE 7.24 Isothermal titration calorimetry for inclusion complexation between an α-cyclodextrin-based molecular tube and sodium dodecyl sulfonate at 298 K. (A) Signal of titration. (B) Binding isotherm. (From Ikeda, T. et al., *Lamgmuir*, 17, 234, 2001, with permission.)

7.9 KINETICS

Kinetic analysis is briefly introduced. In early studies, temperature-jump[98] or stopped flow measurement[99] was often used. The time course change of physical property, e.g., absorbance, toward an equilibrium state was measured and analyzed. In an equilibrium reaction like Equation(5), the relaxation time (τ) is expressed as Equation (6).

$$\text{Host} + \text{Guest} \underset{}{\overset{k_a}{\rightleftharpoons}} \text{Complex} \tag{5}$$

$$\tau^{-1} = k_a([\text{Host}] + [\text{Guest}]) + k_d \tag{6}$$

where [Host] and [Guest] are the concentration of host and guest molecules in the equilibrium state, respectively, k_a and k_d association and dissociation rate constants, respectively. When [Host] is much higher than [Guest], Equation (6) can be simplified as follows:

$$\tau^{-1} = k_a[\text{Host}]_t + k_d \tag{7}$$

From k_a and k_d, one can obtain the association constant:

$$K_a = k_a / k_d \tag{8}$$

When it is possible to obtain the different chemical shifts for two identical states, NMR line shape analysis is a useful method to estimate the exchange rate.

$$A \longleftrightarrow B \tag{9}$$

The relationship between the exchange rate constant at coalescence temperature (k_c) and the frequency difference ($v_A - v_B$) can be approximated as follows:[100]

$$k_c = \pi(v_A - v_B)/(2)^{1/2} \tag{10}$$

This equation is applicable only when the population of each site is equal ($p_A = p_B = 0.5$) and $v_A - v_B$ is large compared with the half-height line widths of each peak attributed to A and B. By using the Eyring equation, the free energy of activation for exchange process ($\Delta G^{\ddagger}$) can be obtained from T_c and k_c.

$$k = K \frac{k_B T}{h} \exp\left(-\frac{\Delta G^{\ne}}{RT}\right) \tag{11}$$

$$\Delta G^{\neq} = 4.57\, T_c (10.32 + \log T_c - \log k_c)\, (\text{at } T_c) \tag{12}$$

in which K, k_B, h, T_c and R denote a constant ($K \approx 1$), Boltzmann constant, Planck constant, coalescence temperature, and gas constant, respectively. The exchange rate constant at a temperature can be calculated from the $\Delta G^{\neq}$ obtained by the Eyring equation.

Stopped-flow measurement was used to determine the diffusion of the cyclodextrin-based molecular tube on the polymer.[101] The diffusion of the cyclodextrin-based molecular tube on the polymer is 10^{1-2} times smaller than diffusion in water. The NMR line-shape method has been used to estimate the exchange rates between two stations in the molecular shuttle. The exchange rate of the molecular shuttle in Figure 7.18 was found to be 3.0×10^5 sec^{-1} (298K).[78]

7.10 CONCLUSION

Although interlocked molecules have been studied as promising functional materials in recent years, most of their properties are unknown. The studies of the relationship of the structures and properties of interlocked molecules are important and should open the door to their application in various fields including biomaterials. As with biological systems, the hierarchical organization of the molecular assembly is essential for achieving sophisticated functionality. Thus, the organization of the interlocked molecule will be an important area of research. The micelle or bilayer systems consisting of amphiphilic molecules are promising candidates for organization of interlocked molecules. The liquid crystal system or self-assembled monolayers at interfaces (solid–liquid, liquid–air, etc.) are also useful. Supramolecular systems expand the possibilities of designing new biomaterials. The highly organized interlocked supramolecular systems should exhibit various fascinating characteristics and properties, mimicking the sophisticated systems in nature.

REFERENCES

1. Pedersen, C.J., Cyclic polyethers and their complexes with metal salts, *J. Am. Chem. Soc.*, 89, 7017, 1967.
2. Bradshaw, J.S. et al., Crown ethers, *Compr. Supramolecular Chem.*, 1, 35, 1996.
3. Szejtli, J., Introduction and general overview of cyclodextrin chemistry, *Chem. Rev.*, 98, 1743, 1998.
4. Odashima, K. and Koga, K., Cyclophanes and related synthetic hosts for recognition and discrimination of nonpolar structures in aqueous solutions and at membrane surfaces, *Compr. Supramolecular Chem.*, 2, 143, 1996.
5. Pochini, A. and Ungaro, R., Calixarenes and related hosts, *Compr. Supramolecular Chem.* 2, 103, 1996.
6. Lehn, J.M., *Supramolecular Chemistry*, VCH, Weinheim, 1995.
7. Wenz, G., Cyclodextrins as building blocks for supramolecular structures and functional units, *Angew. Chem. Int. Ed. Engl.*, 33, 803, 1994.

8. Gibson, H.W., Bheda M.C., and Engen, P.T., Rotaxanes, catenanes, polyrotaxanes, polycatenanes and related materials, *Prog. Polym. Sci.*, 19, 843, 1994.

9. Harada, A., Preparation and structures of supramolecules between cyclodextrins and polymers, *Coord. Chem. Rev.*, 148, 115, 1996.

10. Harada, A., Polyrotaxanes, *Acta Polym.*, 49, 3, 1998.

11. Amabilino, D.A. and Stoddart, J.F., Interlocked and intertwined structures and super-structures, *Chem. Rev.*, 95, 2725, 1995.

12. Raymo, F.M. and Stoddart, J.F., Interlocked macromolecules, *Chem. Rev.*, 99, 1643 1999.

13. Hubin, T.J. and Busch, D.H., Template routes to interlocked molecular structures and orderly molecular entanglements, *Coord. Chem. Rev.*, 200, 5, 2000.

14. Nepogodiev, S.A. and Stoddart, J.F., Cyclodextrin-based catenanes and rotaxanes, Chem. Rev., 98, 1959, 1998.

15. Connors, K.A., The stability of cyclodextrin complexes in solution, *Chem. Rev.* 97, 1325, 1997.

16. Rekharsky, M.V. and Inoue, Y., Complexation thermodynamics of cyclodextrins, *Chem. Rev.*, 98, 1875, 1998.

17. Harada, A., Li, J., and Kamachi, M., Non-ionic [2]rotaxanes containing methylated α–cyclodextrins, *Chem. Commun.*, 1413, 1997.

18. Watanabe, M., Nakamura, H., and Matsuo, T., Formation of through-ring α-cyclodextrin complexes with α, ω-alkanedicarboxylate anion, *Bull. Chem. Soc. Jpn.*, 65, 164, 1992.

19. Murakami, H. et al., A light-driven molecular shuttle based on a rotaxane, *J. Am. Chem. Soc.*, 119, 7605, 1997.

20. Ashton, P. R. et al., Pseudorotaxanes formed between secondary dialkylammonium salts and crown ethers, *Chem. Eur. J.*, 2, 709, 1996.

21. Kolchinski, A.G., Busch, D.H., and Alcock, N.W., Gaining control over molecular threading: benefits of second coordination sites and aqueous-organic interfaces in rotaxane synthesis, *J. Chem. Soc. Chem. Commun.*, 1289, 1995.

22. Ashton, P.R. et al., Self-assembling [2]- and [3]rotaxanes from secondary dialkylammonium salts and crown ethers, *Chem. Eur. J.*, 2, 729, 1996.

23. Rowan, S.J., Cantrill, S.J., and Stoddart, J.F., Triphenylphosphonium-stoppered [2]rotaxanes, *Org. Lett.*, 1, 129, 1999.

24. Cantrill, S.J. et al., The influence of macrocyclic polyether constitution upon ammonium ion/crown ether recognition process, *Chem. Eur. J.*, 6, 2274, 2000.

25. Kawasaki, H., Kihara, N., and Takata, T., High yielding and practical synthesis of rotaxanes by calmative end-capping catalyzed by tributylphosphine, *Chem Lett.*, 1015, 1999.

26. Ashton, P.R. et al., Isostructural, alternately-charged receptor stacks. The inclusion complexes of hydroquinone and catechol dimethyl ethers with cyclobis(paraquat-*p*-phenylene), *Angew. Chem. Int. Ed. Engl.*, 27, 1550, 1988.

27. Amabilino, D.B., Raymo, F.M., and Stoddart, J.F., Donor-acceptor template-directed synthesis of catenanes and rotaxanes, *Compr. Supramolecular Chem.*, 9, 85, 1996.

28. Anelli, P.-L. et al., Toward controllable molecular shuttles, *Chem. Eur. J.*, 3, 1113, 1997.

29. Preece, J.A. and Stoddart, J.F., Concept transfer from biology to materials, *Nanobiology*, 3, 149, 1994.

30. Hunter, C.A., Synthesis and structure elucidation of a new [2]-catenane, *J. Am. Chem. Soc.*, 114, 5303, 1992.

31. Deleuze, M.S., Leigh, D.A., and Zerbetto, F., How do benzylic amide [2]catenane rings rotate? *J. Am. Chem. Soc.*, 121, 2364, 1999.

32. Johnston, A.G. et al., Facile synthesis and solid-state structure of a benzylic amide [2]catenane, *Angew. Chem. Int. Ed. Engl.* 34, 1209, 1995.

33. Johnston, A.G. et al., Structually diverse and dynamically versatile benzylic amide [2]catenanes assembled directly from commercially available precursors. *Angew. Chem. Int. Ed. Engl.*, 34, 1212, 1995.

34. Leigh, D.A. et al., Glycylglycine rotaxanes — The hydrogen bond-directed assembly of synthetic peptide rotaxanes, *Angew. Chem. Int. Ed. Engl.*, 36, 728, 1997.

35. Leigh, D.A. et al., Controlling the frequency of macrocyclic ring rotation in benzylic amide [2]catenanes, *J. Am. Chem. Soc.*, 120, 6458, 1998.

36. Bermudez, V. et al., Influencing intramolecular motion with an alternating electric field, *Nature*, 406, 608, 2000.

37. Buchecker, C.O., Sauvage, J.-P., and Kern, J.-M., Templated synthesis of interlocked macrocyclic ligands: the catenanes, *J. Am Chem. Soc.*, 106, 3043, 1984.

38. Chambron, J.-C., Buchecker, C., and Sauvage, J.-P., Transition metals as assembling and templating species: synthesis of catenanes and molecular knots, *Compr. Supramolecular Chem.*, 9, 43, 1996.

39. McWhinnie, W.R. and Miller, J.D., Chemistry of complexes containing 2,2'-bipyridyl, 1,10-phenanthroline, or 2,2',6',2''-terpyridyl as ligands, *Adv. Inorg. Chem. Radiochem.*, 12, 135, 1969.

40. Nord, G., Some properties of 2, 2'-bipyridine, 1,10-phenanthroline and their metal complexes, *Comments Inorg. Chem.*, 4, 193, 1985.

41. Ogino, H., Relatively high yield synthesis of rotaxanes. Synthesis and properties of compound consisting of cyclodextrins threaded by α, ω-diaminoalkanes coordinated to cobalt (III) complexes, *J. Am. Chem. Soc.*, 103, 1303, 1981.

42. Fujita, M. et al., Quantitative self-assembly of a [2]catenane from two preformed molecular rings, *Nature*, 367, 720, 1994.

43. Ogata, N., Sanui, K., and Wada, J., Nobel synthesis of inclusion polyamides, *J. Polym. Sci., Polym. Lett. Ed.*, 14, 459, 1976.

44. Maciejewski, M. et al., Polymer inclusion compounds by polymerization of monomers in β-cyclodextrin matrix in DMF solution, *J. Macromol. Sci., Chem.*, A13, 77, 1979.

45. Wenz, G., Steinbrunn, M.B., and Landfester, K., Solid state polycondensation within cyclodextrin channels leading to water soluble polyamide rotaxanes, *Tetrahedron*, 53, 15575, 1997.

46. Yamaguchi, I., Osakada, K., and Yamamoto, T., Polyrotaxane containing a blocking group in every structural unit of the polymer chain. Direct synthesis of poly(alkylenebenzimidazole) rotaxane from Ru complex–catalyzed reaction of 1,12-dodecanediol and 3, 3'-diaminobenzimidine in the presence of cyclodextrin, *J. Am. Chem. Soc.*, 118, 1811, 1996.

47. Yamaguchi, I. et al., Preparation and characterization of polyurethane–cyclodextrin pseudopolyrotaxane, *Macromolecules*, 32, 2051, 1999.

48. Wenz, G. and Keller, B., Threading cyclodextrin rings on polymer chains, *Angew. Chem., Int. Ed. Engl.*, 31, 197, 1992.

49. Wenz, G. and Keller, B., Speed control for cyclodextrin rings on polymer chains, *Macromol. Symp.*, 87, 11, 1994.

50. Meier, L.P. et al., Adsorption of polymeric inclusion compounds on Muscovite mica, *Macromolecules*, 29, 718, 1996.

51. Li, J., Harada, A., and Kamachi, M., Sol-gel transition during inclusion complex formation between α–cyclodextrin and high molecular weight poly(ethylene glycol)s in aqueous solution, *Polym. J.*, 26, 1019, 1994.

52. Harada, A., Li, J., and Kamachi, M., Double-stranded inclusion complexes of cyclodextrin threaded on poly(ethylene glycol), *Nature*, 370, 126, 1994.

53. Harada, A. et al., Preparation and characterization of inclusion complexes of poly(ethylene glycol) with cyclodextrins, *Macromolecules*, 28, 8406, 1995.

54. Harada, A. and Kamachi, M., Complex formation between cyclodextrin and poly(propylene glycol), *J. Chem. Soc., Chem. Commun.*, 1322, 1990.

55. Harada, A. et al., Preparation and characterization of inclusion complexes of polyisobutylene with cyclodextrins, *Macromolecules*, 29, 5611, 1996.

56. Harada, A. et al., Preparation and characterization of inclusion complexes of aliphatic polyesters with cyclodextrins, *Macromolecules*, 30, 7115, 1997.

57. Weickenmeier, M. and Wenz G., Threading of cyclodextrins onto a polyester of octanedicarboxylic acid and polyethylene glycol, *Macromol. Rapid. Commun.*, 18, 1109, 1997.

58. Kawaguchi, Y. et al., Complex formation of poly(e–caprolactone) with cyclodextrins, *Macromolecules*, 33, 4472, 2000.

59. Huh, K.M., Ooya, T., and Yui, N., Polymer inclusion complex consisting of poly(ε-lysine) and α–cyclodextrin, *Macromolecules*, in press, 2001.

60. Okumura, H. et al., Complex formation between poly(dimethylsiloxane) and cyclodextrins: New pseudo-polyrotaxanes containing inorganic polymers, *Macromolecules*, 33, 4297, 2000.

61. Yoshida, K. et al., Inclusion complex formation of cyclodextrin and polyaniline, *Langmuir*, 15, 910, 1999.

62. Harada, A., Li, J., and Kamachi, M., The molecular necklace: a rotaxane containing many threaded α–cyclodextrins, *Nature*, 356, 325, 1992.

63. Harada, A., Li, J., and Kamachi, M., Preparation and characterization of polyrotaxanes consisting of monodisperse poly(ethylene glycol) and α–cyclodextrins, *J. Am. Chem. Soc.*, 116, 3192, 1994.

64. Harada, A., Li, J., and Kamachi, M., Synthesis of a tubular polymer from threaded cyclodextrins, *Nature*, 364, 516, 1993.

65. Amabilino, D.B. et al., Oligocatenanes made to order, *J. Am. Chem. Soc.*, 120, 4295, 1998.

66. Muscat, D. et al., Synthesis and characterization of poly[2]-catenanes containing rigid catenane segments, *Macromolecules*, 32, 1737, 1999.

67. Weidmann, J.-L. et al., Poly[2]-catenanes containing alternating topological and covalent bonds, *Chem. Commun.*, 1243, 1996.

68. Menzer, S. et al., Self-assembly of functionalized [2]catenanes bearing a reactive functional group on either one or both macrocyclic components — from monomeric [2]catenanes to polycatenanes, *Macromolecules*, 31, 295, 1998.

69. Hamers, C., Raymo, F.M., and Stoddart, J.F., Main-chain and pendant poly([2]catenane)s incorporating complementary π-electron-rich and -deficient components, *Eur. J. Org. Chem.*, 9, 2109, 1998.

70. Lehn, J.-M., Supramolecular chemistry — molecular information and the design of supramolecular materials, *Macromol. Chem., Macromol. Symp.*, 69, 1, 1993.

71. Amiel, C. and Sébille, B., Association between amphiphilic poly(ethylene oxide) and β–cyclodextrin polymers: aggregation and phase separation, *Adv. Colloid Interface Sci.*, 79, 105, 1999.

72. Okumura, Y. et al., Self-assembling dendritic supramolecule of molecular nanotubes and starpolymers, *Langmuir*, 16, 10278, 2000.

73. Ikeda, T., Ooya, T., and Yui, N., Supramolecular network formation through inclusion complexation of an α-cyclodextrin-based molecular tube, *Macromol. Rapid. Commun.*, 21, 1257, 2000.

74. Hirotsu, K. et al., Polymeric inclusion compound derived from β-cyclodextrin, *J. Org. Chem.*, 47, 1143, 1982.

75. Yamaguchi, N., Nagvekar, D.S., and Gibson, H.W., Self-organization of a heteroditopic molecule to linear polymolecular arrays in solution, *Angew. Chem., Int. Ed. Engl.*, 37, 2361, 1998.

76. Hoshino, T. et al., Daisy chain necklace: tri[2]rotaxane containing cyclodextrins, *J. Am. Chem. Soc.*, 122, 9876, 2000.

77. Ichi, T. et al., Controllable erosion time and profile in poly(ethylene glycol) hydrogels by supramolecular structure of hydrolyzable polyrotaxane, *Biomacromolecules*, 2, 204, 2001.

78. Anelli, P.L., Spencer, N., and Stoddart, J.F., A molecular shuttle, *J. Am. Chem. Soc.*, 113, 5131, 1991.

79. Mock, W.L. and Pierpont, J., A cucurbituril-based molecular switch, *J. Chem. Soc., Chem. Commun.*, 1509, 1990.

80. Ashton, P.R. et al., Acid–base controllable molecular shuttles, *J. Am. Chem. Soc.*, 120, 11932, 1998.

81. Jun, S.I. et al., Rotaxane-based molecular switch with fluorescence signaling, *Tetrahedron Lett.*, 41, 471, 2000.

82. Lane, A.S., Leigh, D.A., and Murphy, A., Peptide-based molecular shuttles, *J. Am. Chem. Soc.*, 119, 11092, 1997.

83. Ashton, P.R. et al., A photochemically driven molecular-level abacus, *Chem. Eur. J.*, 6, 3558, 2000.

84. Livoreil, A., Buchecker, C.O., and Sauvage, J.P., Electrochemically triggered swinging of a [2]–catenate, *J. Am. Chem. Soc.*, 116, 9399, 1994.

85. Collin, J.–P., Gavina, P., and Sauvage, J.-P., Electrochemically induced molecular motions in a copper (I) complex pseudorotaxane, *J. Chem. Soc., Chem. Commun.*, 2005, 1996.

86. Balzani, V. et al., Switching of pseudorotaxanes and catenanes incorporating a tetrathiafulvalene unit by redox and chemical imputs, *J. Org. Chem.*, 65, 1924, 2000.

87. Collier, C.P. et al., A [2]catenane–based solid state electronically reconfigurable switch, *Science*, 289, 1172, 2000.

88. Jiménez, M.C., Buchecker, C., and Sauvage, J.-P., Towards synthetic molecular muscles: contraction and stretching of a linear rotaxane dimer, *Angew. Chem., Int. Ed.* 39, 3284, 2000.

89. Fujita, H., Ooya, T., and Yui, N., Thermally–induced localization of β-cyclodextrins in a polyrotaxane consisting of β-cyclodextrins and poly(ethylene glycol)-poly(propylene glycol) triblock copolymer, *Macromolecules*, 32, 2534, 1999.

90. Ooya, T. and Yui, N., Synthesis and characrerizaiton of biodegradable polyrotaxane as a novel supramolecular-structured drug carrier *J. Biomater. Sci. Polym. Ed.*, 8, 437, 1997.

91. Ooya, T. and Yui, N., Supramolecular dissociation of biodegradable polyrotaxanes by terminal hydrolysis, *Macromol. Chem. Phys.*, 199, 2311, 1998.

92. Ooya, T. and Yui, N., Polyrotaxanes: synthesis, structure,and potential in drug delivery, *Crit. Rev. Ther. Drug Deliv. Syst.*, 16, 289, 1999.

93. Ooya, T. and Yui, N., Synthesis of theophylline–polyrotaxane conjugates and their drug release via supramolecular dissociation, *J. Controlled Release,* 58, 251, 1999.

94. Connors, K.A., Measurement of cyclodextrin complex stability constants, *Compr. Supramolecular Chem.,* 3, 205, 1996.

95. Schneider, H.-J. and Yatsimirsky, A., *Principles and Methods in Supramolecular Chemistry,* John Wiley & Sons, New York, 137, 2000.

96. Ikeda, T., Hirota, E., Ooya, T., and Yui, N., Thermodynamic analysis of inclusion complexation between α–cyclodextrin–based molecular tube and sodium alkyl sulfonate, *Langmuir,* 17, 234, 2001.

97. Izatt, R.M. et al., Thermodynamic and kinetic data for cation–macrocycle interaction, *Chem. Rev.,* 85, 271, 1985.

98. Cramer, F., Saenger, W., and Spatz, H.–C., Inclusion compounds. XIX. The formation of inclusion compounds of α–cyclodextrin in aqueous solutions. Thermodynamics and kinetics, *J. Am. Chem. Soc.,* 89, 14, 1967.

99. Yoshida, N., Seiyama, A., and Fujimoto, M., Dynamic aspects in host–guest interactions. Mechanism for molecular recognition by α–cyclodextrin of alkyl–substituted hydroxyphenylazo derivatives of sulfanilic acid, *J. Phys. Chem.,* 94, 4246, 1990.

100. Sutherland, I.O., The investigation of the kinetics of conformational changes by nuclear magnetic resonance spectroscopy, *Annu. Rep. NMR Spectrosc.,* 4, 71, 1971.

101. Tachibana, J. et al., Inclusion dynamics of molecular nanotube and linear polymer chain as studied by stopped–flow circular dichroism method, *Phys. Rev. Lett.,* submitted.

SECTION II

*Biological Applications of
Supramolecular Architectures*

8 Biodegradable Polymers

Nobuhiko Yui and Tooru Ooya

CONTENTS

8.1 INTRODUCTION

Biodegradable polymers have been extensively studied for various applications in the medical, pharmaceutical, and agricultural fields. "Biodegradation" has been defined broadly as (1) simple hydrolysis with or without acid/base catalysis, and (2) enzymatically catalyzed hydrolysis in the interaction between a polymer and living organisms or microorganisms.[1] Concerning the mechanism of biodegradation (hydrolytic degradation), labile linkages should be included in the polymers. A lot of reviews and books discuss classification and degradation properties of polymers.[1-13] According to Baker,[10] factors affecting biodegradation are:

1. Chemistry of biodegradable polymers: the types of labile linkages used in the biodegradable polymers and the positions of the linkages in relation to molecular structure are important to control hydrolysis rate.
2. Mode and kinetics of hydrolysis: the method of hydrolysis in relation to water intrusion and enzymatic catalysis yields different profiles of biodegradation behavior.
3. Design of devices: physicochemical parameters including dimensions of devices and crystallinities are related to biodegradability.

0-8493-0965-4/02/$0.00+$1.50

Biodegradable polymers have been designed to degrade *in vivo* in a controlled manner over a predetermined period to serve as matrices for controlled drug delivery. Historically, *controlled release* of bioactive compounds in the field of agriculture was proposed in the 1960s.[10] By the late 1960s, biodegradable polymers were used in injections and implants. The most favorable characteristic of biodegradable polymers is that they do not have to be removed when they are no longer needed. If injections and implants are fabricated from nonbiodegradable polymers, the polymers have to be removed when the release of the agents is complete. In the early development of biodegradable drug delivery formulations, researchers believed they could achieve degradation-controlled drug release by developing a polymeric matrix in which active agents would be dispersed. However, the dispersed agents were usually released by diffusion prior to degradation. Because of this unfavorable characteristic, the development of biodegradable formulations has been much more difficult than anticipated. One key parameter is how the drug release is controlled by the degradation behavior of the polymer matrices. Degradation-controlled drug release is one approach to achieve zero-order drug release. Heller proposed degradation-controlled drug release using poly(ortho ester)s that can be hydrolyzed from the surface due to the regulated rate of water intrusion into the matrices.[14]

Biodegradable polymers have been used as scaffolds for tissue engineering. Tissue engineering is the application of principles and methods of engineering and life sciences toward the fundamental understanding of structure–function relationships in normal and pathological mammalian tissues and development of biological substitutes that restore, maintain, or improve tissue function.[15] Scaffolds are mainly used as templates for growth of tissue in the body or as delivery vehicles for drugs or transplanted cells. The time to use scaffolds is limited until tissue regeneration is complete. These temporary scaffolds cannot be removed if tissue grows in the scaffolds. Scaffolds should be made of biodegradable polymers whose degradation rates can be synchronized to the extent of tissue regeneration. Most biodegradable scaffold materials were not tailor-made for tissue regeneration. Commercially available biodegradable polymers were simply applied for fabricating tissue scaffolds. Two problems arose: (1) uncontrolled degradation independent of tissue regeneration, and (2) inflammatory reaction due to residues of incomplete degradation of semicrystalline polymers. Incorporating peptide sequences, which can be hydrolyzed by enzymes derived from regenerated tissue, into polymeric devices is one suggested approach.[16] However, the high costs of peptides may be a problem if one considers clinical applications. In addition, the inflammatory reactions can be avoided by complete degradation of polymeric matrices.

The supramolecular architectures of biodegradable polymers may be exploited in another way to control biodegradation, for example, new molecular structures with spatial specificities and/or hierarchical orders. In this chapter, the recent development of biodegradable polymers with supramolecular architectures is overviewed.

8.2 CLASSIFICATION OF BIODEGRADABLE POLYMERS WITH SUPRAMOLECULAR ARCHITECTURES

8.2.1 TERMINOLOGY

Figure 8.1 shows biodegradable polymers with supramolecular architectures and degradation images. Biodegradable polymeric micelles (Figure 8.1a) consist of amphiphilic block copolymers including multiblock copolymers, AB type di-block copolymers, and ABA type tri-block copolymers with hydrophobic cores (A or B segment) and hydrophilic shells (A or B segment). Polylactide (PLA) and PLA-*co*-polyglycolide (PLGA) are usually used as a hydrophobic segment. Branched biodegradable polymers can include comb-type copolymers (Figure 8.1b), star-

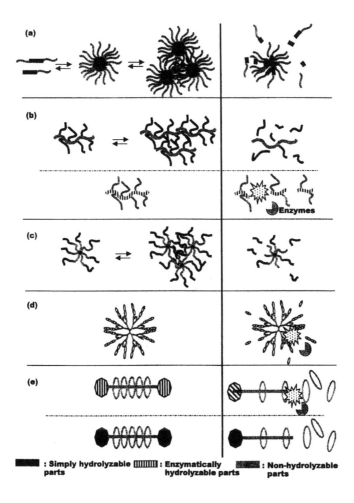

FIGURE 8.1 Biodegradable supramolecular architectures and biodegradation images.

shaped copolymers (Figure 8.1c), and dendrimers (Figure 8.1d). Comb-type copolymers are comprised of blocks of one chain grafted onto the backbone of another as branches. As for the biodegradable polymeric chains, comb-type copolymers are divided into two types: biodegradable polymeric parts as the grafts and main chains. The definition of star-shaped copolymers has not been clearly established. According to studies on star-shaped copolymers, single terminals of several biodegradable polymers are covalently or noncovalently bound at one point like stars.

Dendrimer is derived from the Greek words *dendron* (tree) and *meros* (part). Another category is polymer networks, which take the idea of polymer branching to its extreme. Biodegradable interpenetrating polymer networks (IPNs) have mechanically entangled structures. The basic concepts and stimuli-responsive properties of polymer networks including biodegradation are introduced in Chapters 6 and 9, respectively. Biodegradable polyrotaxanes (Figure 8.1e) are defined as interlocked molecules in which many cyclic molecules such as cyclodextrins (CDs) are threaded onto a linear polymeric chain capped with bulky end-groups via nonenzymatically or enzymatically degradable bonds.[17,18] The biodegradable polyrotaxanes can be used as cross-linkers to prepare hydrogels. Hydrolyzable chains thread into the cavities of CDs, hydroxyl groups of which are covalently bound with a bifunctional poly(ethylene gylocol). Such mechanical locking between CDs and hydrolyzable chains can act as cross-linked points in the hydrogels.

8.2.2 CHEMISTRY

The majority of biodegradable-polymeric chains are PLA and PLGA, in which ester linkages are readily hydrolyzed with or without acid/base catalysis. The preparation of PLA and PLGA is conventionally carried out by ring-opening polymerization of a cyclic dimer of lactic acid (lactide) or glycolic acid (glycolide) in the presence of stannous octoate as a catalyst. Hydroxyl groups of PEG,[19-21] polysaccharides,[22] depsipeptide,[23] and poly(vinyl alcohol)[24] have been used as initiating groups to synthesize block copolymers for polymeric micelles, star-shaped copolymers, and comb-type copolymers (Figure 8.2). Other approaches to synthesize the comb-type copolymers include coupling reactions between hydroxyl groups of polysaccharides and L- or D-lactide using an activating agent (N,N'-carbonyldiimidazole) (Figure 8.3).[25] When polysaccharides are used as biodegradable chains, the hydroxyl groups of the polysaccharides are activated by p-nitrophenyl chloroformate and then coupled with functional polymeric chains such as semitelechelic poly(N-isopropylacrylamide)[26] and amino-terminated PEG.[27] If the polysaccharides have functional groups, for example hyaluronic acid, the polymeric chain can be directly coupled with the polysaccharides using condensation agents such as dicyclohexylcarbodiimide (DCC).[28]

Biodegradable polymeric micelles of di-block copolymers such as PEG-*b*-PLA,[20] poly(β-maleic acid)-*b*-poly(β-alkylmaleic acid alkyl ester),[29] and tri-block copolymers such as PEG-*b*-PLGA-*b*-PEG[19,30] are prepared by mixing the polymers in aqueous solution or by dialysis of organic solutions such as dimethylformamide against water. Films and microspheres are prepared by general film casting methods and

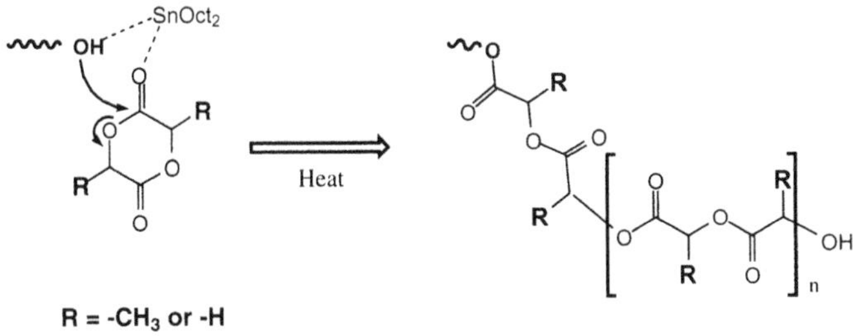

R = -CH₃ or -H

FIGURE 8.2 Synthetic schemes of various copolymers by ring-opening polymerization of lactide and/or glycolide. (From Breitenbach, A. and Kissel, T., *Polymer*, 39, 3261, 1998, with permission.)

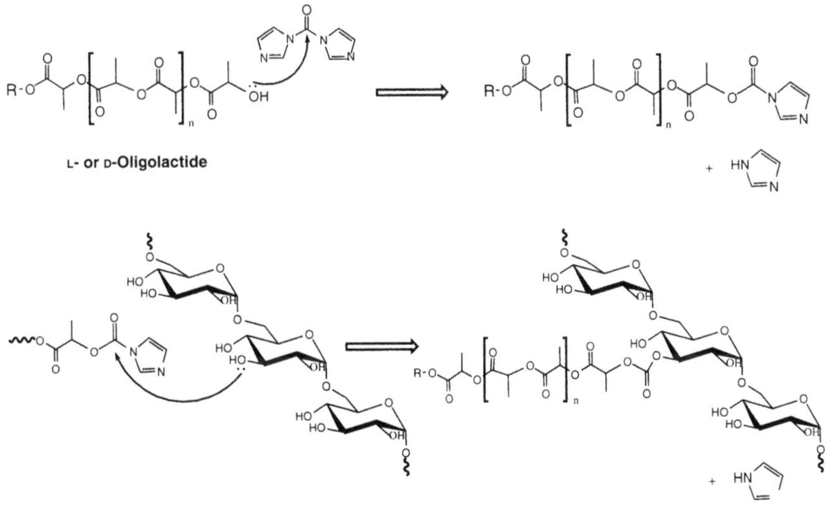

L- or D-Oligolactide

FIGURE 8.3 Synthetic scheme of a comb-type copolymer by coupling reactions. (From de Jong, S.J. et al., *Macromolecules*, 33, 3680, 2000. With permission.)

W/O/W double-emulsion technique, respectively. Physical hydrogels with stereo-complexes of oligo(L- and D-lactide)s in comb-type copolymers[25] or with inclusion complexation with poly(β-maleic acid-*co*-β-maleic acid alkyl ester) and β-cyclodextrin copolymer can be prepared by mixing the two aqueous solutions containing each copolymer.[31,32]

Star-shaped copolymers prepared by ion chelation methods are quite new. Self-assembling between bipyridine (bpy) ligands incorporating PLA and iron (II) or ruthenium (II) has been introduced (Figure 8.4).[33] The microligands were prepared by stannous octoate catalyzed ring-opening polymerization of DL-lactide using bis(hydroxymethyl)-2,2′-bipyridine as an initiator. The bpy–PLA ligands are

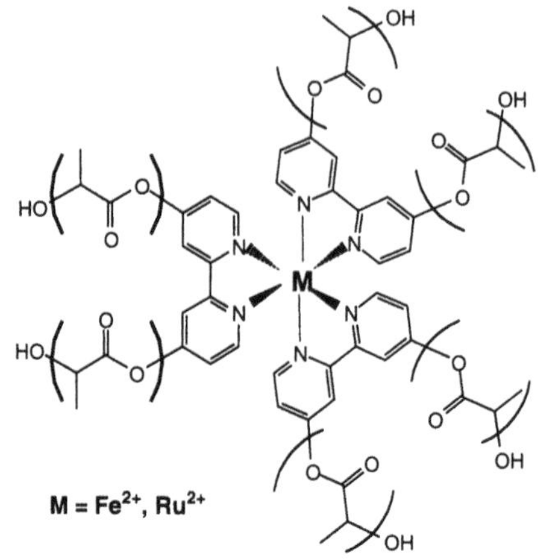

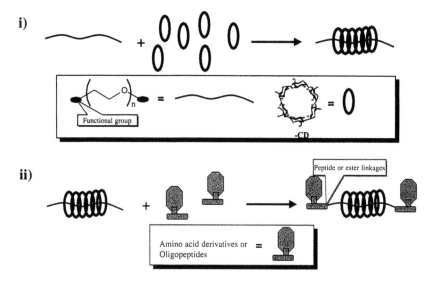

OH
OH
HO
HO
N
M
OH
M = Fe^{2+}, Ru^{2+}
OH

FIGURE 8.4 Star-shaped copolymer based on ion chelation. (From Corbin, P.S. et al., *Biomacromolecules*, 2, 223, 2001. With permission.)

i)
Functional group
n
-CD
ii)
Peptide or ester linkages
Amino acid derivatives or
Oligopeptides

FIGURE 8.5 Synthetic schemes of biodegradable polyrotaxanes: (i) preparation of inclusion complexes and (ii) capping both terminals of the inclusion complexes.

chelated to the ions to afford six-armed and ion-centered star-shaped polymers in some organic solvents.

Biodegradable polyrotaxanes are prepared in two steps: (1) preparing inclusion complexes between α-CDs and bifunctional PEG, the principle of which is described in Chapter 7, and (2) capping both terminals of PEG using amino acid derivatives or oligopeptides via peptide or ester linkages (Figure 8.5).[34-37] The solvent for polyrotaxanes is limited to dimethylsulfoxide (DMSO). However, hydrophilic modifications such as hydroxypropylation[35] and hydrophobic modifications such as acetylation[37] change the solubility. Another type of biodegradable polyrotaxane is the combination of α-CDs and poly(ε-lysine) that is degradable by some hydrolytic enzymes.[38] The preparation is simply mixing of α-CD saturated aqueous solution and poly(ε-lysine) dissolved in water. The number of α-CDs threaded onto poly(ε-lysine) is controllable by pH due to the ionization of α-amino groups of the poly(ε-lysine) (pKa = 8.5) and hydroxyl groups of α-CDs (p$_{Ka}$ = 12.2).

Hydrogels cross-linked by biodegradable polyrotaxanes having ester linkages at the PEG terminals are prepared by activating the hydroxyl groups in the polyrotaxanes using N,N'-carbonyldiimidazole and a coupling reaction between the activated hydroxyl groups (N-acylimidazole) and amino-terminated PEG (Figure 8.6).[39] By changing the molar ratio of the polyrotaxane and the amino-terminated PEG, the water content of the

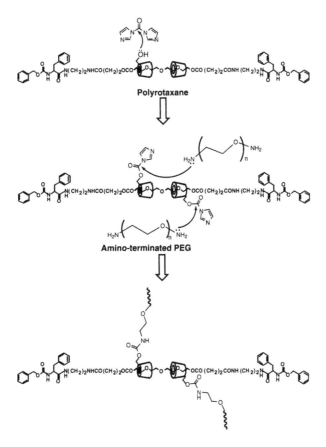

FIGURE 8.6 Preparation of hydrogels cross-linked by hydrolyzable polyrotaxanes. (From Ichi, T et al., *Biomacromolecules*, 2, 204, 2001. With permission.)

hydrogels can be controlled. Inclusion complexation of polysaccharide (dextran) grafted with PEG and α-CDs can produce hydrogels. The comb-type copolymer is synthesized by a coupling reaction using *p*-nitrophenyl choloroformate as mentioned above. The obtained copolymer dissolved in water is then mixed with α-CD saturated solution. The inclusion complex is hydrophobic due to hydrogen bonding between hydroxyl groups of α-CDs, and is aggregated to act as physical cross-link points.

IPN-structured biodegradable hydrogels consisting of gelatin and dextran are prepared by sequential cross-linking reactions below and above the sol–gel transition temperature of gelatin.[40] Methacrylated dextran and gelatin are dissolved in water containing ammonium peroxodisulfate as an initiator, and then the solution is photoirradiated to cross-link the methacrylated dextran. The obtained semi-IPN is immersed in a formaldehyde solution to cross-link the gelatin in the semi-IPN. The IPN-structured hydrogels prepared below and above sol–gel transition temperature of gelatin shows homogeneous and phase-separated structures, respectively.

8.2.3 MOLECULAR CHARACTERIZATION

The micellization of di- or tri-block copolymer is usually characterized by the following methods:

1. Dye solubilization methods using 1,6-diphenyl-1,3,5-hexatriene (DPH) and pyrene, including determination of critical micelle concentration (CMC)
2. Static and dynamic light scattering measurements
3. Gel permeation chromatography

As for the dye solubilization methods, for instance, DPH is preferentially partitioned into the hydrophobic cores of micelles with the formation of micelles, which causes an increase in the absorbance of the dyes. When the concentration of the block copolymers changes, CMC can be determined as a cross-point of extrapolating the change in absorbance in a wide range of the concentration.[30] Weight average molecular weight (M_W) of micelles is calculated by the results of static light scattering (SLS) measurements using a Debye plot:

$$K(C\text{-CMC})/(R\text{-}R_{CMC}) = 1/M_W + 2A_2 (C\text{-CMC}) \qquad (1)$$

where K indicates $4\pi^2(dn/dc)^2/N_A\lambda^4$, R and R_{CMC} the excess Rayleigh ratios at concentrations C and CMC, n is the refractive index of the solution at CMC, dn/dc is the refractive index increment, N_A is the Avogadro number, λ is the wavelength of laser light, and A_2 is the second virial coefficient. Hydrodynamic radii (R_H) of micelles can be determined by dynamic light scattering (DLS) measurements using the Stokes–Einstein equation:

$$R_H = k_B T / (3\pi\eta D)$$

$$D = \Gamma / K^2 \qquad (2)$$

where k_B is Boltzmann constant, T is the absolute temperature, η is the solvent viscosity, D is the diffusion coefficient obtained from Γ (average characteristic line width), and K^2 is the magnitude of the scattering vector. Since polymeric micelles are spherical assemblies, the diffusion coefficients should be independent of detection angle due to the undetectable rotational motions.

The branched structure of a comb-type copolymer is usually confirmed by the following methods:

1. ^{1}H and ^{13}C NMR spectroscopies
2. SLS measurements
3. Determination of intrinsic viscosities

From the ^{1}H NMR spectra of the copolymers, new signals of the terminal graft chains that are quite different chemical shifts from those for linear polymers, can be observed. If the graft chains connect to hydroxyl groups of the polymer backbone such as polysaccharides and poly(vinyl alcohol), the connecting ester bonds and methylene groups in the vicinity of the hydroxyl groups can be confirmed on ^{13}C NMR spectra. Conventional GPC analysis is not suitable for the determination of M_w of the comb-type copolymers, since it always underestimates the M_w due to their smaller hydrodynamic volumes in solution compared with linear polymer references such as polystyrene.

The combination of GPC and SLS (GPC–SLS) is a powerful method to characterize both real M_w and hydrodynamic volume. SLS measurements give the M_w and the root-mean-square radii of gyration (R_g) using the Zimm plot. R_g represents physical properties depending on molecular architecture and molecular weight, and this relation is proposed by the following equation:[24]

$$R_g = A\ M_w^{\ \alpha} \tag{3}$$

where A is a constant and α is correlated to the polymeric structure. Generally, stiff polymers are likely to be rod-like structures, so that R_g and α values become larger. A random coil structure leads to smaller R_g and α values although these values are larger than those of spherical molecules in solutions. Comb-type copolymers show lower values for R_g and α. Both the R_g and α values decrease upon increasing the number of the graft L-PLA chain, thus indicating the structures of comb-type copolymers. Values of intrinsic viscosity also show the evidence of the comb-type copolymers.

In a similar manner to comb-type copolymers, SLS with or without GPC measurements is useful for the characterization of star-shaped copolymers or dendrimers. The R_g of star-shaped PEG-*co*-PLA and PEG-*co*-PLGA is significantly reduced with increasing the number of star arms, although their molecular weights increase according to the number of the polyester star arms.[41] This is due to the reduced intermolecular interactions in relation to their steric architectures.

Polymer networks are characterized by rheological experiments such as measuring the shear storage modulus (G′) and the loss modulus (G″) using a rheometer,[25] thermal transition change by means of differential scanning calorimeter (DSC)[19] and viscosity measurements.[31] Molecular characterizations of biodegradable polyrotaxanes are followed by the characterization methods described in Chapter 7.

8.3 BIODEGRADATION PROPERTIES

8.3.1 MODE, KINETICS, AND PROFILE OF BIODEGRADATION

The degradation mode of water-insoluble polymeric devices of polyesters have been extensively studied. The two kinds of biodegradation modes are bulk and surface degradation.[10] Bulk degradation is a homogeneous degradation process in which degradation of labile bonds of the polymer occurs at a uniform rate throughout the polymer matrix. Surface degradation is a heterogeneous process in which degradation is confined to a thin layer of polymer at the exposed surface of the polymer.[10] In principle, polymeric chain does not dissolve under physiological conditions until the chain cleavage reaches critical phase on bulk degradation. This is due to slow rates of degradation in comparison with water solubilization of the polymer matrix. The kinetics of nonenzymatic hydrolysis can be explained by random cleavage of labile linkages. When the cleavage of hydrolyzable bonds such as ester groups occurs at random, the concentration of cleaved bonds, C_n, at a lower conversion ratio can be determined from:[3]

$$C_n = k_{H_2O} \, c^\circ \, c^\circ_{H_2O} t \qquad (4)$$

where k_{H_2O} is the rate constant of cleavage of hydrolyzable bonds, c°_{H2O} is the water solubility in the polymer, and c° is the concentration of hydrolyzable bonds in the polymer.

The kinetics of surface degradation have been established[10] and the rate of degradation is proportional to the surface degradation rate, the density of the polymer matrix and surface are as follows when the device is slab-shaped;

$$dM_t/dt = B \, \rho \, A \qquad (5)$$

where M_t is the amount of polymer degraded, B is the surface degradation rate, ρ is the density of the polymer matrix, and A is the surface area of the slab.

PLA and PLGA are to be hydrolyzed under physiological conditions, and the degradation products (lower molecular weight fragments) are ultimately metabolized to carbon dioxide and water and likely to be excreted via the kidneys. Degradation of PLA and PLGA is influenced by the degree of crystallinity (melting point), molecular weight, and packing order (equivalent repeating units of PLGA). Generally, regularity of arrangement of repeating units in PLA and PLGA determines crystallization, making the hydrolyzable groups impermeable to water entry. Degradation of semicrystalline polyesters shows that the crysallinity of the polymer during degradation increases rapidly at first and then levels off to a much smaller rate. This is attributed to preferential ester hydrolysis of amorphous portions of the polymers.

Enzymatically catalyzed hydrolysis has been studied for polysaccharides, polypeptides, their derivatives, and synthetic polymers in order to achieve site-specific degradation in the living body.[1] The enzymatic hydrolysis of biodegradable polymers is known to depend predominantly on their chemical structures and environments (e.g., living organisms). The most important point of degradation involves interactions between enzymes and susceptible bonds in the polymers. There are two kinds of controllable factors: the ease with which the enzyme–substrate complex is formed and the rate of hydrolysis. The former depends on the supramolecular structures of the polymers such as protein folding, and the latter on the sequence in the vicinity of the susceptible bonds.[1] Further, the extent of cross-linking density is known to affect the susceptibility of enzymes. The kinetics of the enzymatic hydrolysis is usually followed by classical Michaelis–Menten kinetic model.

8.3.2 RELATION TO SUPRAMOLECULAR STRUCTURE

Table 8.1 summarizes the effect of supramolecular architectures on the hydrolysis of ester linkages. Kissel et al. reported the effect of grafting a PLGA chain to a PVA backbone on degradation and erosion properties of the PVA-*g*-PLGA film.[42] The erosion of the film with high molecular weight PLGA followed a bulk erosion mechanism that is comparable to linear PLGA. An initial lag time phase, typical of bulk erosion, became shorter in comparison with linear PLGA (Figure 8.7a). This suggests that the PVA backbone contributes to an increase in hydrophilicity, and rapid water penetration leads to accelerating rates of ester hydrolysis. On the contrary, the low-molecular weight PVA-*g*-PLGA (M_n below 1,000 kg/mol) did not show the lag time phase, indicating surface erosion of the film (Figure 8.7b).

A hypothetical degradation mechanism is direct cleavage of the grafted PLG chain in both cases, and water solubility of the cleaved PLGA chain is a dominant factor in changing the erosion mechanism. Ohya et al. also reported the effect of grafting PLA to pullulan backbone.[22] Increasing hydrophilicity due to the backbone accelerates the degradation rate.

Star-shaped PEG-*co*-PLA and PEG-*co*-PLG exhibit smaller hydrodynamic radii compared to linear compounds. Such an architectural modification significantly affects its degradation properties due to the differences in chain length, crystallinity, and morphology.[43] Kissel et al. reported the effect of star-shaped architecture on the erosion of PEG-*co*-PLGA film.[41] This erosion behavior follows the bulk erosion mechanism as well as the linear ABA type block copolymer of PEG and PLGA, but the rate of decreasing molecular weight and mass loss in the initial 2 to 3 weeks is significantly slower. This is due to retaining PEG in the initial degradation phase, leading to the swollen state of the film. Thus, hydrophilic environments in the film or microspheres may be maintained during the erosion period, which is not achieved in the linear block copolymer.

TABLE 8.1
Effects of Supramolecular Architectures on the Hydrolysis of Ester Linkages

Types of biodegradable polymers	Polymer components	Usage form	Advantage for hydrolysis of ester linkages	References
Comb-type	Backbone: PVA, polysaccharides Graft: PLGA, PLA	Film, Microsphere	Controlling erosion mechanism from bulk to surface Acceleration of degradation rate	24,42
Star-shaped or dendritic	Core: multiarm PEG Outer region: PLGA, PLA	Film, Microsphere	Maintaining hydrophilicity during degradation period	41,43
Star-shaped or dendritic	Core: luminescent and cleavable metal Outer region: PLA	Solution, Film	Biodegradability with chemical responsiveness such as acid, base, peroxides, and ammonia	33
Comb-type with stereocomplex	Backbone: dextran Graft: L-PLA and D-PLA	Hydrogel	Fully degradable properties of PLA chain Controllable erosion time	44
Polyrotaxane	α-cyclodextrin, PEG, L-phenylalanine	Hydrogel	Controllable erosion time and profile in highly swollen conditions	18,39

(a)

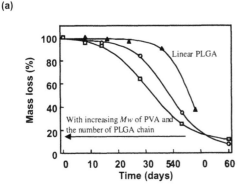

(b)

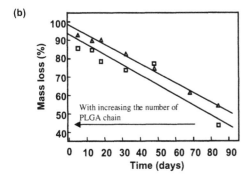

FIGURE 8.7 Effect of grafting PLGA to PVA backbone on film erosion. (a) High molecular weight of PVA-G-PLGA. Open circle: M_w of PVA = 15 kg/mol; M_n of PVA-g-PLGA = 1254 kg/mol, Open square: M_w of PVA = 20 kg/mol; M_n of PVA-g-PLGA = 1135 kg/mol, Closed triangle: linear PLGA with M_w of 40 kg/mol. (b) Low molecular weight of PVA-g-PLGA. Open square: M_w of PVA = 15 kg/mol; M_n of PVA-g-PLGA = 134 kg/mol. Open triangle: M_w of PVA = 15 kg/mol; M_n of PVA-g-PLGA = 238 kg/mol. (From Breitenbach, A. et al., *Polymer*, 41, 4781, 2000. With permission.)

Hennink et al. studied degradation of physically cross-linked dextran hydrogels by stereocomplex formation of oligo(L- and D-lactide)s (Figure 8.8) and found the effect of the stereocomplex formation on the hydrolytic behavior.[44] The stereocomplex formation reduced water solubility in comparison with L- and D-lactide oligomers, and the rate-determining factor in the degradation of the stereocomplex is the dissolution rate of the oligomers. The degradation of hydrogels follows bulk degradation, and the time to complete erosion of the hydrogels becomes longer with increasing either the number of oligolactide side chains or degree of polymerization of lactide. Low polydispersity of the L- and D-lactide oligomers is important for stabler and stronger network formation and prolonged degradation time. Since PLA with high molecular weight stereocomplexes is highly resistant to degradation and erosion,[45] the resulting crystalline fragments cause adverse foreign body reactions. In this sense, fully degradable properties may be advantageous for *in vivo* use.

Yui et al. proposed a unique degradation and erosion mechanism using PEG-based hydrogels cross-linked by a hydrolyzable polyrotaxane.[39] α-CDs as cross-linkers in the polyrotaxane are covalently bound to other PEG chains (M_n values of 600, 2000, and 4000). Gel erosion experiments show that the time to reach complete hydrogel erosion is prolonged by decreasing the polyrotaxane content and increasing

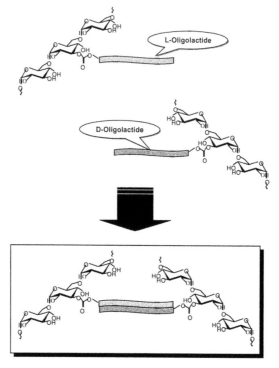

FIGURE 8.8 Preparation of hydrogels cross-linked by stereocomplex formation.

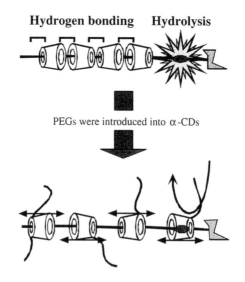

FIGURE 8.9 Proposed mechanism of the enhanced stability of ester linkages by inclusion complexation.

the number of the PEG chains linked with one α-CD molecule in the polyrotaxane (PEG/α-CD ratio). Since the water content of these hydrogels increases with decreasing the polyrotaxane content, the hydrogel network in a highly water-swollen state is more stably maintained. Presumably, intermolecular hydrogen bonds among α-CDs in the polyrotaxane may be eliminated by linking α-CDs with PEG chains, which may enhance the stability of ester linkages via inclusion complexation of α-CDs (Figure 8.9).

Supramolecular architectures also affect enzymatic degradation and enzymatic-degradation controlled drug release behavior, especially, enzyme–substrate complexation. Kopeček et al. reported the effect of star-shaped architecture on cathepsin B-catalyzed degradation of Gly–Phe–Leu–Gly–doxorubicin bound to poly(2-hydroxypropyl)methacrylamide (PHPMA) main chain.[46] By drug conjugations, doxorubicin (DOX) can be released via enzymatic degradation. The result of *in vitro* release of DOX shows that the release rate from the star-shaped PHPMA copolymer–DOX conjugate is lower in comparison with linear polymer–DOX conjugate. Because of the smaller hydrodynamic volumes of star-shaped copolymers, the formation of the enzyme (cathepsin B)-substrate (Gly–Phe–Leu–Gly–DOX) complex may be more difficult.

On the other hand, Yui et al. found enhanced accessibility of peptide substrates toward endo-type proteinase[47] and exopeptidase[48] using the polyrotaxane structure. Polyrotaxanes form loosely packed associations due to their rod-like structures under physiological conditions, which maintains enzymatic accessibility to terminal peptide moieties. A typical example is degradation of the terminal oligopeptides in the polyrotaxane by aminopeptidase M. An L-phenylalanlylglycylglycine (H-L-PheGlyGly)-terminated polyrotaxane in which many α-CDs were threaded onto poly(ethylene oxide) (PEO) was synthesized to evaluate the effect of α-CD threading on the degradation of the terminal H-L-PheGlyGly by a membrane-bound metalloexopeptidase (aminopeptidase M). The Michaelis-Menten constant (K_m) value of the polyrotaxane was 1/22 of H-L-PheGlyGly-terminated PEO. Presumably, the terminal H-L-PheGlyGly is exposed to the aqueous environment due to expansion of the linear backbone by the threading of α-CDs (Figure 8.10).

The complete drug release behavior can be synchronized with the hydrolysis pattern of the polyrotaxanes, i.e., drug-immobilized α-CDs in the polyrotaxane can be completely released.[49] In this case, the immobilized drug molecules associate with each other in physiological conditions, and the terminal peptide moieties are considered still exposed to the aqueous environment.

The polymer chain entanglements composed of comb-type copolymers seen in IPN-structured hydrogels affect enzymatic degradation. Yui et al. demonstrated dual stimuli-responsive degradation of hydrogels in relation to miscibility in an IPN consisting of gelatin and dextran.[37] Physical chain entanglement was observed for the IPN-structured hydrogels prepared below the sol–gel transition temperature of a gelatin with a homogeneous structure. The hydrogels were not degraded in the presence of α-chymotrypsin or dextranase, whereas they were completely degraded by the action of both enzymes. These phenomena were not observed for hydrogels showing phase-separated structures prepared above the sol–gel transition temperature. Thus,

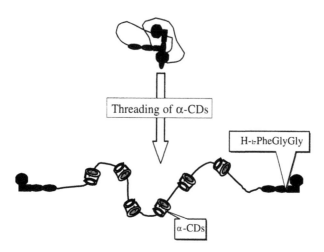

FIGURE 8.10 The expanded structure of H-L-PheGlyGly-terminated PEG by threading of α-CDs.

the two polymer networks (gelatin and dextran) are hydrolyzed sequentially in the presence of both enzymes(α-chymotrypsin and dextranase), leading to a total degradation of the IPN-structured hydrogels. In the presence of both enzymes, one of the two polymer networks (e.g., gelatin) at the outermost surface may be hydrolyzed, then another network (e.g., dextran) exposed at the outer surface may be hydrolyzed.

8.4. APPLICATIONS

8.4.1 DRUG DELIVERY SYSTEMS

Drug release from these biodegradable supramolecular materials can be modulated in comparison with linear polymers. Drug release from biodegradable matrices occurs based on diffusion in the early phase, and the final release phase is governed by degradation and erosion of biodegradable polymer devices. Because of this characteristic, continuous drug release profiles from biodegradable matrices are difficult to achieve for protein drugs.

Kissel et al. studied protein drug release from hydrolyzable microspheres consisting of hydrophilic polymers such as polysaccharides grafted with PLA or PLGA.[41] When bovine serum albumin (BSA) is loaded in the microspheres, BSA can be continuously released by diffusion without any drug burst. Formation of a porous, water-filled structure through surface erosion leads to zero-order release profiles. Such a supramolecular effect on drug release is also observed when star-shaped PEG-*co*-PLGA is used. Retaining PEG chains during the initial two to three weeks, which is not observed in linear PEG-*co*-PLGA, leads to swelling of the microspheres in that period. Kissel also reported that cumulative release of FITC–dextran as a model protein from the star-shaped block copolymers was higher than that of linear copolymers.[41] Such a continuous release of protein drugs may be advantageous for advanced therapeutics using bioengineered proteins.[50]

Kim et al. studied release of hydrophilic and hydrophobic drugs incorporated into PEG-*b*-PLGA-*b*-PEG-based polymeric micelles that become a physical hydrogel at body temperature.[51] A model hydrophilic drug is released with a first-order profile, indicating diffusion-controlled drug release. On the other hand, a model hydrophobic drug is released with a sigmoidal release profile, suggesting that the drug release is initially governed by diffusion, followed by degradation of the micelles. This biphasic drug release is consistent with a simulation model of hydrophobic drug release from a core-shell structure of matrix in which the hydrophobic drug is partitioned in two different domains. Since the polymeric micelles become a hydrogel at body temperature, such biodegradable and thermosensitive hydrogel formulations may be fascinating techniques for injectable drug delivery systems.[52]

Hennink et al. studied protein (lysozyme, BSA, and IgG) release from dextran hydrogels physically cross-linked by stereocomplex formation of oligo(L- and D-lactide)s.[44] The release of proteins with larger diameters, e.g., IgG (10.7 μm), is governed by both Fickian diffusion and degradation. Significant properties of these proteins include quantitative release, which depends on the physicochemical characteristics of the stereocomplex hydrogels such as initial water content and stability of the stereocomplex. Thus, IgG release is controlled by the choice of comb-type copolymers and polydispersity of the oligo(lactide) grafts.

8.4.2 SCAFFOLDS FOR TISSUE ENGINEERING

Biodegradable polymers used for pharmaceutical applications include matrices (scaffolds) for tissue engineering. For example, a patient's cells are incorporated into three-dimensional scaffolds of biodegradable polymers, and then the scaffolds are transplanted to the desired site. A number of the scaffolds including porous sponges, fibrous meshes, and hydrogels have been studied. Hydrogels are potentially feasible for tissue reconstruction and regeneration; swollen hydrogels provide a microenvironment that allows the exchange of metabolites and nutrients. The desirable properties of the components in polymer networks should include good biocompatibility, biodegradability for eventual disappearance, and reactivity for chemical modifications to immobilize specific cell ligands.

Yui et al. studied cell adhesion properties on polyrotaxane hydrogels.[53] The number of cell adhesions on the hydrogels cross-linked by the polyrotaxane was larger than those cross-linked by α-CDs in spite of similar surface hydrophobicity. These results suggest that the cells recognize the surface heterogeneity due to the polyrotaxane structure, and the amount of cell adhesion and proliferation is controllable by the polyrotaxane content. Yui et al. recently prepared microporous scaffolds using this hydrogel by means of salt leaching and gas forming techniques.[54] The resultant hydrogel scaffolds have well interconnected microporous structures, and chondrocytes are found to adhere and spread in the scaffolds. In addition, mucopolysaccharides, the representative cartilaginous extracellular matrices produced by cultured chondrocytes, are observed by Alcian Blue staining. Considering the controllable erosion of the hydrogels in highly swollen states, the cell growth on and/or in the PEG hydrogels cross-linked by the hydrolyzable polyrotaxane may be a promising approach to reconstruct damaged tissues.

8.5 CONCLUDING REMARKS

Biodegradation function in biomaterials is considered essential for biomedical use. Chemical modification and design of linear biodegradable polymers have been studied to achieve degradation-controlled drug release and tissue regeneration. Such approaches were "conventional" in the last century. Supramolecular architectures such as polymeric micelles, branched copolymers, polyrotaxanes, and polymer networks have unique physical and physicochemical characteristics and morphology that will allow us to modulate biodegradation. Controlled degradation by the stereocomplex formation of comb-type oligolactide copolymers and modulated hydrolysis of polyrotaxane hydrogels described above are examples of supramolecular design of biodegradable polymers. In controlled degradation, selection of the length and polydispersity of oligolactide can lead to the modulation of hydrolysis rate. The modulated hydrolysis of ester linkages located at the terminals of polymeric chains can be prolonged by inclusion complexation with CDs. Good biocompatibility is required even for the supramolecular-structured biodegradable polymers, and is an important issue when considering polymer design. A biomimetic approach to biocompatibility may be a good method. For instance, sulfonation of hundreds of hydroxyl groups in biodegradable polyrotaxanes mimicking heparin is significantly effective for improving blood compatibilities.[55] The control of water structures surrounding biodegradable polymers may be an important factor related to both biocompatibility and biodegradability. Supramolecular-structured biodegradable polymers will play important parts in many biological applications in the coming decades.

REFERENCES

1. Kopeček, J. and Ulbrich, K., Biodegradation of biomedical polymers, *Prog. Polym. Sci.,* 9, 1–58 (1983).
2. Zaikov, G.E., Quantitative aspects of polymer degradation in the living body, *JMS-Rev. Macromol. Chem. Phys.,* C25, 551–597 (1985).
3. Pierre, St. T. and Chiellini, E., Biodegradability of synthetic polymers used for medical and pharmaceutical applications; I. Principles of hydrolysis mechanisms, *J. Bioact. Comp. Polym.,* 1, 467–497 (1986).
4. Pierre, St. T. and Chiellini, E., Biodegradability of synthetic polymers used for medical and pharmaceutical applications; II. Backbone hydrolysis, *J. Bioact. Comp. Polym.,* 2, 4–30 (1987).
5. Kamath, K.R. and Park, K., Biodegradable hydrogels in drug delivery, *Adv. Drug Deliv. Rev.,* 11, 59–84 (1993).
6. Piskin, E., Biodegradable polymers as biomaterials, *J. Biomater. Sci. Polym. Edn.,* 6, 775–795 (1994).

7. Okada, H. and Toguchi, H., Biodegradable microspheres in drug delivery, *Crit. Rev. Ther. Drug Carrier Syst.*, 12, 1–99 (1995).

8. Ogawa, Y., Injectable microcapsules prepared with biodegradable poly(α-hydroxy) acids for prolonged release of drugs, *J. Biomater. Sci. Polym. Edn.*, 8, 391–409 (1997).

9. Chadra, R. and Rustgi, R., Biodegradable polymers, *Prog. Polym. Sci.*, 23, 1273–1335 (1998).

10. Baker, R.W., Ed., *Controlled Release of Biologically Active Agents*, John Wiley & Sons, New York, 1987.

11. Park, K., Shalaby, W.S.W., and Park, H., Eds., *Biodegradable Hydrogels for Drug Delivery*, Technomic Publishing, Basel, 1993.

12. Otthnbrite, R.M., Huang, S.J., and Park, K., Eds., *Hydrogels and Biodegradable Polymers for Bioapplications,* American Chemical Society, Washington, 1996.

13. Dumb, A.J., Kost, J., and Wiseman, D.M., Eds., *Handbook of Biodegradable Polymers,* Vol. 7, Drug Targeting and Delivery, Harwood Academic, Amsterdam, 1997.

14. Heller, J., Biodegradable polymers in controlled drug delivery, *CRC Crit. Rev. Ther. Drug Carrier Syst.*, 1, 39–90 (1984).

15. Partric, C., Jr., Mikos, A.G. and McLutire, V., Eds., *Frontiers in Tissue Engineering*, Pergamon, Oxford, 1998.

16. West, J.L. and Hubell, J.A., Polymeric biomaterials with degradation sites for proteases involved in cell migration, *Macromolecules*, 32, 241–244 (1999).

17. Ooya, T. and Yui, N., Polyrotaxanes; synthesis, structure and potential in drug delivery, *Crit. Rev. Ther. Drug Carrier Syst.,* 16, 289–330 (1999).

18. Watanabe, J. et al., Design of polyrotaxane-based hydrolyzable materials for tissue engineering, in *Biomaterials and Drug Delivery: Toward New Millennium,* Park, K.D. et al., Eds., Han Rim Won, Seoul, 2000, pp. 565–577.

19. Jeong, B. Bae, Y.H., and Kim, S.W., Thermoreversible gelation of PEG-PLGA-PEG triblock copolymer aqueous solutions, *Macromolecules*, 32, 7064–7069 (1999).

20. Yasugi, K. et al., Preparation and characterization of polymer micelles from poly(ethylene glycol)-poly(D.L-lactide) block copolymers as potential drug carrier, *J. Contr. Rel.*, 62, 89–100 (1999).

21. Choi, Y.K., Bae, Y.H., and Kim, S.W., Star-shaped poly(ether-ester) block copolymers: synthesis, characterization, and their physical properties, *Macromolecules*, 31, 8766–8774 (1998).

22. Ohya, Y., Mruhashi, S., and Ouchi, T., Graft polymerization of L–lactide on pullulan through the trimethylsilyl protection method and degradation of the graft copolymers, *Macromolecules*, 31, 4662–4665 (1999).

23. Tasaka, Y. et al., Synthesis of comb-type biodegradable polylactide through depsipeptide–lactide copolymer containing serine residues, *Macromolecules*, 32, 6386–6389 (1999).

24. Breitenbach, A. and Kissel, T., Biodegradable comb polyesters. I. Synthesis, characterization and structural analysis of poly(lactide) and poly(lactide-*co*-glycolide) grafted onto water-soluble poly(vinyl alchol) as back bone, *Polymer,* 39, 3261–3271 (1998).

25. de Jong, S.J. et al., Novel self-assembled hydrogels by stereocomplex formation in aqueous solution of enantiomeric lactic acid oligomers grafted to dextran, *Macromolecules*, 33, 3680–3686 (2000).

26. Huh, K.M., Kumashiro, Y., Ooya, T., and Yui, N., A new synthetic route for dextran graft copolymers containing thermo-responsive polymers, *Polym. J.*, 33, 103–106 (2001).

27. Huh, K.M. et al., Supramolecular-structured hydrogel showing a reversible phase transition by inclusion complexation between poly(ethylene glycol) grafted dextran and α–cyclodextrin, *Macromolecules*, 34, 8657–8662, 2002.

28. Moriyama, K., Ooya, T., and Yui, N., Hyaluronic acid grafted with poly(ethylene glycol) as a novel peptide formulation, *J. Contr. Rel.*, 59, 77–86 (1999).

29. Bear, M.M. et al., New degradable macromolecular micelles based on degradable amphiphilic block-copolymers, *J. Contr. Rel.*, 64, 270–273 (2000).

30. Jeong, B. Bae, Y. H., and Kim, S. W., Biodegradable thermoresponsive micelles of PEG–PLGA–PEG triblock copolymers, *Colloids and Surfaces B: Biointerfaces*, 16, 185–193 (1999).

31. Moine, L. et al., New pH sensitive network: combination of an amphiphilic degradable polyester with a β–cyclodextrin copolymer, *Macromol. Symp.*, 130, 45–52 (1998).

32. Cammas, S. et al., Polymers of malic acid and 3-alkymalic acid as synthetic PHAs in the design of biocompatible hydrolyzable devices, *Int. J. Biol. Macro.*, 25, 273–282 (1999).

33. Corbin, P.S. et al., Biocompatibile polyester microligands: new subunits for the assembly of star-shaped polymers with luminescent and cleavable metal cores, *Biomacromolecules*, 2, 223–232 (2001).

34. Ooya, T. and Yui, N., Synthesis and characterization of biodegradable polyrotaxane as a novel supramolecular-structured drug carrier, *J. Biomater. Sci. Polym. Edn.* 8, 437–456 (1997).

35. Watanabe, J., Ooya, T., and Yui, N., Preparation and characterization of a polyrotaxane with non-enzymatically hydrolyzable stoppers, *Chem. Lett.*, 1031–1032 (1998).

36. Ooya, T., Arizono, K., and Yui, N., Synthesis and characterization of an oligopeptide-terminated polyrotaxane as a drug carrier, *Polym. Adv. Tech.*, 11, 642–651 (2000).

37. Watanabe, J., Ooya, T., and Yui, N., Effect of acetylation of biodegradable polyrotaxanes on its supramolecular dissociation via terminal ester hydrolysis, *J. Biomater. Sci. Polym. Edn.*, 10, 1275–1288 (1999).

38. Huh, K.M. et al., Polymer inclusion complex consisting of poly(ε-lysine) and α-cyclodextrin, *Macromolecules*, 34, 2402–2404 (2001).

39. Ichi, T., Watanabe, J., Ooya, T., and Yui, N., Controllable erosion time and profile in poly(ethylene glycol) hydrogels by supramolecular structure of hydrolyzable polyrotaxane, *Biomacromolecules*, 2, 204–210 (2001).

40. Kurisawa, M. and Yui, N., Gelatin/dextran intelligent hydrogels for drug delivery: dual-stimuli-responsive degradation in relation to miscibility in interpenetrating polymer networks, *Macromol. Chem. Phys.*, 199, 1547–1554 (1998).

41. Breitenbach, A., Li, Y., and Kissel, T., Branched biodegradable polyesters for parenteral drug delivery systems, *J. Contr. Rel.*, 64, 167–178 (2000).

42. Breitenbach, A., Pistel, K.F., and Kissel, T., Biodegradable comb polyesters. II. Erosion and release properties of poly(vinyl alcohol)-g-poly(lactic-co-glycolic acid), *Polymer*, 41, 4781–4793 (2000).

43. Jeong, B. et al., New biodegradable polymers for injectable drug delivery, *J. Contr. Rel.*, 62, 109–114 (1999).

44. de Jong, S.J. et al., Physically crosslinked hydrogels by stereocomplex formation of lactic acid oligomers: degradation and protein release behavior, *J. Contr. Rel.*, 71, 261–275 (2001).

45. Li, S. and Vert, M., Morphological changes resulting from the hydrolytic degradation of stereocopolymers derived from L- and DL-lactide, *Macromolecules*, 27, 3107–3110 (1994).

46. Wang, D. et al., Synthesis of star-like *N*-(2-hydroxypropyl)methacrylamide copolymers: potential drug carriers, *Biomacromolecules*, 1, 313–319 (2000)

47. Ooya, T. and Yui, N., Supramolecular dissociation of biodegradable polyrotaxanes by terminal hydrolysis, *Macromol. Chem. Phys.*, 199, 2311–2320 (1998).

48. Ooya, T., Eguchi, M., and Yui, N., Enhanced accessibility of peptide substrate toward a membrane-bound metalloexopeptidase by supramolecular structure of polyrotaxane, *Biomacromolecules*, 2, 200–203 (2001).

49. Ooya, T. and Yui, N., Synthesis of a theophylline–polyrotaxane conjugate and its drug release via supramolecular dissociation, *J. Contr. Rel.*, 58, 251–269 (1999).

50. Jung, T. et al., Biodegradable nanoparticles for oral delivery of peptides: is there a role for polymers to affect mucosal uptake? *Eur. J. Pharm. Biopharm.*, 50, 147–160 (2000).

51. Jeong, B. Bae, Y.H., and Kim, S.W., Drug release from biodegradable injectable thermosensitive hydrogel of PEG-PLGA-PEG triblock copolymers, *J. Contr. Rel.*, 63, 155–163 (2000).

52. Jeong, B. et al., Biodegradable block copolymers as injectable drug-delivery systems, *Nature*, 388, 860–862 (1997).

53. Watanabe, J. et al., Fibroblast adhesion and proliferation on poly(ethylene glycol) hydrogels crosslinked by hydrolyzable polyrotaxane, submitted, *Biomaterials*, 2001.

54. Lee, W.K. et al., Novel biodegradable polymer scaffolds containing polyrotaxane for cartilage tissue engineering, *Polym. Preprints*, 42, 137–138 (2001).

55. Park, H.D. et al., Anticoagulant activity of sulfonated polyrotaxanes as blood compatible materials, *J. Biomed. Mater. Res.*, in press, 2001.

9 Stimuli-Responsive Polymers and Gels

Takashi Miyata

CONTENTS

9.1 INTRODUCTION

The most important biosystems that sustain life are closely associated with natural feedback system functions such as homeostasis. For example, hormone release from secretory cells is regulated by physiological cycles or specific input signals. In such natural feedback systems, cell membranes perceive specific ions or biological molecules like hormones, and induce conformational changes or rearrangements of their biomolecules to allow them to function biologically. A natural feedback system consists of a sensor to sense a stimulus as a signal, a processor to judge the magnitude of the signal, and an effector to alter function in direct response to the stimulus. In biomolecules, cell, and various biological systems, the functions of the sensor, processor, and effector are associated through hierarchical structures on the basis of covalent or noncovalent bonds. Therefore, combining their functions in polymeric materials can lead to mimicking the natural feedback systems. Such mimicking will be an integral part of the next generation of biomaterials and drug delivery systems.

When dissolved in a solvent, polymer chains undergo conformational changes by varying environmental conditions, as their affinity for the solvent is strongly dependent upon the conditions (Figure 9.1a). For example, polymer chains of poly(*N*-isopropylacrylamide) change dramatically from an expanded state to a collapsed state by a temperature rise over 32°C due to a change in chain hydrophilicity. Polymers that can change their properties or structures in response to environmental stimuli such as pH, temperature, etc. are called stimuli-responsive polymers. Similarly, some gels have a unique ability to undergo abrupt changes in their volume in response to environmental changes (Figure 9.1b). Since this unique property called volume phase transition was discovered[1,2] (see Chapter 6), many researchers have focused on gels as stimuli-responsive materials.[3-11] Such stimuli-responsive polymers and gels mimic natural feedback system since they have sensor, processor, and effector functions. The fascinating properties of stimuli-responsive polymers and gels suggest that they have potential as suitable intelligent materials for mimicking biomolecules and smart systems in the biochemical and biomedical fields. They have been used to construct switches, sensors, actuators, bioreactors, separation systems, and drug delivery systems.

The unique behaviors of stimuli-responsive polymers and gels are governed by the affinity of polymer chains for solvent and/or other chains (Figure 9.1).[12] Such affinity of polymer chains is based on fundamental interactions such as van der Waals interaction, hydrophobic interaction, hydrogen bonding, and electrostatic interaction. Therefore, molecular architectures and gel structures must be designed from the viewpoint of fundamental interactions.

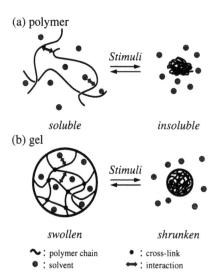

(a) polymer

Stimuli

soluble   *insoluble*

(b) gel

Stimuli

swollen   *shrunken*

〜 : polymer chain   ● : cross-link
● : solvent   ⬌ : interaction

FIGURE 9.1 Unique behaviors of stimuli-responsive polymers and gels.

For instance, pH-responsive polymers that induce conformational changes by varying pH can be synthesized by introducing ionizable groups into the polymers. The temperature-responsiveness of some polymers results from the architectural balance between hydrophilic and hydrophobic parts in constitutional components. To summarize, the development of stimuli-responsive polymers and gels requires architectural designs of molecular and gel structures that control fundamental interactions. In addition, swelling behaviors of gels are influenced by not only the affinities of polymer chains and cross-linking structures (Figure 9.1). This means that stimuli-responsive gels can be prepared by introducing reversible cross-linking points that can be formed and dissociated in response to environmental changes. Reversible complex formation by fundamental interactions such as hydrogen bonding and electrostatic interaction is useful in constructing such stimuli-responsive cross-linking structures. A few stimuli-responsive gels have been prepared by applying complex formation and dissociation to a gel cross-linking. Based on these synthetic strategies, a variety of stimuli-responsive polymers and gels have been synthesized as intelligent materials and have attracted considerable attention in the biochemical and biomedical fields.

This chapter provides a short overview of important research on the synthesis and applications of stimuli-responsive polymers and gels. The polymers and gels reviewed in this chapter have contributed significantly to the development of the next generation of biomaterials and drug delivery systems.

9.2 PHYSICOCHEMICAL STIMULI-RESPONSIVE POLYMERS AND GELS

9.2.1 TEMPERATURE-RESPONSIVE POLYMERS AND GELS

Temperature is an important factor for determining the states of polymers and gels. There are many potential applications of temperature-responsive polymers and gels that induce structural changes in response to temperature changes. Most temperature-responsive polymers and gels are based on poly(N-alkylacrylamide),[13-15] poly(vinyl methyl ether),[16] poly(ethylene oxide)-poly(propylene oxide)-poly(ethylene oxide),[17] and poly(N-vinylisobutylamide).[18] The poly(N-isopropylacrylamide) (PNIPAAm) of a representative temperature-responsive polymer is very unique in that its solubility in water changes abruptly at a lower critical solution temperature (LCST). It is soluble in water at temperatures below LCST (about 32°C), but becomes insoluble above LCST due to strong intermolecular interaction between the hydrophobic groups. Therefore, most researchers have used PNIPAAm as a temperature-responsive component in the development of temperature-responsive materials. Temperature-responsive polymers and gels containing PNIPAAm are currently of great interest in biochemical and biomedical fields.

Hoffman et al.[19,20] prepared cross-linked PNIPAAm gels that show temperature-responsive swelling behavior, and discussed the possibility of their application to drug delivery systems. The PNIPAAm gels shrunk in aqueous solution due to their hydrophobic chains when the temperature was raised through their LCST. They

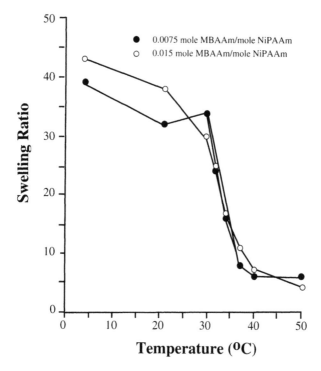

FIGURE 9.2 Effect of temperature on the swelling ratios of PNIPAAm hydrogels with different cross-linker concentrations in water.[19]

reswelled when cooled below the LCST (Figure 9.2). They demonstrated that the temperature-responsive PNIPAAm gels might be used to absorb and release biologically and industrially important substances in response to environmental temperature changes. In addition, enzymes such as asparaginase and β-galactosidase have been immobilized in a temperature-responsive gel in order to prepare the novel gel system that can control enzymatic activity by temperature.[21, 22] The activity of β-galactosidase immobilized in the temperature-responsive gels was turned on and off by temperature changes as thermal cycling through LCST changed their pore sizes. Mass transfer within the gels and substrate conversion efficiency were enhanced by a pumping action resulting from the temperature-responsive collapse and reswelling of the gel.

Kim and Okano et al.[23-25] synthesized a temperature-responsive gel consisting of NIPAAm and butyl methacrylate (BMA) to improve the mechanical properties of the cross-linked PNIPAAm gels. Pulsatile release of a model drug in response to stepwise temperature changes was achieved by using the temperature-responsive gels. The temperature-responsive swelling behavior of some cross-linked poly(*N*,*N*'-alkyl substituted acrylamide) gels was studied from the viewpoint of enthalpic and entropic contributions.[26] The studies revealed that the temperature-responsive swelling behavior of the gels is attributed to the delicate hydrophilic/hydrophobic balance of their polymer chains, which is influenced by the size, configuration, and mobility of alkyl side groups. In addition, the studies on the shrinking kinetics of the temperature-responsive gels clarified that the shrinking rates of the gels from swollen to collapsed states at several different temperatures are dramatically influenced by gel surface structural changes and formation of a collapsed polymer skin layer which prevents the gel from shrinking rapidly.[27-29] Okano et al.[30-33] enhanced the shrinking rates of the PNIPAAm temperature-responsive gels by introducing comb-type grafted structures, based on the concept of tailoring gel architecture. The comb-type grafted PNIPAAm gels showed much larger shrinking rates during the deswelling beyond LCST than the conventional cross-linked PNIPAAm gel (Figure 9.3). This was attributed to rapid hydrophobic aggregation of freely mobile PNIPAAm graft chains and intrinsic elastic forces of polymer networks. These results suggest that the molecular architecture of the gel must be designed for development of useful temperature responsiveness based on the purpose.

The negatively temperature-responsive gels that are swollen at low temperatures and shrunken at high temperatures can be easily prepared by using PNIPAAm as a temperature-responsive component. Many researchers have studied the negatively temperature-responsive gels from the viewpoints of fundamental gel science and

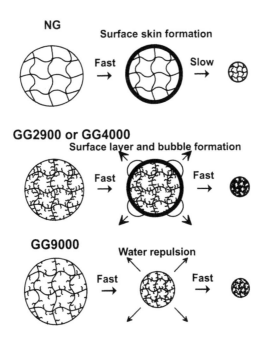

FIGURE 9.3 Deswelling mechanism of comb-type grafted PNIPAAm gels having different lengths of grafted chains above their phase transition temperatures.[31]

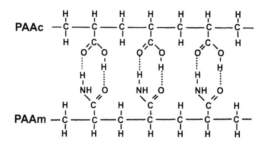

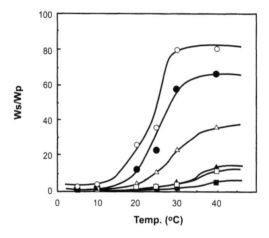

FIGURE 9.4 Temperature dependence of equilibrium swelling ratios of PAAc/PAAm IPN gels with various BMA contents: ○, 0 wt%; ●, 5 wt%; △, 10 wt%; ▲, 20 wt%; □, 30 wt%; ■, 50 wt%.[34]

potential applications. However, very few studies of the positively temperature-responsive gels that swell at higher temperatures have been reported. Okano et al.[34-36] focused on complex formation between acrylamide (AAm) or *N,N*-dimethylacrylamide (DMAAm) as hydrogen-bonding acceptors and PAAc as a hydrogen-bonding donor, and utilized the temperature dependence of their complex formation to synthesize positively temperature-responsive gels. Their complex interpenetrating polymer networks (IPNs) prepared by a sequential method showed lower swelling ratios at lower temperatures and higher swelling ratios at higher temperatures (Figure 9.4). This is due to the fact that the hydrogen bond between AAm and AAc is formed at a lower temperature and dissociated at a higher temperature. Comparison between random copolymers and IPNs of PAAc and PAAm revealed that introducing the IPN structure is very effective for improving the sensitivities of the positively temperature-responsive gels. Okano's result clearly shows the importance of designing gel architecture. Moreover, the positively temperature-responsive IPN gels enabled a model drug to be released at a high temperature and prevented its release at a lower temperature.

A temperature-responsive gel consisting of biodegradable blocks of poly(ethylene oxide) and poly(L-lactic acid) (PEG-PLGA-PEG triblock copolymer) was shown to be a fascinating sustained-release matrix for drugs.[37-40] An aqueous solution of the triblock copolymer exhibited reversibly temperature-responsive sol–gel transition in that the sol (at low temperature) formed a gel (at body temperature). The sol–gel transition is based on micelllar growth and intra- and intermicelle phase mixing and packing. The critical gelation temperature can be controlled by the molecular architectures of the triblock such as composition and block length. An injectable sol of the triblock copolymer containing drugs was changed to a biodegradable gel by subcutaneous injection and subsequent rapid cooling to body temperature. Sustained release of drugs was achieved by the degradation of the triblock copolymer gel with a core-shell structure. These studies revealed that the temperature-responsive PEG-PLGA-PEG triblock copolymer has great advantages for sustained injectable drug delivery systems.

Recently, unique temperature-responsive gels were synthesized by assembling from water-soluble synthetic polymers and a well-defined protein-folding motif, the coiled coil.[41] In the hybrid gels, a linear hydrophilic copolymer of N-(2-hydroxypropyl)-methacrylamide and a metal-chelating monomer formed a metal complex with Ni^{2+} and terminal histidine residues (His tags) of the coiled-coil protein through the pendant metal-chelating ligand. The hybrid gels were collapsed at a temperature above 35°C owing to temperature-induced cooperative conformational transition of the coiled-coil protein domain. This result suggests that novel gels having unusual physicochemical and biological properties can be created by tailoring the coiled coils using the techniques of molecular biology. Furthermore, positively temperature-responsive hybrid gels were also synthesized by cross-linking AAm copolymer through metal coordination bonding between its metal chelating nitrilotriacetic acid-containing side chains and His tags of the I28 immunoglobulin (Ig)-like module of human cardiac titin, an elastic muscle protein (Figure 9.5).[42] The hybrid gel cross-linked with the I28 module was swollen to three times its initial volume at temperatures above the melting temperature of the module. These studies on hybrid gels prepared from well-characterized protein modules provide a practical strategy to create stimuli-responsive materials having unique properties that can be predicted during gel structure design.

Covalent conjugates of biomolecules and soluble synthetic polymers like poly(ethylene glycol) (PEG) have attracted much attention for applications in drug delivery, affinity separations, diagnostics, and bioprocesses. Some researchers used PNIPAAm to develop intelligent polymer–biomolecule conjugates that can control the functions of biomolecules like proteins and DNA by temperature. Hoffman et al.[43-47] and Okano et al.[48-52] synthesized conjugates of PNIPAAm–enzyme, PNIPAAm–antibody, and PNIPAAm–streptavidin that show their activity in aqueous solution below their LCST and can be separated from the solution by their precipitation above the LCST. For example, temperature-reversible soluble-insoluble conjugates of PNIPAAm and enzymes like β-D-glucosidase,[45] lipase,[51] and trypsin[46,47,52] were prepared by the reaction of a terminal carboxyl group on the NIPAAm oligomer with amino groups on the enzymes. Their PNIPAAm–enzyme conjugates can

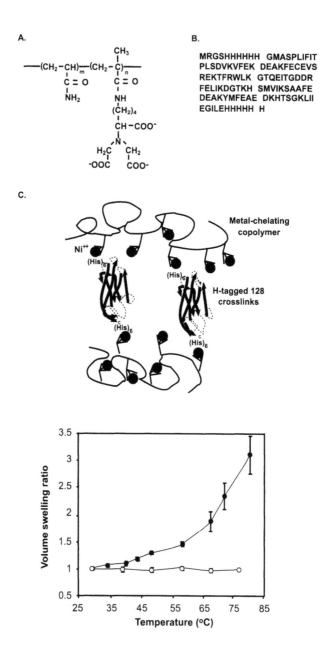

A.

B.

MRGSHHHHHH GMASPLIFIT
PLSDVKVFEK DEAKFECEVS
REKTFRWLK GTQEITGDDR
FELIKDGTKH SMVIKSAAFE
DEAKYMFEAE DKHTSGKLII
EGILEHHHHH H

C.

Metal-chelating copolymer

Ni++

(His)₆

(His)₆

(His)₆

(His)₆

H-tagged 128 crosslinks

FIGURE 9.5 Bottom: Effect of temperature on swelling ratios of gels cross-linked with titin I28 (●) and without titin I28 (○). Top: Assembly of the I28 cross-linked hydrogel. (A) Chemical structure of metal-chelating copolymer. (B) Protein sequence of the recombinant titin I28 cross-linker H-I28-H. (C) Structure of the hybrid hydrogel.[42]

catalyze enzymatic reaction in solution below their LCST and then can be separated from the solution by precipitation above their LCST.

Okano et al.[52] investigated the effects of the molecular architectures of poly(*N*-isopropylacrylamide)–trypsin conjugates on their solution and enzymatic properties. The trypsin conjugate in which PNIPAAm chains were attached by single-point conjugation was more stable than that produced by multipoint conjugation during repeated temperature cycling. Furthermore, Hoffman et al.[53-55] reported the site-specific conjugation of a temperature-responsive PNIPAAm by its terminal active groups to a genetically engineered site on streptavidin. The site-specific conjugation of the temperature-responsive PNIPAAm near the biotin binding site of the streptavidin enabled binding of biotin to the modified streptavidin below the LCST and prevented the biotin from binding with the modified streptavidin above its LCST (Figure 9.6).

These studies suggest that molecular designs are of great importance in the development of stimuli-responsive bioconjugates having controllable biofunctions. Maeda et al.[56,57] synthesized PNIPAAm–DNA conjugates by photochemically binding psoralen-terminated PNIPAAm to double-stranded DNA and by copolymerizing NIPAAm with vinyl derivative of a single-stranded DNA. The PNIPAAm–DNA conjugates were used for the one-pot separation of the target molecules. For example, the conjugates of PNIPAAm and single-stranded DNA hybridize with the target sequence below their LCST, and their target sequences can be separated from

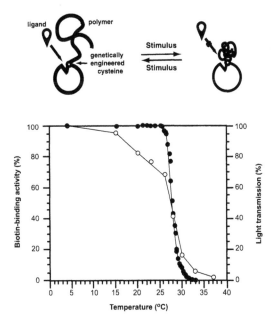

FIGURE 9.6 Temperature dependence of the biotin-blocking activity (○) of the PNIPAAm-streptavidin conjugate, and temperature-stimulated cloud-point behavior (●) of free PNIPAAm. Schematic illustration shows the molecular 'gate' created by conjugating a stimuli-responsive polymer to a genetically engineered site near the receptor binding pocket of a protein.[53]

mismatched DNAs by their precipitation above the LCST.[56] Thus, the conjugation of PNIPAAm with biomolecules can lead to intelligent bioconjugates with controllable functions and easy separation.

Temperature-responsive PNIPAAm is applicable as an intelligent component to develop a molecular separation system. Cussler et al.[58-60] reported that a cross-linked PNIPAAm gel could be used to extract water and low molecular weight solutes from macromolecular solutions. The PNIPAAm gel absorbed water and small solutes, and excluded large solutes on the basis of its network size below its LCST. The gel could be regenerated by a slight increase in temperature above its LCST owing to the release of the absorbed water. Kim et al.[61] revealed that a temperature-responsive gel membrane consisting of NIPAAm and BMA could separate molecules of different sizes. Swelling changes of the copolymer gel membranes by temperature strongly influenced the permeability of the molecules with the different sizes.

PNIPAAm-modified surfaces demonstrated a unique property: temperature changes induce wettability changes.[62] This unique property was used to control attachment and detachment of cultured cells.[63,64] Cells cultured on a hydrophobic PNIPAAm-modified surface at 37°C were easily detached from the surface by lowering the incubation temperature without any deterioration of the cellular function. Silica beads with PNIPAAm-modified surfaces are intelligent column-packing materials for high-performance liquid chromatography (HPLC) that can control separation and solute-surface partitioning by temperature.[65-68] The temperature-responsive surfaces control the function and properties of the stationary phase of HPLC by changing aqueous mobile phase temperature because the hydrophilic–hydrophobic property changes in response to external temperature changes. Such intelligent chromatography systems are very effective in biological and biomedical separations of peptides and proteins.

9.2.2 pH-Responsive Polymers and Gels

A change in pH is one of the most important stimuli that strongly influence the states of polymers and gels. Therefore, most initial stimuli-responsive materials were pH-responsive polymers or gels. Polymers with ionizable groups are promising candidates as pH-responsive polymers since an environmental change in pH as a stimulus induces their conformational changes due to ionization of the polymer chains. Many studies on pH-responsive polymers and gels based on polymers with ionizable groups, such as carboxyl, sulfonic, and amino groups have been reported. This subsection focuses on some studies of pH-responsive polymers and gels synthesized from monomers with such ionizable groups.

Tanaka et al.[69,70] found that ionized poly(acrylamide) (PAAm) gels undergo a discrete phase transition in equilibrium volume upon varying the salt concentration in the solution. The ionized PAAm gels were collapsed in response to varying pH (Figure 9.7). Experiments revealed that the ionization of the polymer network plays an essential role in the volume phase transition of gels.

Siegel et al.[71-74] investigated the swelling behavior of lightly cross-linked hydrophobic polyelectrolyte gels of methyl methacrylate (MMA) and *N,N*-dimethy-

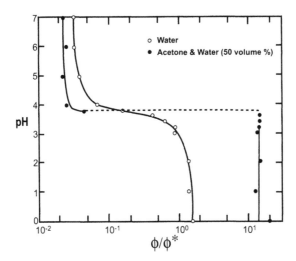

FIGURE 9.7 Effect of pH on the swelling ratios of ionized PAAm gels in water (○) and 50% acetone–water mixture (●).[69]

laminoethyl methacrylate (DMA). Their gels with amino groups were swollen under acidic conditions but shrunken above neutral pH because ionization of the amino groups was governed by environmental pH. In addition, pH-responsive release of caffeine was realized by using the gels with amino groups. On the other hand, Peppas et al.[75,76] focused on carboxyls as an ionizable group, and prepared gels with carboxyl groups by copolymerizing 2-hydroxyethyl methacrylate (HEMA) with methacrylic acid (MAAc) or by forming IPNs of poly(vinyl alcohol) (PVA) and poly(acrylic acid) (PAAc). A change from acidic to neutral pH resulted in an increase in the swelling ratios of gels with carboxyl groups.

Hoffman et al.[77,78] proposed a novel approach for preparation of pH-responsive polymers and gels by introducing temperature-responsive NIPAAm. Their gels were sensitive to both temperature and pH, and responded to the pH change to a much greater extent than normal gels with carboxyl groups, as they were composed of pH-responsive PAAc and temperature-responsive PNIPAAm. The studies by Peppas et al.[79,80] also revealed that random copolymer or IPN gels of MAAc and NIPAAm showed sharp swelling transition with small changes in pH. Besides, Kim et al.[81,82] also synthesized copolymer gels composed of PNIPAAm as the temperature-responsive component, (diethylamino)ethyl methacrylate as the pH-responsive component, and BMA as a hydrophobic component to improve the mechanical properties of the gels. The pH-responsive swelling behavior of the copolymer gels can be controlled by temperature because the ionization of pH-responsive components is influenced by temperature-responsive PNIPAAm.

As the acidic phosphate group is very important, a few gels with phosphate groups were prepared by copolymerization of a monomer with a phosphate group and various monomers.[83,84] The swelling ratios of the gels with the phosphate groups increased strongly at pH 5 and 10 because of the action of the phosphates as acidic charged divalent groups. The gels with phosphate groups also underwent swelling changes in response to changes in temperature and solvent composition; the changes were strongly dependent upon the kind of comonomer and the composition of the copolymers.

Some studies manifested that the gels with phosphate groups were promising supports to immobilize physiologically active compounds that can be applied to novel drug delivery systems. The lysozyme of a cationic protein was efficiently immobilized within negatively charged gels that were synthesized by copolymerization of NIPAAm and the monomer with a phosphate group.[85,86] The lysozyme release from the gels with phosphate groups could be controlled by environmental conditions such as pH and ionic strength because of environmental stimuli-responsive complex formation between the phosphate groups and lysozyme. In particular, the studies on the pH-responsive lysozyme release suggested that lysozyme could be released at pH 7.4 (enteric conditions) and resists release at pH 1.4 (gastric conditions).[86]

Intelligent polymer membranes with pH-responsive molecular valves have been prepared by grafting pH-responsive polymers such as PAAc onto porous membranes. Iwata et al.[87,88] investigated the filtration characteristics of porous membranes on which PAAc was grafted by plasma treatment. The filtration characteristics of the membrane changed reversibly from ultrafilter to microfilter in response to environmental pH, reflecting the configuration of the grafted PAAc chains. Ito et al.[89] prepared a porous membrane with ionizable polypeptides as a pH-responsive gate. The permeation rate of water through the porous membrane was high at high pH and became low at low pH due to pH-responsive conformational change of the polypeptide chains. Thus, grafting pH-responsive polymer chains onto porous membranes might enable us to prepare stimuli-responsive materials with fast responses.

Nagasaki and Kataoka et al.[90,91] synthesized unique poly(silamine) comprising alternating units of N,N'-diethylethylenediamine and 3,3-dimethyl-3-silapentamethylene. The poly(silamine) showed pH-responsive stiffness changes in the polymer chain by protonation due to rotation hindrance around protonated ethylenediamine units. The poly(silamine) LCST can be controlled by environmental pH. A pH-responsive poly(silamine) gel exhibited reproducible swelling/deswelling behavior in response to the protonation degree (α) of the network (Figure 9.8).[92] The shear moduli of the poly(silamine) gel increased abruptly at the phase transition point ($\alpha = 0.5$) because the network became expanded and rigid due to the amine protonation along with the anion binding. Consequently, as the poly(silamine) and its gel showed reversible rod–globule transitions and unique phase transition properties in response to environmental pH changes, they have many potential applications as intelligent materials in biomedical fields.

Superstructures of proteins and polypeptides, which are closely associated with their functions, are influenced by external stimuli such as pH and temperature. Some researchers exploited reversibly stimuli-responsive conformation changes of proteins or polypeptides to design novel stimuli-responsive materials. For example, a poly(butyl methacrylate)-poly(L-aspartic acid) graft copolymer having a polypeptide

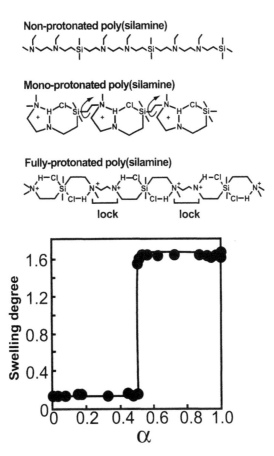

FIGURE 9.8 Bottom: Changes in gel swelling as a function of degree of protonation of poly(silamine) gel in 5.0 M NaCl solution. Top: Plausible poly(silamine) conformations on protonation and anion binding.[92]

branch was synthesized as a new type of biomembrane model.[93,94] In the graft copolymer membrane prepared by the solvent casting method, poly(L-aspartic acid) domain formed continuous phases to function as channels for solute transport. Its reversible conformation changes in response to pH changes regulated the transport of ion and sugars through the membrane.

Tirrell et al.[95] created unique pH-responsive triblock proteins that consisted of 230 amino acids containing a leucine zipper helix repeat and an alanylglycine-rich repeat using recombinant DNA methods (Figure 9.9). The triblock protein formed disulfide-linked dimers through their COOH terminal cysteine residues. Gelation of the triblock proteins occurred by the formation of coiled-coil aggregates of the terminal leucine zipper peptide domains in a low pH solution. The polyelectrolyte segments in the proteins played important roles by retaining solvent and preventing the

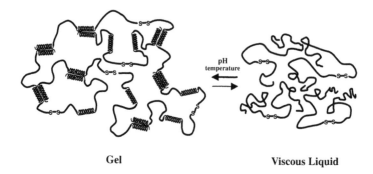

Gel   **Viscous Liquid**

FIGURE 9.9 Proposed physical gelation of monodisperse triblock copolymer. The chains are shown as disulfide-linked dimers joined through their COOH terminal cysteine residues.[95]

precipitation of the chain. However, increasing pH resulted in a change from a protein gel to a viscous polymer solution because the coiled-coil aggregates were dissociated by the repulsive electrostatic interactions between predominantly negatively charged end blocks at high pH. These results mean that stimuli-responsive conformation changes of proteins or polypeptides are valuable in designing intelligent polymers and gels with predetermined physical, chemical, and biological properties.

9.2.3 ELECTRIC FIELD-RESPONSIVE GELS

Electric field-responsive gels have the most potential to serve as actuators or artificial muscles in several applications since the electric field is one of the most controllable stimuli. Research on the collapse of gels under an electric field by Tanaka et al.[96] is the pioneer study related to development of electric field-responsive gels. Partially hydrolyzed poly(acrylamide) gels in an acetone-water mixture were collapsed by the application of an electric field. This is due to the fact that the electric field produced a force on the negatively charged acrylic acid groups in the polymer network. The mean field theory of Flory and Huggins explains that the phase transition of a polyelectrolyte gel is induced by an electric field. Such discrete volume transition of the gel induced by an electric field is useful for designing switches, memories, and mechanochemical transducers.

Osada et al.[97] reported that polyelectrolyte gels swollen in water shrink under an electric field and recover their original size without the electric field. By using a variety of polyelectrolyte gels, electrically modulated release of biomolecules such as pilocarpine hydrochloride, insulin, and glucose was achieved.[98] The electric field-responsive release of the biomolecules was based on swelling changes of the polyelectrolyte gels in response to switching the electric field on and off. In principle, the velocity and amount of release can be controlled by the intensity of the electric field applied. Unique electric field-responsive gel systems were also developed by using reversible and cooperative complexing of positively charged surfactant

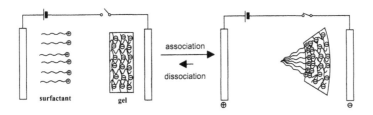

FIGURE 9.10 Bending mechanism produced by anisotropic association of surfactant molecules under an electric field.[99]

molecules with the anionic networks of weakly cross-linked polymers with sulfonic acid groups in an electric field.[99-103] The complexation of the surfactant molecules with the gel network can induce local shrinkage by changes in osmotic pressure between the gel interior and the solution outside. Therefore, anisotropic contraction and bending of the gel occurred by the application of an electric field to cause surfactant binding selectively to one side of the gel (Figure 9.10). The "gel-looper" prepared on the basis of this system moved with a constant velocity in the solution.[99] These suggest the potential applications of the electric field-responsive gels as actuators and artificial muscles.

Kim et al.[104] reported a novel polymeric complex system that rapidly changes from a solid state to a solution in response to small electric currents. Poly(ethyloxazoline) formed a polymer complex with poly(methyacrylic acid) below pH 5.0, but the complex disintegrated to two water-soluble polymers above pH 5.4. Therefore, the polymer complex facing the cathode was dissolved by the application of an electric current because the hydrogen bonding was disrupted in the presence of hydroxyl ions produced by electrolysis of water on the cathode. A stepwise weight loss of the polymeric complex gels was observed under step-function electric current. Consequently, the surface erosion of this polymer system can be controlled by electric current. In addition, the electrically erodible polymer complex gels enable a stepwise release of loaded insulin with the application of step-function electric current.

9.2.4 PHOTO-RESPONSIVE GELS

Very few studies on photo-responsive gels have been reported even though light is a useful stimulus for fabricating switching or memory devices. Most studies on photo-responsive gels utilized photo-dependence of temperature responsiveness of copolymers consisting of PNIPAAm and photo-responsive components like azo compounds.[105] For example, the azobenzene chromophore is a popular photo-responsive component as it isomerizes from the *trans* to the *cis* form upon UV irradiation and the *cis* form returns to the *trans* form by visible irradiation. The LCST of PNIPAAm copolymer with pendant azobenzene groups before UV irradiation was quite different from that after UV irradiation because the *cis* form is more hydrophilic than the *trans* form. As a result, the solubility of the PNIPAAm copolymer with pendant azobenzene groups in water changed through alternate irradiation with UV and visible light. Moreover, the photo-induced LCST changes were applied to prepare photo-responsive gels that undergo a volume phase transition in response to photo-irradiation. A PNIPAAm copolymer gel with pendant triphenylmethane leuconitrile groups, which change the polarity by the ionic photo-dissociation of the C–CN bond, showed a change in volume phase transition temperature after UV irradiation (Figure 9.11).[106,107] Therefore, the copolymer gels underwent a discontinuous swelling/shrinking switching in response to UV irradiation at fixed appropriate temperatures.

Photo-responsive polymer gels that exhibited volume phase transition by visible light were prepared by combining the temperature-responsive NIPAAm with a photo-responsive chromophore, the trisodium salt of copper chlorophyllin.[108] The polymer gels underwent a continuous volume change in response to temperature without light irradiation, but showed a discontinuous volume phase transition under

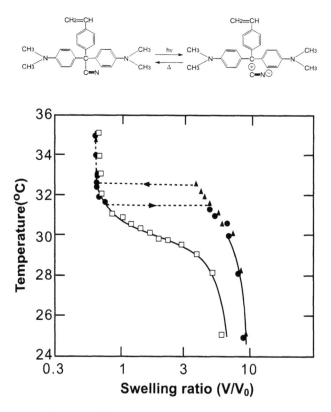

FIGURE 9.11 Bottom: Effect of temperature on swelling ratios of copolymer gels of NIPAAm and the leuco derivative in water without ultraviolet irradiation (◇); under ultraviolet irradiation on raising the temperature (▲); and under ultraviolet irradiation on lowering the temperature, (●). Top: Chemical structural change of the leuco derivative in response to UV irradiation.[107]

light irradiation. At a fixed temperature, the gels underwent a discontinuous volume phase transition as a function of light intensity, based on local heating of polymer chains due to the absorption and subsequent thermal dissipation of light energy by the chromophore. These photo-responsive polymer gels might be used as switching and memory devices.

A photo-responsive gel whose degradation can be controlled by visible light was prepared by complex formation of cross-linked hyaluronic acid (HA) gels and methylene blue (MB) as a photosensitizer.[109] The MB-complexed HA gel was degraded in an aqueous H_2O_2 solution in response to visible light, mediated by the photochemical reaction of MB with H_2O_2. Furthermore, the visible light-induced degradation enabled photo-responsive release of lipid microspheres from the MB-complexed HA gel. Such visible light-responsive gels can be useful for a pulsatile release of hypothalamic regulatory hormones to control endocrine networks.

9.2.5 MAGNETIC FIELD-RESPONSIVE GELS

Few papers have described magnetic field-responsive gels. Zrinyi et al.[110-113] prepared magnetic field-responsive polymer gels, ferrogels, by introducing nanosized magnetic particles into chemically cross-linked poly(vinyl alcohol) gels homogeneously. When an external magnetic field was applied or removed, significant shape distortion of the ferrogels occurred instantaneously and disappeared abruptly. A thermodynamic analysis of the shape transition based on the elasticity of the network chains and magnetic interactions of the magnetic particles revealed that the noncontinuous shape transition was due to a shift of equilibrium state from one local minimum to another one, similar to a first-order phase transition. Mitwalli et al.[114] also developed gels that underwent volume changes in response to an alternating magnetic field. They described practical techniques for using closed-loop feedback to control the positions of magnetically responsive polymer gels. These magnetic field-response gels might serve as actuators in servomechanisms.

9.3 BIOLOGICAL STIMULI-RESPONSIVE POLYMERS AND GELS

9.3.1 GLUCOSE-RESPONSIVE POLYMERS AND GELS

The inability of the pancreas to control blood glucose concentration causes diabetes. In the treatment of diabetes, blood glucose concentration must be monitored and a necessary amount of insulin (a hormone that controls glucose metabolism and is secreted by the islets of Langerhans of the pancreas) must be administered. Many studies have been undertaken to develop delivery systems that can release insulin in response to blood glucose concentration. Glucose-responsive materials are attractive candidates as artificial pancreas to administer necessary amounts of insulin and monitor blood glucose concentration.

Combining glucose oxidase to sense glucose with pH-responsive gels to regulate the release rate of insulin has been the most common approach to a glucose-responsive insulin delivery system. In the glucose-responsive systems, glucose is converted to gluconic acid by glucose oxidase in the gels, and a decrease in pH by the produced gluconic acid induces the pH-responsive swelling of the gels to release insulin. Ishihara et al.[115,116] combined a copolymer membrane of N,N-diethylaminoethyl methacrylate (DEA) and 2-hydroxypropyl methacrylate (HPMA) with a cross-linked poly(acrylamide) membrane in which glucose oxidase was immobilized. The presence of glucose enhanced the permeability of insulin through the complex membrane containing glucose oxidase (Figure 9.12). Glucose that diffused into the membranes was converted to gluconic acid by catalytic action of glucose oxidase. As the result, a decrease in pH induced by the gluconic acid resulted in an increase in the permeability of insulin through the membrane swollen in response to lowering pH.

Polymer capsules containing insulin and glucose oxidase were prepared from a polyelectrolyte with tertiary amino groups by a conventional interfacial precipitation method, and the insulin release from the capsules was investigated. The release rate was very low in the absence of glucose, but was strongly enhanced by its presence.

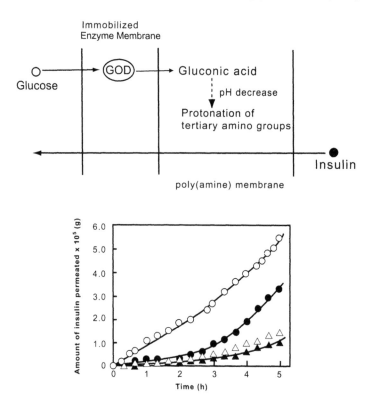

FIGURE 9.12 Permeation profile of insulin through a glucose-responsive polymer membrane consisting of a poly(amine) and a glucose oxidase-immobilized membrane. Glucose concentrations: (▲) 0 M; (●) 0.1 M; (○) 0.2 M; (△) 0.2 M without glucose oxidase.[115]

Horbett et al.[117-119] entrapped glucose oxidase within hydroxyethyl methacrylate-N,N-dimethylaminoethyl methacrylate copolymer membranes to construct a glucose-responsive insulin delivery system. They developed a mathematical model to describe the steady-state behavior of the glucose-responsive membranes using glucose oxidase and pH-responsive polymers. Thus, the studies by Ishihara et al. and Horbett et al. revealed that glucose-responsive insulin release can be achieved by combining a pH-responsive polymer with the enzymatic reaction of glucose oxidase.

Lectins, which are carbohydrate-binding proteins, interact with glycoproteins and glycolipids on cell surfaces, and induce various effects such as cell agglutination, cell adhesion to surface, and hormone-like action. The unique properties of lectins have been applied to the design of glucose-responsive systems. Brownlee et al.[120] and Kim et al.[121-123] were pioneers in the development of glucose-responsive insulin release systems using concanavalin A (ConA) as a lectin. Their strategy was to synthesize a stable, biologically active glycosylated insulin derivative that can form a complex with Con A and be released in the presence of free glucose. They reported that the glycosylated insulin forming a complex with Con A can be released as a function of the free glucose concentration, based on the concept of competitive and complementary binding properties of glycosylated insulin and glucose to Con A. Their studies indicated that the complex formation of glucose and Con A is available for fabricating glucose-responsive materials.

A variety of polymers with pendant saccharides have been synthesized because of their potential as promising materials for biochemical and biomedical applications.[124] Nakamae et al.[125] showed that a polymer with pendant glucose groups, poly(2-glucosyloxyethyl methacrylate) (PGEMA), can form a complex with Con A. The PGEMA–Con A complex was dissociated in the presence of free glucose or mannose by their complex exchange between PGEMA and monosaccharide, but was not dissociated in the presence of free galactose. These results indicated that the PGEMA–Con A complex has monosaccharide recognition functions and can respond to a specific monosaccharide.

The PGEMA–Con A complex formation was used to prepare a glucose-responsive gel that contained the complex as a glucose-responsive cross-linking point.[126,127] The PGEMA–Con A complex gels were prepared by copolymerization of a monomer with a pendant glucose (GEMA) and methylenebisacrylamide (MBAM) in the presence of Con A. The PGEMA–Con A complex gels were swollen in the buffer solution with a free glucose and mannose, but did not change in the presence of galactose (Figure 9.13). This is due to the fact that the cross-linking density of the gels decreased by the competitive exchange of a pendant glucose with a free glucose or mannose. Park et al.[128-130] revealed that an aqueous solution containing Con A and polymers with pendant glucose, vinylpyrrolidinone-allylglucose copolymer, or acrylamide-allylglucose undergoes sol–gel phase-reversible transition by changes in the environmental glucose concentration. The glucose-responsive sol–gel transition is also based on the complex formation between pendant glucose and ConA as a function of a free glucose concentration.

The releases of lysozyme and insulin as model protein drugs were investigated by using glucose-responsive gel membranes based on the complex formation

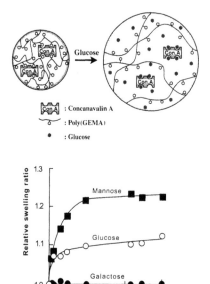

FIGURE 9.13 Bottom: Swelling ratio changes of PGEMA-Con A gel as a function of time after the gel was immersed in a buffer solution containing 1 wt% of monosaccharide: (○), glucose; (■), mannose; (●), galactose. Top: Saccharide-responsive swelling behavior of the PGEMA–Con A gel.[126]

between polymer-bound glucose and ConA.[130] The glucose-responsive gel membranes regulated the release of model drugs in response to the environmental glucose concentration. Thus, the complex formation and dissociation between ConA and polymers with pendant glucose groups are attractive phenomena for constructing glucose-responsive systems.

In a study on saccharide-responsive phase transition of a Con A-loaded gel using temperature-responsive PNIPAAm,[131] the Con A-loaded PNIPAAm gel showed a volume phase transition at an LCST of 34°C. The Con A-loaded PNIPAAm gel was swollen in the presence of ionic saccharide dextran sulfate at a temperature close to LCST because the complex formation between Con A and the ionic saccharide gave rise to increasing ionic osmotic pressure. However, the Con A-loaded PNIPAAm gel was collapsed by replacing the ionic saccharide with a nonionic saccharide. This is an example of the preparation of a saccharide-responsive gel by combining a temperature-responsive property with the complex formation between lectin and saccharide.

All the preceding studies utilized proteins like glucose oxidase or lectin for fabricating glucose-responsive materials. However, Kataoka et al.[132-137] synthesized glucose-responsive polymers and gels without biological components such as proteins, by using the complex formation between a phenylboronic acid group and glucose. Phenylboronic acid and its derivatives can form complexes with polyol compounds such as glucose, but the complexes are dissociated in the presence of competing polyol compounds that can form complexes more strongly. It became clear that the formation and dissociation of the complex between poly(vinyl alcohol) (PVA) and copolymers with phenylboronic acid moieties are strongly influenced by free glucose.[132,133] Therefore, the complexes of PVA and the copolymers with phenylboronic acid moieties are promising candidates for novel glucose-responsive systems.

For example, the complex of PVA and the copolymers with phenylboronic acid moieties was applied to prepare a glucose-responsive electrode in which the presence of free glucose resulted in current changes due to increasing diffusivity of ion species in the gel swollen in response to the glucose.[134] The copolymers with phenylboronic acid that have glucose-responsive LCSTs were synthesized by copolymerization of *N,N*-dimethylacrylamide or NIPAAm with 3-(acrylamido)phenylboronic acid (APBA).[135,136] Their glucose-responsive changes of LCSTs were based on the shift in the equilibrium between the uncharged and charged forms of phenylboronic acid moieties in the polymer chain through complex formation with glucose. Kataoka et al.[137] utilized such glucose-responsive LCST changes to synthesize glucose-responsive gels and achieved on–off regulation of insulin release. The copolymer gels of NIPAAm with APBA exhibited a sharp change in their swelling ratios in response to glucose concentration (Figure 9.14). The glucose-responsive swelling behavior of the copolymer gels repeatedly regulated insulin release in response to stepwise changes in glucose concentration.

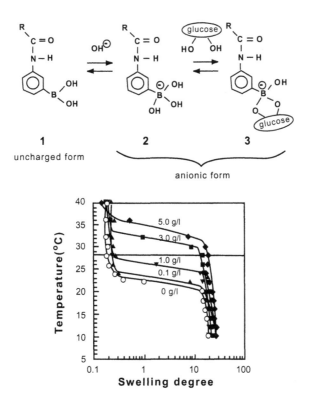

FIGURE 9.14 Bottom: Temperature dependence of swelling curves for PNIPAAm copolymer gel with APBA at different glucose concentrations. Top: Equilibria of (alkylamido)phenyl boronic acid.[137]

9.3.2 Antigen-Responsive Gels

An antibody recognizes a specific antigen and forms an antigen–antibody binding through multiple noncovalent bonds such as electrostatic, hydrogen, hydrophobic, and van der Waals interactions. Such unique features of antibodies are associated with the immune responses that protect an organism from infection. Many biotechnologies using antibodies have been employed as a variety of immunological assays with the specificity and versatility necessary to detect biological substances. These findings suggest that the specific antigen recognition of an antibody can provide the basis for constructing sensors for immunoassay and antigen sensing.

Novel antigen-responsive gels were prepared by the application of an antigen–antibody binding as a stimuli-responsive cross-linking point.[138,139] The antigen-responsive gels with semi-IPN structures were composed of linear PAAm with grafted antibodies (goat anti-rabbit IgG) and PAAm networks with grafted antigens (rabbit IgG). The complexes of the grafted antibodies and grafted antigens played important roles as stimuli-responsive cross-linking points. The addition of rabbit IgG as a free antigen into the buffer solution resulted in a dramatic increase in the swelling ratios of the gels having antigen–antibody bindings, but the addition of free goat IgG did not produce an increase. This means that the gels having antigen–antibody bindings can recognize only rabbit IgG to induce their structural changes. Furthermore, the antigen–antibody gel with a semi-IPN structure was swollen immediately in the presence of a free antigen and shrunken in its absence. Such reversible antigen-responsive swelling behavior of the antigen–antibody semi-IPN gel is due to the fact that its crosslinking density changed reversibly by complex formation and dissociation between grafted antigens and grafted antibody in the absence and presence of a free antigen, respectively. The pulsatile permeation of a model drug in response to a specific antigen concentration can be achieved by using the antigen–antibody semi-IPN gel (Figure 9.15). Thus, the antigen-responsive gels are promising candidates for fabricating intelligent devices to modulate drug release in response to a specific antigen.

9.3.3 Other Biological Stimuli-Responsive Polymers and Gels

The phagocytic cells accumulated at an inflammation site may be activated by immune complexes and other inflammation-generating compounds, and can produce hydroxyl radicals that serve as bactericidal agents. Hyaluronic acid (HA), which is a linear mucopolysaccharide composed of repeating disaccharide subunits of N-acetyl-D-glucosamine and D-glucuronic acid, is mainly degraded by the hyaluronidase enzyme and by hydroxyl radicals. Yui et al.[140,141] focused on hydroxyl radical-responsive biodegradation of HA, and prepared a biodegradable gel composed of hyaluronic acid (HA) cross-linked with glycidylether to develop implantable drug delivery systems that can respond to an inflammatory reaction. The cross-linked HA gels were degraded by hydroxyl radicals on the basis of a surface-controlled degradation mechanism that enabled zero-ordered release of lipid microspheres. *In vivo* implantation experiments demonstrated that drug release in response to inflammation can be

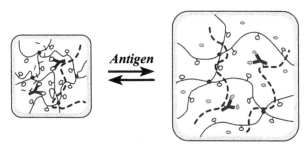

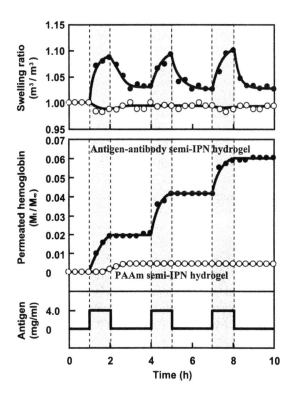

FIGURE 9.15 Bottom: Reversible swelling changes and antigen-responsive permeation profiles of hemoglobin through the PAAm semi-IPN hydrogel (○) and the antigen-antibody semi-IPN hydrogel (●) in response to stepwise changes in the antigen concentration between 0 and 4 mg/ml. Top: Antigen-responsive swelling behavior of the gel.[139]

achieved by using the biodegradability of the HA gel. These studies led to the conclusion that the cross-linked HA gels are inflammation-responsive degradable materials that have potential use as implantable drug delivery systems.

Intelligent biomaterials for drug delivery and medical micromachines will require the ability to sense physiological changes from several diseases at the same time. Yui et al.[142-146] suggested that such multistimuli-responsive materials act as a fail-safe mechanism for guaranteed drug delivery to a certain disease. They prepared biodegradable IPN-structured gels consisting of oligopeptide-terminated poly(ethylene glycol) (PEG) and dextran, and investigated enzymatic degradation by two enzymes as biological stimuli.[142,143] The IPN gel was degraded only in the presence of both papain and dextranase, but was not degraded by one of the two enzymes.

IPN-structured gels prepared by sequential cross-linking reactions of gelatin and methacryloylated dextran below the sol–gel transition temperature (T_{trans}) of gelatin also showed enzymatic degradation in the presence of both α-chymotrypsin and dextranase. However, such specific enzymatic degradation was not observed in the gelatin–dextran IPN gels prepared above T_{trans}.[144] Their studies concluded that the dual-stimuli-responsive degradation is strongly governed by the IPN structure, that is, physical chain entanglements between chemically different polymer networks.

The temperature responsiveness of PNIPAAm was combined with enzymatic degradation to construct intelligent drug delivery devices with multistimuli-responsive functions acting as fail-safe mechanisms.[145,146] The temperature-responsive biodegradable gels consisted of poly(N-isopropylacrylamide-co-N,N-dimethylacrylamide-co-butyl methacrylate) and a novel biodegradable cross-link. The gel was degraded by enzyme at a lower temperature, but was not degraded at a higher temperature. A temperature-dependent change in the cross-linking density permits such an on–off switching degradation of the gel because an increase in the cross-linking density prevents the formation of an enzyme–substrate complex due to steric hindrance. Consequently, such dual stimuli-responsive degradation of gels can be useful as a fail-safe system for guaranteed drug delivery and/or medical micromachines.

Deoxyribonucleic acid (DNA) and ribonucleic acid (RNA) are composed of the nucleotides adenine, cytosine, guanine, thymine and uracil and form double or triple strands with their complementary base pairs by hydrogen bonding and stackings of their bases. Novel stimuli-responsive polymers that sense certain nucleotides can be synthesized by using their complementary hydrogen bonding. Poly(6-(acryloyloxymethyl)uracil) (PAU), having uracil moieties as side chains, was synthesized to utilize complementary hydrogen bonding between uracil and adenine.[147] Because PAU has an upper critical solution temperature (UCST) in water, it is insoluble in water below the UCST due to complex formation between uracil moieties, but it became soluble above the UCST. However, the presence of adenosine in aqueous solutions resulted in a shift of its UCST to a lower temperature as the uracil moieties of PAU form complexes with complementary adenosine. This means that the solubility of PAU in water responds to complementary adenosine. Therefore, it was concluded that PAU is a nucleotide-responsive polymer applicable to intelligent systems for sensing DNA and RNA.

Aoki et al.[148] synthesized a temperature-responsive copolymer that exhibited hydration changes in response to optically active foreign compounds. The copolymer was composed of temperature-responsive NIPAAm and *N-(S)-sec*-butylacrylamide ((*S*)-*sec*-BAAm) with a recognition function for optically active compounds. The LCST of the poly((*S*)-*sec*-BAAm-*co*-NIPAAm) (23.1°C) was shifted to 28.7°C and 34.5°C in the presence of D-tryptophan (D-Trp) and L-Trp, respectively. This is attributed to stereospecific interaction between L-Trp and the optically active (*S*)-*sec*-BAAm in the copolymer. However, LCST of a racemic poly((*R,S*)-*sec*-BAAm-*co*-NIPAAm) was not influenced by the presence of D- and L-Trp. These results imply that temperature-responsive copolymers with optically active moieties might be fascinating enantiomer-responsive materials that can recognize the difference between L- and D-amino acids.

9.4 OTHER STIMULI-RESPONSIVE GELS

9.4.1 MOLECULAR RECOGNITION BY STIMULI-RESPONSIVE GELS

Some proteins such as enzymes and antibodies can recognize specific substrates, proteins, and saccharides, based on fitting guest molecules in their molecular cavities. Molecular imprinting is an attractive technique to create biomimetic polymers having such molecular cavities for molecular recognition.[149-153] In molecular imprinting, some functionalized monomers prearranged around a print molecule by noncovalent interactions are polymerized, and the print molecule is removed from the resultant polymer to form a molecular cavity. The polymer with the molecular cavity can recognize the guest molecule (print molecule) on the basis of a combination of reversible binding and shape complementarity. Recently, molecular imprinting was combined with the temperature-responsiveness of PNIPAAm to prepare stimuli-responsive polymer gels with molecular recognition functions.

Watanabe et al.[154] synthesized temperature-responsive gels consisting of NIPAAm and AAc in the presence of guest molecules as print molecules. The copolymer gels in the swollen state at a low temperature showed no swelling change in the presence of the guest molecule, but the gels in the collapsed state at a high temperature showed an increase in their swelling ratios with increasing guest molecule concentration in water. Since the copolymer gels in the collapsed state might remember the guest molecule during their preparation and exhibit the specific increase in adsorption, they show their specific volume change in response to the guest molecule. The preparation conditions affected the guest molecule-responsiveness of the gels prepared by molecular imprinting. The NIPAAm–AAc copolymer gels prepared using norephedrine as a print molecule were swollen with increasing norephedrine concentration in water, but showed no swelling change with increasing adrenaline concentration in water (Figure 9.16). Thus, the temperature-responsive copolymer gels prepared by molecular imprinting can memorize guest molecules in the collapsed states and undergo their specific volume changes in response to the guest molecules in water.

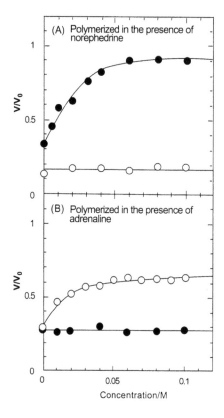

FIGURE 9.16 Equilibrium swelling ratios at 50°C as functions of concentration of norphedrine (●) and adrenaline (○) in water for molecular recognition gels prepared in the presence of norphedrine (A) and adrenaline (B).[154]

Tanaka et al.[155] presented a general approach for creating polymer gels that can recognize and capture a target molecule by multiple-point interaction. The polymer gels consisted of temperature-responsive majority monomers (NIPAAm) and minority monomers (methyacrylamidopropyltrimethylammonium chloride, MAPTAC) that induced multiple-point interaction with the negatively three- and four-charged target molecules. The NIPAAm–MAPTAC copolymer gels recognized and captured a negatively multicharged target molecule through multipoint interaction, and reversibly changed their affinity to the target molecule by more than one order of magnitude. In the shrunken state especially, the NIPAAm–MAPTAC copolymer gel showed a dramatic change in affinity in response to a slight change in volume. These results suggest that the affinity of gels for target molecules can be controlled by varying polymer conformation. In addition, NIPAAm–MAAc gels prepared by molecular imprinting in the presence of lead ions as print molecules adsorbed calcium ions in their shrunken state and desorbed them in the swollen state.[156] In the imprinted gels, pairs of carboxyl groups of MAAc were formed to capture calcium ions in the shrunken state. It was concluded that the pair formation of the carboxyl groups is inhibited in the random gels prepared without molecular imprinting, but is not inhibited in the imprinted gels because the memory of the pair formation is encoded in the primary sequence of NIPAAm, MAAc, and cross-links by molecular imprinting.

9.4.2 SELF-OSCILLATING GELS

Most of the stimuli-responsive gels described above exhibit abrupt volume changes only when they are stimulated by environmental changes. In contrast to the stimuli-responsive swelling or deswelling toward a stable equilibrium state, many physiological systems produce rhythmical oscillations in a nonequilibrium state, e.g., autonomic heartbeat, brain waves, periodic hormone secretions, etc. Yoshida et al. [157,158] developed a novel polymeric gel that swells autonomously and deswells periodically in a closed homogeneous solution without any external stimuli. To prepare the gel, they utilized the Belousov–Zhabotinskii (BZ) reaction — an oscillating reaction accompanying a rhythmical change in the redox potential exhibiting temporal and spatial oscillating phenomena with periodic redox changes of the catalysts. The polymer gel consisted of NIPAAm and ruthenium tris(2,2′-bipyridine) (Ru(bpy)$_3$) that serves as a catalyst for the BZ reaction. The PNIPAAm gel with Ru(bpy)$_3$ swelled and deswelled at the oxidized and reduced states of Ru(bpy)$_3$, respectively. Therefore, the gel underwent an autonomic and periodical swelling–deswelling oscillation by the BZ reaction because the hydrophobicity of the polymer chains changed due to periodic redox changes of Ru(bpy)$_3$ in the reaction within the gel. The self-oscillating gels may have future uses in dynamically oscillating devices such as pacemakers and automobile actuators.

9.5 OUTLOOK

This chapter focused on stimuli-responsive polymers and gels that undergo conformational changes or volume phase transition in response to a variety of environmental stimuli. The fascinating properties of the stimuli-responsive polymers and gels can provide the tools for creating intelligent biomaterials with a wide variety of uses. Fundamental research on their stimuli responsiveness has contributed significantly to our understanding of the biological functions of biomolecules. Even though most stimuli-responsive polymers and gels require further research into possible applications, they are likely to become important biomaterials in the near future. Advances in supramolecular chemistry that allow us to use noncovalent bonds to fabricate well defined and well organized materials will surely lead to better strategies for developing stimuli-responsive biomaterials.

REFERENCES

1. Tanaka, T., Gels, *Sci. Am.*, 244, 123, 1981.
2. Tanaka, T., Collapse of gels and the critical endpoint, *Phys. Rev. Lett.*, 40, 820, 1978.
3. Peppas, N.A., *Hydrogels in Medicine and Pharmacy*, CRC Press, Boca Raton, FL,1987.
4. DeRossi, D. et al., *Polymer Gels: Fundamentals and Biomedical Applications*, Plenum, New York, 1991.
5. Dusek, K., *Responsive Gels, Volume Transitions I*, Advances in Polymer Science, Vol. 109, Springer, Berlin, 1993.

6. Dusek, K., *Responsive Gels, Volume Transitions II*, Advances in Polymer Science, Vol. 110, Springer, Berlin, 1993.

7. Osada, Y. and Ross-Murphy, S.B., Intelligent gels, *Sci. Am.*, 268, 82, 1993.

8. Hoffman, A.S., "Intelligent" polymers in medicine and biotechnology, *Macromol. Symp.*, 98, 645, 1995.

9. Hoffman, A.S., Application of thermally reversible polymers and hydrogels in therapeutics and diagnostics, *J. Controlled Release*, 6, 297, 1987.

10. Okano, T., *Biorelated Polymers and Gels*, Academic Press, Boston, 1998.

11. Langer, R., Drug delivery and targeting, *Nature*, 392, 5, 1998.

12. Flory, P.J., *Principles of Polymer Chemistry*, Cornell University Press, Ithaca, NY, 1953.

13. Hirokawa, Y. and Tanaka, T., Volume phase transition in a nonionic gel, *J. Chem. Phys.*, 81, 6379, 1984.

14. Amiya, T. et al., Reentrant phase transition of N-isopropylacrylamide gels in mixed solvents, *J. Chem. Phys.*, 86, 2375, 1987.

15. Fujishige, S., Kubota, K., and Ando, I., Phase transition of aqueous solutions of poly(N-isopropylacrylamide) and poly(N-isopropylmethacrylamide), *J. Phys. Chem.*, 93, 3311, 1989.

16. Kabra, B.G., Akhtar, M.K., and Gehrke, S.H., Volume change kinetics of temperature-sensitive poly(vinyl methyl-ether) gel, *Polymer*, 33, 990, 1992.

17. Malstom, M. and Lindman, B., Self-assembly in aqueous block copolymer solutions, *Macromolecules*, 25, 5440, 1992.

18. Akashi, M., Nakano, S., and Kishida, A., Synthesis of poly(*N*-vinylisobutyramide) from poly(N-vinylacetamide) and its thermosensitive property. *J. Polym. Sci., Part A, Polym. Chem. Ed.*, 34, 301, 1996.

19. Hoffman, A.S., Afrassiabi, A., and Dong, L.C., Thermally reversible hydrogels: II. Delivery and selective removal of substances from aqueous solutions, *J. Controlled Release*, 4, 213, 1986.

20. Dong, L.-C. and Hoffman, A.S., Synthesis and application of thermally reversible heterogels for drug delivery, *J. Controlled Release*, 13, 21, 1990.

21. Dong, L.-C. and Hoffman, A.S., Thermally reversible hydrogels: III. Immobilization of enzymes for feedback reaction control, *J. Controlled Release*, 4, 223, 1986.

22. Park, T.G. and Hoffman, A.S., Immobilization and characterization of β-galactosidase in thermally reversible hydrogel beads, *J. Biomed. Mater. Res.*, 24, 21, 1990.

23. Bae, Y. H. et al., Thermo-sensitive polymers as on–off switches for drug release, *Makromol. Chem., Rapid Commun.*, 8, 481, 1987.

24. Okano, T. et al., Thermally on–off switching polymers for drug permeation and release, *J. Controlled Release*, 11, 255, 1990.

25. Yoshida, R. et al., Sigmoidal swelling profiles for temperature-responsive poly(N-isopropylacrylamide-co-butyl methacrylate) hydrogel, *J. Membrane Sci.*, 89, 267, 1994.

26. Bae, Y.H., Okano, T., and Kim, S.W., Temperature dependence of swelling of crosslinked poly(N,N'-alkyl substituted acrylamide) in water, J. *Polym. Sci., Polym. Phys.*, 28, 923. 1990.

27. Okano, T. et al., Thermo-responsive polymeric hydrogels and their application to pulsatile drug delivery, in *Polymer Gels*, DeRossi, D., Ed., Plenum Press, New York, 1991, 299.

28. Okano, T. and Yoshida, R., Polymer for pharmaceutical and biomolecular engineering, in *Biomedical Applications of Polymeric Materials*, Tsuruta, T. et al., Eds., CRC Press, Boca Raton, FL, 1993, 407.

29. Kaneko, Y. et al., Temperature-responsive shrinking kinetics of poly(N-isopropylacrylamide) copolymer gels with hydrophilic and hydrophobic comonomers, *J. Membrane Sci.,* 101, 13, 1995.

30. Yoshida, R. et al., Comb-type grafted hydrogels with rapid de-swelling response to temperature changes, *Nature*, 374, 240, 1995.

31. Kaneko, Y. et al., Influence of freely mobile grafted chain length on dynamic properties of comb-type grafted poly(N-isopropylacrylamide) hydrogels, *Macromolecules*, 28, 7717, 1995.

32. Kaneko, Y. et al., Fast swelling/deswelling kinetics of comb-type grafted poly(N-isopropylacrylamide) hydrogels, *Macromol. Symp.,* 109, 41, 1996.

33. Kaneko, Y. et al., Deswelling mechanism for comb-type grafted poly(N-isopropylacrylamide) hydrogels with rapid temperature responses, *Polym. Gels Networks,* 6, 333, 1998.

34. Katono, H. et al., Thermo-responsive swelling and drug release switching of interpenetrating polymer networks composed of poly(acrylamide-co-butyl methacrylate) and poly(acrylic acid), *J. Controlled Release*, 16, 215, 1991.

35. Katono, H. et al., Drug release OFF behavior and deswelling kinetics of thermo-responsive IPNs composed of poly(acrylamide-co-butyl methacrylate) and poly(acrylic acid), *J. Polym.,* 23, 1179, 1991.

36. Aoki, T. et al., Temperature-responsive interpenetrating polymer networks constructed with poly(acrylic acid) and poly(N,N-dimethylacrylamide), *Macromolecules*, 27, 947, 1994.

37. Jeong, B. et al., Biodegradable block copolymers as injectable drug-delivery systems, *Nature*, 388, 860, 1997.

38. Jeong, B. et al., New biodegradable polymers for injectable drug delivery systems, *J. Controlled Release,* 62, 109, 1999.

39. Jeong, B., Bae, Y.H., and Kim, S.W., Thermoreversible gelation of PEG-PLGA-PEG triblock copolymer aqueous solutions, *Macromolecules*, 32, 7064, 1999.

40. Jeong, B., Bae, Y.H., and Kim, S.W., Drug release from biodegradable injectable thermosensitive hydrogel of PEG-PLGA-PEG triblock copolymers, *J. Controlled Release*, 63, 155, 2000.

41. Wang, C., Stewart, R.J., and Kopecek, J., Hybrid hydrogels assembled from synthetic polymers and coiled-coil protein domains, *Nature*, 397, 417, 1999.

42. Chen, L., Kopecek, J., and Stewart, R.J., Responsive hybrid hydrogels with volume transitions modulated by a titin immunoglobulin module, *Bioconjugate Chem.*, 11, 734, 2000.

43. Chen, J.P. and Hoffman, A.S., Polymer-protein conjugates II. Affinity precipitation of human IgG by poly(N-isopropylacrylamide)-protein A conjugates, *Biomaterials*, 11, 631, 1990.

44. Chen, J.P., Yang, H.J., and Hoffman, A.S., Polymer-protein conjugates I. Effect of protein conjugation on the cloud point of poly(N-isopropylacrylamide), *Biomaterials*, 11, 625, 1990.

45. Chen, G. and Hoffman, A.S., Preparation and properties of thermoreversible, phase-separating enzyme-oligo(N-isopropylacrylamide) conjugates, *Bioconjugate Chem.,* 4, 509, 1993.

46. Ding, Z.L., Chen, G.H., and Hoffman, A.S., Synthesis and purification of thermally sensitive oligomer-enzyme conjugates of poly(N-isopropylacrylamide)-trypsin, *Bioconjugate Chem.*, 7, 121, 1996.

47. Ding, Z.L., Chen, G.H., and Hoffman, A.S., Unusual properties of thermally sensitive oligomer–enzyme conjugates of poly(N-isopropylacrylamide)–trypsin, *J. Biomed. Mater. Res.*, 39, 498, 1998.

48. Takei, Y.G. et al., Temperature-responsive bioconjugates. 1. Synthesis of temperature-responsive oligomers with reactive end groups and their coupling to biomolecules, *Bioconjugate Chem.*, 4, 42, 1993.

49. Takei, Y.G. et al., Temperature-responsive bioconjugates. 2. Molecular design for temperature-modulated bioseparations, *Bioconjugate Chem.*, 4, 341, 1993.

50. Takei, Y.G. et al., Temperature-responsive bioconjugates.3. Antibody-poly(N-isopropylacrylamide) conjugates for temperature-modulated precipitations and affinity bioseparations, *Bioconjugate Chem.*, 5, 577, 1994.

51. Matsukata, M. et al., Temperature modulated solubility-activity alterations for poly(N-isopropylacrylamide)–lipase conjugates, *J. Biochem.*, 116, 682, 1994.

52. Matsukata, M. et al., Effect of molecular architecture of poly(N-isopropylacrylamide)-trypsin conjugates on their solution and enzymatic properties, *Bioconjugate Chem.*, 7, 96, 1996

53. Stayton, P.S. et al., Control of protein-ligand recognition using a stimuli-responsive polymer, *Nature*, 378, 472, 1995.

54. Ding, Z. et al., Temperature control of biotin binding and release with a streptavidin–poly(N-isopropylacrylamide) site-specific conjugate, *Bioconjugate Chem.*, 10, 395, 1999.

55. Fong, R.B. et al., Thermoprecipitation of streptavidin via oligonucleotide-mediated self-assembly with poly(N-isopropylacrylamide), *Bioconjugate Chem.*, 10, 720, 1999.

56. Umeno, D., Mori, T., and Maeda, M., Single stranded DNA-poly(N-isopropylacrylamide) conjugate for affinity separation of oligonucleotides, *Chem. Commun.*, 1433, 1998.

57. Umeno, D., Kawasaki, M., and Maeda, M., Water-soluble conjugate of double-stranded DNA and poly(N-isopropylacrylamide) for one-pot affinity precipitation separation of DNA-binding proteins, *Bioconjugate Chem.*, 9, 719, 1998

58. Wang, K.L., Burban, J.H., and Cussler, E.L., Hydrogels as separation agents, *Adv. Polym. Sci.*, 110, 67, 1993.

59. Freitas, R.S. and Cussler, E.L., Temperature-sensitive gels as size-selective adsorbants, *Sep. Sci. Technol.*, 22, 911, 1987.

60. Freitas, R.S. and Cussler, E.L., Temperature-sensitive gels as extraction solvents, *Chem. Eng. Sci.*, 42, 97, 1987.

61. Feil, H. et al., Molecular separation by thermosensitive hydrogel membranes, *J. Membrane Sci.*, 64, 283, 1991.

62. Yakushiji, T. et al., Graft architectural effects on thermoresponsive wettability changes of poly(N-isopropylacrylamide)-modified surfaces, *Langmuir*, 14, 4657, 1998.

63. Yamada, N. et al., Thermo-responsive polymeric surfaces; control of attachment and detachment of cultured cells, *Makromol. Chem., Rapid Commun.*, 11, 571, 1990.

64. Okano, T. et al., Mechanism of cell detachment from temperature-modulated, hydrophilic–hydrophobic polymer surfaces, *Biomaterials*, 16, 297, 1995.

65. Kikuchi, A., Sakurai, Y., and Okano, T., Temperature-responsive chromatography using poly(N-isopropylacrylamide)-modified silica, *Anal. Chem.*, 68, 100, 1996.

66. Kikuchi, A., Sakurai, Y., and Okano, T., Temperature-responsive liquid chromatography.2. Effects of hydrophobic groups in N-isopropylacrylamide copolymer-modified silica, *Anal. Chem.*, 69, 823, 1997.

67. Yakushiji, T. et al., Effects of cross-linked structure on temperature-responsive hydrophobic interaction of poly(N-isopropylacrylamide) hydrogel-modified surfaces with steroids, *Anal. Chem.*, 71, 1125, 1999.

68. Kanazawa, H. et al., Temperature-responsive chromatographic separation of amino acid phenylthiohydantions using aqueous media as the mobile phase, *Anal. Chem.*, 72, 5961, 2000.

69. Tanaka, T. et al., Phase transitions in ionic gels, *Phys. Rev. Lett.*, 45, 1636, 1980.

70. Ohmine, I. and Tanaka, T., Salt effects on the phase transition of ionic gels, *J. Chem. Phys.*, 77, 5725, 1982.

71. Firestone, B.A. and Siegel, R.A., Dynamic pH-dependence swelling properties of a hydrophobic polyelectrolyte gel, *Polym. Commun.*, 29, 204, 1988.

72. Siegel, R. A. et al., pH-controlled release from hydrophobic/polyelectrolyte copolymer hydrogels, *J. Controlled Release*, 8, 179, 1988.

73. Siegel, R.A. and Firestone, B.A., pH-dependent equilibrium swelling properties of hydrophobic polyelectrolyte copolymer gels, *Macromolecules*, 21, 3254, 1988.

74. Siegel, R.A., Hydrophobic weak polyelectrolyte gels: studies of swelling equilibria and kinetics, *Adv. Polym. Sci.*, 109, 233, 1993.

75. Brannon-Peppas, L. and Peppas, N.A., Dynamic and equilibrium swelling behavior of pH-sensitive hydrogels containing 2-hydroxyethyl methacrylate, *Biomaterials*, 11, 635, 1990.

76. Gudeman, L.F. and Peppas, N.A., pH-sensitive membranes from poly(vinyl alcohol)/poly(acrylic acid) interpenetrating networks, *J. Membrane Sci.*, 107, 239, 1995.

77. Dong, L.-C. and Hoffman, A.S., A novel approach for preparation of pH-sensitive hydrogels for enteric drug delivery, *J. Controlled Release*, 15, 141, 1991.

78. Chen, G. and Hoffman, A.S., Graft copolymers that exhibit temperature-induced phase transitions over a wide range of pH, *Nature*, 373, 49, 1995.

79. Brazel, C.S. and Peppas, N.A., Synthesis and characterization of thermo- and chemomechanically responsive poly(N-isopropylacrylamide-co-methacrylic acid) hydrogels, *Macromolecules*, 28, 8016, 1995.

80. Zhang, J. and Peppas, N.A., Synthesis and characterization of pH- and temperature-sensitive poly(methacrylic acid)/poly(N-isopropylacrylamide) interpenetrating polymeric networks, *Macromolecules*, 33, 102, 2000.

81. Kim, Y.H., Bae, Y.H., and Kim, S.W., pH/temperature sensitive polymers for macromolecular drug loading and release, *J. Controlled Release*, 28, 143, 1994.

82. Feil, H. et al., Mutual influence of pH and temperature on the swelling of ionizable and thermosensitive hydrogels, *Macromolecules*, 25, 5528, 1992.

83. Nakamae, K., Miyata, T., and Hoffman, A.S., Swelling behavior of hydrogels containing phosphate groups, *Makromol. Chem.*, 193, 983, 1992.

84. Miyata, T. et al., Stimuli-sensitivities of hydrogels containing phosphate groups, *Macromol. Chem. Phys.*, 195, 1111, 1994.

85. Nakamae, K. et al., Lysozyme loading and release from hydrogels carrying pendant phosphate groups, *J. Biomater. Sci. Polym. Ed.*, 9, 43, 1997.

86. Nakamae, K. et al., Stimuli-sensitive release of lysozyme from hydrogel containing phosphate groups, in *Advanced Biomaterials in Biomedical Engineering and Drug Delivery Systems*, Ogata, N. et al., Eds., Springer, Tokyo, 1996, 313.

87. Iwata, H. and Matsuda, T., Preparation and properties of novel environment-sensitive membranes prepared by graft polymerization onto a porous membrane, *J. Membrane Sci.*, 38, 185, 1988.

88. Iwata, H., Hirata, I., and Ikada, Y., Atomic force microscopic analysis of a porous membrane with pH-sensitive molecular valves, *Macromolecules*, 31, 3671, 1998.

89. Ito, Y. et al., pH-sensitive gating by conformational change of a polypeptide brush grafted onto a porous polymer membrane, *J. Am. Chem. Soc.*, 119, 1619, 1997.

90. Nagasaki, Y. et al., Novel stimuli-sensitive telechelic oligomers: pH and temperature sensitivities of poly(silamine) oligomers, *Macromolecules*, 27, 4848, 1994.

91. Nagasaki, Y. et al., Rubber elasticity transition of poly(silamine) induced by ionic interactions, *Macromolecules*, 28, 8870, 1995.

92. Luo, L. et al., Stimuli-sensitive polymer gels that stiffen upon swelling, *Macromolecules*, 33, 4992, 2000.

93. Higuchi, S. et al., pH-induced regulation of the permeability of a polymer membrane with a transmembrane pathway prepared from a synthetic polypeptide, *Macromolecules*, 19, 2263, 1986.

94. Chung, D. W. et al., pH-induced regulation of permselectivity of sugars by polymer membranes from polyvinyl–polypeptide graft copolymer, *J. Am. Chem. Soc.*, 108, 5823, 1986.

95. Petka, W.A. et al., Reversible hydrogels from self-assembling artificial proteins, *Science*, 281, 389, 1998.

96. Tanaka, T. et al., Collapse of gels in an electric field, *Science*, 218, 467, 1982.

97. Osada, Y. and Hasebe, M., Electrically activated mechanochemical devices using polyelectrolyte gels, *Chem. Lett.*, 1285, 1985.

98. Sawahata, K. et al., Electrically controlled drug delivery system using polyelectrolyte gels, *J. Controlled Release*, 14, 253, 1990.

99. Osada, Y., Okuzaki, H., and Hori, H., A polymer gel with electrically driven motility, *Nature*, 355, 242, 1992.

100. Okuzaki, H. and Osada, Y., Electro-driven chemomechanical polymer gel as an intelligent soft material, *J. Biomater. Sci.-Polym. Ed.*, 5, 485, 1994.

101. Okuzaki, H. and Osada, Y., Electro-driven polyelectrolyte gel with biomimetic motility, *Electrochimica Acta*, 40, 2229, 1995.

102. Okuzaki, H. and Osada, Y., Electro-driven polymer gels with biomimetic motility, *Polym. Gels Networks*, 2, 267, 1994.

103. Ueoka, Y., Gong, J., and Osada, Y., Chemomechanical polymer gel with fish-like motion, *J. Intell. Mater. Syst. Struct.*, 8, 465, 1997.

104. Kwon, I.C., Bae, Y.H., and Kim, S.W., Electrically erodible polymer gel for controlled release of drugs, *Nature*, 354, 291, 1991.

105. Irie, M., Stimuli-responsive poly(N-isopropylacrylamide). Photo- and chemical-induced phase transitions, *Adv. Polym. Sci.*, 110, 49, 1993.

106. Irie, M. and Kunwatchakun, D., Photoresponsive polymers.8. Reversible photostimulated dilation of polyacrylamide gels having triphenylmethane leuco derivatives, *Macromolecules*, 19, 2476, 1986.

107. Maeda, A. et al., Photoinduced phase transition of gels, *Macromolecules*, 23, 1517, 1990.

108. Suzuki, A. and Tanaka, T., Phase transition in polymer gels induced by visible light, *Nature*, 346, 345, 1990.

109. Yui, N., Okano, T., and Sakurai, Y., Photo-responsive degradation of heterogeneous hydrogels comprising crosslinked hyaluronic acid and lipid microspheres for temporal drug delivery, *J. Controlled Release*, 26, 141, 1993.

110. Zrinyi, M., Magnetic-field-sensitive polymer gels, *Trends Polym. Sci.*, 5, 280, 1997.

111. Zrinyi, M., Barsi, L., and Buki, A., Ferrogels: a new magneto-controlled elastic medium, *Polym. Gels Networks*, 5, 415, 1997.

112. Zrinyi, M., Szabo, D., and Kilian, H.G., Kinetics of the shape change of magnetic field sensitive polymer gels, *Polym. Gels Networks*, 6, 441, 1998.

113. Szabo, D., Szeghy, G., and Zrinyi, M., Shape transition of magnetic field sensitive polymer gels, *Macromolecules*, 31, 6541, 1998.

114. Mitwalli, A. H. et al., Closed-loop feedback control of magnetically-activated gels, *J. Intell. Mater. Syst. Struct.*, 8, 596, 1997.

115. Ishihara, K. et al., Glucose-induced permeation control of insulin through a complex membrane consisting of immobilized glucose oxidase and a poly(amine), *Polym. J.*, 16, 625, 1984.

116. Ishihara, K., and Matsui, K., Glucose-responsive insulin release from polymer capsule, *J. Polym. Sci., Polym. Lett. Ed.*, 24, 413, 1986.

117. Albin, G., Horbett, T.A., and Ratner, B.D., Glucose sensitive membranes for controlled delivery of insulin: insulin transport studies, *J. Controlled Release*, 2, 153, 1985.

118. Albin, G. W. et al., Theoretical and experimental studies of glucose sensitive membranes, *J. Controlled Release*, 6, 267, 1987.

119. Cartier, S., Horbett, T.A., and Ratner, B., Glucose-sensitive membrane coated porous filters for control of hydraulic permeability and insulin delivery from a pressurized reservoir, *J. Membrane Sci.*, 106, 17, 1995.

120. Brownlee, M. and Cerami, A., A glucose-controlled insulin delivery system: semisynthetic insulin bound to lectin, *Science*, 206,1190, 1979.

121. Seminoff, L.A., Olsen, G.B., and Kim, S.W., A self-regulating insulin delivery system. I. Characterization of a synthetic glycosylated insulin derivative, *Int. J. Pharm.*, 54, 241, 1989.˙

122. Kim, S. W. et al., Self-regulated glycosylated insulin delivery, *J. Controlled Release*, 11, 193, 1990.

123. Makino, K. et al., A microcapsule self-regulating delivery system for insulin, *J. Controlled Release*, 12, 235, 1990.

124. Miyata, T. and Nakamae, K., Polymers with pendant saccharides — 'glycopolymers,' *Trends Polym. Sci.*, 5, 198, 1997.

125. Nakamae, K. et al., Formation of poly(glucosyloxyethyl methacrylate)-concanavalin A complex and its glucose-sensitivity, *J. Biomater. Sci., Polym. Ed.*, 6, 79, 1994.

126. Miyata, T. et al., Preparation of poly(2-glucosyloxyethyl methacrylate)–concanavalin A complex hydrogel and its glucose-sensitivity, *Macromol. Chem. Phys.*, 197, 1135, 1996.

127. Miyata, T. et al., Preparation of glucose-sensitive hydrogels by entrapment or copolymerization of concanavalin A in a glucosyloxyethyl methacrylate hydrogel, in *Advanced Biomaterials in Biomedical Engineering and Drug Delivery Systems*, Ogata, N. et al., Eds., Springer, Tokyo, 1996, 237.

128. Lee, S.J. and Park, K., Synthesis and characterization of sol–gel phase-reversible hydrogels sensitive to glucose, *J. Molecular Recognition*, 9, 549, 1996.

129. Obaidat, A.A. and Park, K., Characterization of glucose dependent gel–sol phase transition of the polymeric glucose–concanavalin A hydrogel system, *Pharm. Res.*, 13, 989, 1996.

130. Obaidat, A.A. and Park, K., Characterization of protein release through glucose-sensitive hydrogel membranes, *Biomaterials*, 18, 801, 1997.

131. Kokufuta, E., Zhang, Y.-Q., and Tanaka, T., Saccharide-sensitive phase transition of a lectin-loaded gel, *Nature*, 351, 302, 1991.

132. Kitano, S. et al., Glucose-responsive complex formation between poly(vinyl alcohol) and poly(N-vinyl-2pyrrolidone) with pendant phenylboronic acid moieties, *Makromol. Chem., Rapid Commun.*, 12, 227, 1991.

133. Kitano, S. et al., A novel drug delivery system utilizing a glucose responsive polymer complex between poly(vinyl alcohol) and poly(N-vinyl-2-pyrrolidone) with a phenyl-boronic acid moiety, *J. Controlled Release*, 19, 162, 1992.

134. Kikuchi, A. et al., Glucose-sensing electrode coated with polymer complex gel containing phenylboronic acid, *Anal. Chem.*, 68, 823, 1996.

135. Kataoka, K. et al., Sensitive glucose-induced change of the lower critical solution temperature of poly[N,N-dimethylacrylamide-co-3-(acrylamido)phenylboronic acid] in physiological saline, *Macromolecules*, 27, 1061, 1994.

136. Aoki, T. et al., Glucose-sensitive lower critical solution temperature changes of copolymers composed of N-isopropylacrylamide and phenylboronic acid moieties, *Polym. J.*, 28, 371, 1996.

137. Kataoka, K. et al., Totally synthetic polymer gels responding to external glucose concentration: their preparation and application to on–off regulation of insulin release, *J. Am. Chem. Soc.*, 120, 12694, 1998.

138. Miyata, T., Asami, N., and Uragami, T., Preparation of an antigen-sensitive hydrogel using antigen–antibody bindings, *Macromolecules*, 32, 2082, 1999.

139. Miyata, T., Asami, N., and Uragami, T., A reversibly antigen-responsive hydrogel, *Nature*, 399, 766, 1999.

140. Yui, N., Okano, T., and Sakurai, Y., Inflammation responsive degradation of crosslinked hyaluronic acid gels, *J. Controlled Release*, 22, 105, 1992.

141. Yui, N. et al., Regulated release of drug microspheres from inflammation-responsive degradable matrices of crosslinked hyaluronic acid, *J. Controlled Release*, 25, 133, 1993.

142. Yamamoto, N., Kurisawa, M., and Yui, N., Double-stimuli-responsive degradable hydrogels: interpenetrating polymer networks consisting of gelatin and dextran with different phase separation, *Makromol. Rapid Commun.*, 17, 313, 1996.

143. Kurisawa, M., Terano, M., and Yui, N., Double-stimuli-responsive degradation of hydrogels consisting of oligopeptide-terminated poly(ethylene glycol) and dextran with an interpenetrating polymer network, *J. Biomater. Sci. Polym. Edn.*, 8, 691, 1997.

144. Kurisawa, M. and Yui, N., Dual-stimuli-responsive drug release from interpenetrating polymer network-structured hydrogels of gelatin and dextran, *J. Controlled Release*, 54, 191, 1998.

145. Kurisawa, M., Matsuo, Y., and Yui, N., Modulated degradation of hydrogels with thermo-responsive network in relation to their swelling behavior, *Macromol. Chem. Phys.*, 199, 705, 1998.

146. Huh, K. M. et al., Synthesis and characterization of dextran grafted with poly(N-iso-propylacrylamide-co-N, N-dimethylacrylamide), *Macromol. Chem. Phys.*, 201, 613, 2000.

147. Aoki, T. et al., Adenosine-induced changes of the phase transition of poly(6-(acryloy-loxymethyl)uracil) aqueous solution, *Polym. J.*, 31, 1185, 1999.

148. Aoki, T. et al., Phase-transition changes of poly(N-(S)-sec-butylacrylamide-co-N-iso-propylacrylamide) in response to amino acids and its chiral recognition, *React. & Functional Polym.*, 37, 299, 1998.

149. Wulff, G., Sarhan, A., and Zabrocki, K., Enzyme-analogue built polymers and their use for the resolution of racemates, *Tetrahedron Lett*, 44, 4329, 1973.

150. Sellergren, B., Lepisto, M., and Mosbach, K., Highly enantioselective and substrate-selective polymers obtained by molecular imprinting utilizing noncovalent interactions. NMR and chromatographic studies on the nature of recognition, *J. Am. Chem. Soc.*, 110, 5853, 1988.

151. Mosbach, K., Molecular imprinting, *Trends Biochem. Sci.*, 19, 9,1994.
152. Shea, K., Molecular imprinting of synthetic network polymers: the *de novo* synthesis of macromolecular binding and catalytic sites, *Trends Polym. Sci.*, 2, 166, 1994.
153. Wulff, G., Molecular imprinting in cross-linked materials with the aid of molecular templates — a way towards artificial antibodies, *Angew. Chem., Int. Ed. Engl.*, 34, 1812, 1995.
154. Watanabe, M. et al., Molecular specific swelling change of hydrogels in accordance with the concentration of guest molecules, *J. Am. Chem. Soc.*, 120, 5577, 1998.
155. Oya, T. et al., Reversible molecular adsorption based on multiple-point interaction by shrinkable gels, *Science*, 286, 1543, 1999.
156. Alvarez-Lorezo, C. et al., Polymer gels that memorize elements of molecular conformation, *Macromolecules*, 33, 8693, 2000.
157. Yoshida, R. et al., Self-oscillating gel, *J. Am. Chem. Soc.*, 118, 5134, 1996.
158. Yoshida, R. et al., In-phase synchronization of chemical and mechanical oscillations in self-oscillating gels, *J. Phys. Chem. A*, 104, 7549, 2000.

10 Modulated Drug Delivery

Yong Qiu and Kinam Park

CONTENTS

10.1 INTRODUCTION

Drug delivery systems can be classified into two broad systems: conventional dosage forms and controlled-release dosage forms. Since the introduction of controlled-release dosage forms about half a century ago, controlled drug delivery technologies advanced to the point where drug release can continue for years at predictable release rates. The controlled drug delivery technologies have focused on continuous release at or near zero-order. A large number of commercial controlled-release dosage forms have substantially improved convenience and patient compliance. While long-term continuous delivery at a constant rate is desirable, many drugs such as insulin do not require continuous release. While continuous release of a small amount of insulin may be acceptable to maintain baseline insulin levels, a bolus of insulin needs to be administered to control the increase in glucose level after a meal. Long-term maintenance of glucose levels in diabetic patients requires pulsatile deliveries of exact doses at specific times. Furthermore, intermittent delivery of some drugs at certain times of day appears to be more beneficial than continuous delivery throughout the day,[1,2] and non-continuous drug delivery systems are urgently needed.

The ideal drug delivery system would be able to sense the signal caused by a disease, judge the magnitude of the signal, and release the correct amount of a drug when needed. Such a system is called a modulated or self-regulated drug delivery system. As more protein drugs are developed as a result of the human genome project, more modulated delivery systems will be required, and modulated drug delivery will be the dominant mode of administration in the future. The concept has been explored for almost two decades. One of the pioneers in modulated drug delivery is Jorge Heller, who defined modulated drug release systems as devices that are capable of adjusting drug output in response to a physiological need.[3,4] Materials that can respond to environmental changes are often used. Because they perform additional functions, they are often called "smart" (or "intelligent") materials.[5,6] Smart materials are the keys to successful modulated drug delivery systems.

10.1.1 SMART MATERIALS

Smart materials can adapt themselves to changes in environmental factors by altering their structures and other properties in a reversible way.[6] Since most drug delivery systems are made of polymers, we will focus on smart polymers. To adapt to the changes in environment and act accordingly, a smart polymer must have the abilities to function as a sensor, as a signal (or information) processor, and as an actuator (or effector).[6] These abilities come from the chemical groups that provide additional properties beyond the inherent structural properties of the polymers. Examples are polymers sensitive to pH, temperature, light, and/or electricity, polymers with shape memories,[7,8] and those that recognize specific biomolecules.[9,10] Stimuli-responsive polymers and gels are described in detail in Chapter 9. Smart polymers are incorporated into drug delivery systems so that the systems can respond to changes in factors found inside the body or factors that can be easily transported into the body. The actuator is important because it controls the drug release. Most smart polymers used in the body can function in the presence of water, and thus smart hydrogels are most frequently used for modulated drug delivery. In many cases, the drug release is controlled by changes in the size of hydrogels (they can swell and shrink) or by changes in their physical states (transition between the gel and sol states or degradation).

10.2 MECHANISMS OF MODULATED DRUG RELEASE

The types of modulated drug delivery systems vary greatly due to the diversity of the smart polymers and hydrogels. For convenience, modulated drug delivery systems can be further divided into externally modulated and self-modulated drug delivery systems.[11]

10.2.1 TYPES OF MODULATED DRUG DELIVERY

10.2.1.1 Externally Modulated Drug Delivery

Externally modulated drug delivery systems utilize signals generated outside of the body either manually or automatically via computer. Examples of signals that can be applied to the body are shown in Figure 10.1. All the signals shown are generated by specific devices. Despite widespread miniaturization and micro/nano technologies, such devices are still too bulky for daily use. As technologies improve, however, all these approaches are expected to be practical. Another improvement required for effective externally modulated drug delivery is to make all aspects of operation automatic. The advantages of modulated drug delivery will not be fully realized if external signals must be generated manually by the user. Miniaturized automatic signal generators are essential for making these approaches practical. Of the signals shown in Figure 10.1, application of electric current presents the most challenging hurdles. For external applications, such as iontophoresis, applying electric current does not pose a big difficulty, but for devices designed to be used inside the body, it presents a dilemma. It will not be easy to apply electric current to electricity-responsive polymers and hydrogels,[12-14] electrically erodible polymer gels,[15] microchip systems,[16,17] and other electronically controlled delivery systems[18] for use inside the body.

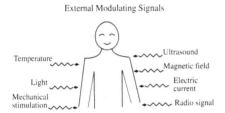

FIGURE 10.1 External signals that can be applied to the body to modulate drug delivery.

10.2.1.2 Self-Modulated Drug Delivery

Unlike externally modulated drug delivery systems, self-modulated drug delivery systems utilize internal body signals such as small changes in pH, disease-induced temperature increases, and activities of specific molecules found in the body (Figure 10.2). Significant changes in pH are observed in many parts of the body. The dramatic difference in pH levels in the stomach and intestine is well known, and pH-sensitive hydrogels have been used for modulating drug delivery.[19,20] The extracellular pH level in tumors is lower than that around normal cells.[21] The modulated delivery systems can be designed to respond to concentration changes of specific molecules, such as glucose.[9,22-33] It is also possible to have the system triggered by the introduction of a specific molecule, such as naltrexon, using antibody–enzyme conjugates.[34] This type of approach is the most desirable, although it requires more engineering and will involve higher cost.

10.2.2 Mechanisms of Modulated Drug Delivery

Various modulated drug delivery systems utilize different smart polymers and hydrogels, but only a few mechanisms been used. The mechanisms are classified into three groups: diffusion-controlled release; dissolution-controlled release; and

Internal Modulating Signals

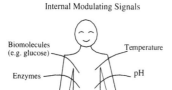

FIGURE 10.2 Internal stimuli that can be used to modulate drug delivery.

A. Polymer chains extend or collapse on the pore surface

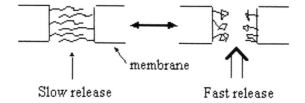

Slow release   Fast release

B. A hydrogel matrix swells or shrinks inside a device

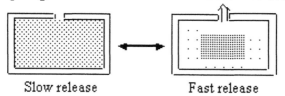

Slow release   Fast release

C. Hydrogel changes a phase between sol and gel

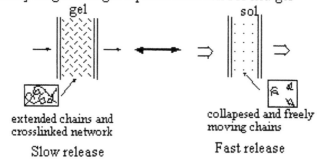

extended chains and crosslinked network

Slow release

collapesed and freely moving chains

Fast release

FIGURE 10.3 Examples of a diffusion-controlled modulated delivery system. (From Ito, Y. et al., *J. Controlled Release*, 10, 195, 1989; Bae, Y.H. et al., U.S. Patent 5,226,902, 1993; and Obaidat, A.A. et al., *Biomaterials*, 18, 801, 1997. With permission.)

exchange-controlled release. In diffusion-controlled systems, the drug release can be modulated by altering the drug diffusion through blocking/opening of the pores using smart polymers grafted to the surface (Figure 10.3A). Diffusion through pores can also be controlled by smart hydrogels that undergo swelling/deswelling depending on environmental signals, such as pH and temperature changes (Figure 10.3B).[35,36] Diffusion of drugs through the hydrogel layer is much slower than diffusion through the sol layer, and sol–gel phase-reversible hydrogel membranes can be used to modulate drug release (Figure 10.3C). The thermodynamics and kinetics of diffusion in hydrogels are discussed extensively in Chapter 6.

In dissolution-controlled modulated drug delivery (Figure 10.4), water-soluble smart polymers are usually made into water-insoluble complexes such as hydrogels. In the presence of signal molecules, polymer chains in the complexes become dissociated to release embedded drugs. The dissolution-controlled modulated systems are, of course, not reversible. Thus, this type of system is ideal for implantation, and the use of biodegradable and biocompatible polymers is essential.

Another widely used mechanism for modulated drug delivery is exchange-controlled release (Figure 10.5). Drugs to be delivered are usually attached to the signal molecules and then attached to other matrices. Upon introduction of signal molecules, the bound signal–drug conjugates are dissociated from the matrix by competitive binding of individual signal molecules. This mechanism is the same as the ion-exchange mechanism for the delivery of charged drug molecules from ion-exchange resins. Since the mechanism depends on competitive binding, the amount of release is in direct proportion to the concentration of the signal molecules.

10.3   POLYMERS USED IN MODULATED DRUG DELIVERY

All the polymers and hydrogels used in modulated drug delivery systems have sensing and actuator functions. Smart polymers and hydrogels are classified by their abilities to respond to specific environmental factors.

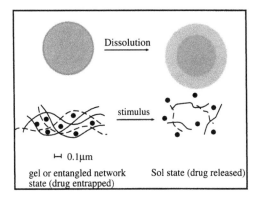

FIGURE 10.4 An example of a dissolution-controlled modulated delivery system.

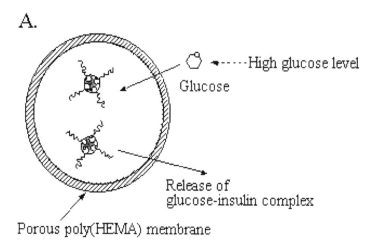

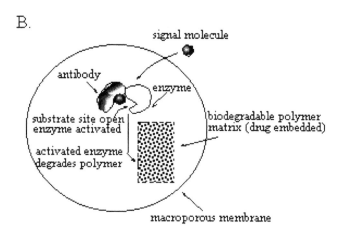

FIGURE 10.5 An example of an exchange-controlled modulated delivery system. (From Kim, S.W. et al., *J. Controlled Release*, 11, 193, 1990; and Makino, K. et al., *Biomater. Artif. Cells Immobiliation Biotechnol.*, 19, 219, 1991. With permission.)

10.3.1 pH-Sensitive Polymers and Hydrogels

pH-sensitive polymers and hydrogels possess ionizable groups, such as carboxyl or amine groups, which become charged depending on the pH of the environment. Two examples of ionizable polymers are shown in Figure 10.6. Ionized polymers increase their water solubility, and ionized hydrogels swell much more than in the

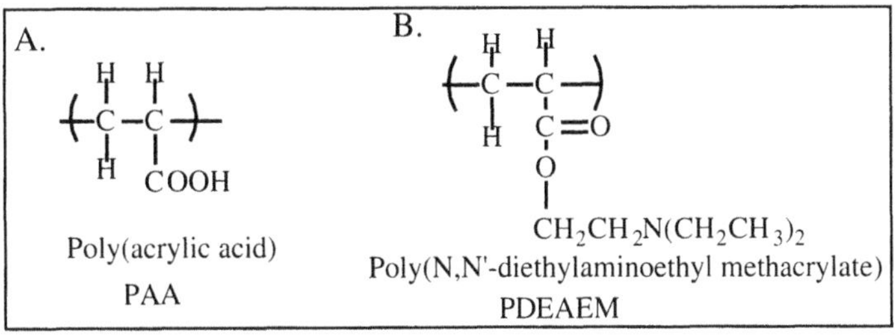

FIGURE 10.6 Examples of anionic (A) and cationic (B) polymers.

neutral state. The extent of swelling is influenced by conditions that alter electrostatic repulsion, such as ionic strength and type of counterion. Adding neutral comonomers can also adjust the swelling extent and pH-responsive behavior by providing different hydrophobicity to the polymer chain. Such changes in water-solubility and swelling ability are the main driving forces for controlling drug release as a function of the environmental pH. When water-soluble polymers are grafted to a surface, the grafted polymer layer creates a two-dimensional hydrogel layer. Thus, stretching of the grafted polymer chains upon ionization is the same as more swelling of hydrogels in the ionized state. pH-sensitive polymers and hydrogels have been used quite extensively in the diffusion-controlled modulated drug delivery systems shown in Figure 10.3.

For sensing molecules that do not affect the pH of the environment, e.g., glucose, additional components need to be added to generate hydrogen ions. Thus, glucose oxidase is commonly added to transform glucose to gluconic acid and lower the pH of the medium. For anionic polymers and hydrogels, lowering pH results in collapse of the polymers and hydrogels. This may open the pores (Figures 10.3A and 10.3B).[30] Cationic polymers are also used to increase the release rate since more swelling of cationic hydrogels at lower pH leads to increased pore size.[28,37,38] This is true as long as the thickness of the hydrogel layer remains the same. Since the swelling of hydrogels is the same in all three directions, an increase in thickness, i.e., path length for the drug to migrate, can counterbalance the increased pore size. Thus, it appears safer to rely on anionic polymers that precipitate or hydrogels that collapse at lower pH. If a drug is incorporated inside the hydrogel matrix, the anionic polymer matrix tends to "squeeze" the incorporated drugs for faster release.[31] pH-sensitive polymers can also be used to make dissolution-controlled modulated release systems. In a system where insulin-containing pH-sensitive erodible polymer was surrounded by a hydrogel layer with embedded glucose oxidase, pH lowering was used to control the polymer erosion, and thus insulin release.[32] To ensure a useful swelling/shrinking ratio by small pH changes for reliable insulin delivery, the activity of the immobilized enzymes must be maintained. In most cases, however, the enzyme activity is significantly reduced due to harsh conditions used for enzyme immobilization and polymerization.

10.3.2 TEMPERATURE-SENSITIVE POLYMERS AND HYDROGELS

Temperature-sensitive polymers used for modulated drug delivery are mainly inverse thermosensitive polymers.[39,40] Inverse thermosensitivity is due to the increased solubility at lower temperatures. This is opposite to normal polymers that increase their solubility at higher temperatures. The inverse thermosensitivity comes from the presence of hydrophobic groups, and the delicate balance between functional groups capable of hydrogen bonding and hydrophobic groups decides the temperature of the sol–gel phase transition. As the hydrophobicity increases, the phase transition temperature is lowered,[41] and this hydrophilic and hydrophobic balance can be achieved by using different monomers to form copolymers.[42-45] Detailed discussion of the force balance involving fundamental molecular interactions in the gel network can be found in Chapter 6. Thermosensitive polymers and hydrogels have been used extensively for modulated drug delivery,[46,47] but in most cases, local body temperature must be increased by external heat sources. It is possible to utilize the natural increase in body temperature that occurs with bacterial and virus infections and colds, but the extent and kinetics of the temperature increase are not easily controllable. Examples of thermosensitive polymers are shown in Figure 10.7.

Temperature-dependent modulated drug delivery systems can be further classified into three categories. The first is the negatively thermoresponsive drug delivery system in which the drug release is on at low temperature and off at high temperature.[48,49] Those studies used cross-linked P(NIPAAm-co-BMA) hydrogels,[40,50,51] interpenetrating polymer networks (IPNs) of P(NIPAAm), and polytetramethylene ether glycol. The modulating mechanism in this system is the formation of a dense, less permeable surface layer of gel, described as a skin barrier, upon a sudden

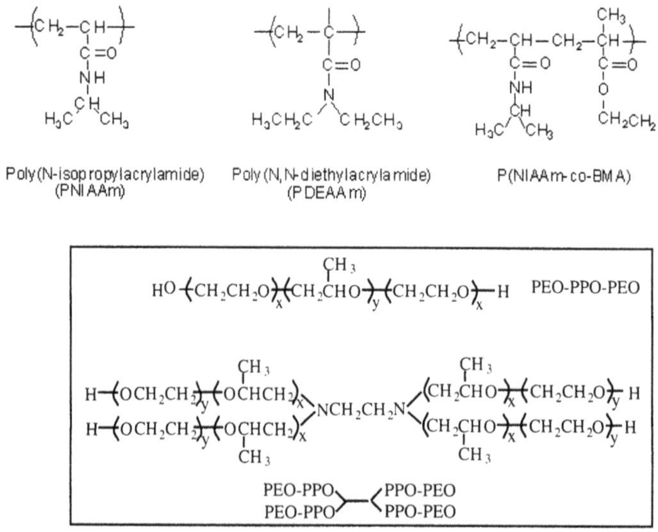

Poly(N-isopropylacrylamide) (PNIAAm)

Poly(N,N-diethylacrylamide) (PDEAAm)

P(NIAAm-co-BMA)

PEO-PPO-PEO

PEO-PPO / PEO-PPO — PPO-PEO / PPO-PEO

FIGURE 10.7 Examples of inverse thermosensitive polymers.

temperature change due to the faster collapse of the gel surface than the interior. This surface shrinking process can be regulated by the length of the methacrylate alkyl side-chain, i.e., the hydrophobicity of the comonomer.[52,53]

The second type is the positively thermoresponsive drug delivery system. This type of system can be formed by IPNs that show positive thermosensitivity, i.e., swelling at high temperature and shrinking at low temperature. More information on synthesis, structures, and characterization of IPNs can be found in Chapter 6. IPNs of poly(acrylic acid), polyacrylamide (PAAm), and P(AAm-co-BMA) are good examples.[54] The transition temperature can be adjusted by controlling the BMA content in the polymer. The swelling of those hydrogels was reversible; they respond to stepwise temperature changes. An on–off temperature modulated delivery system could therefore be achieved by loading model drugs in this system.

The last type of system is the thermally reversible gel, e.g., Pluronics© and Tetronics©. For parenteral application thermoreversible gels should be biodegradable. To increase biodegradability, the poly(propylene oxide) (PPO) segments of PEO–PPO–PEO block copolymers can be replaced by biodegradable poly(L-lactic acid) segments.[55-57] The molecular architecture is not limited to the A–B–A type block copolymer, but can be expanded into three-dimensional hyperbranched structures, such as star-shaped structures.[56] Proper combinations of molecular weight and polymer architecture resulted in gels with different lower critical solution temperatures (LCSTs).

10.3.3 Biomolecule-Sensitive Hydrogels

Hydrogels can be made to respond to specific molecules. To do so they should contain receptors for the target molecule. To make a glucose-specific delivery system, glucose binding molecules should be present. The system can be used for diffusion-controlled, dissolution-controlled, and exchange-controlled devices (Figures 10.3–10.5) for modulated insulin delivery. The only difference between the diffusion-controlled and dissolution-controlled systems is that the glucose-sensitive hydrogel is placed inside the two membranes to prevent loss of components during the sol state. Glucose-containing polymers can be mixed with glucose-binding proteins, e.g., concanavalin A (Con A) to form a gel.[9,58,59] Since Con A exists as a tetramer at physiological pH and each subunit has a glucose binding site, Con A can function as a cross-linking agent for glucose-containing polymer chains.

In the absence of free glucose, the system forms a gel as shown in Figure 10.8A. When the external glucose molecules diffuse into the hydrogel, individual free glucose molecules can compete with the polymer-attached glucose molecules to replace them from the Con A binding sites, and a sol is formed. Insulin diffusion through the gel is much slower than through the sol; therefore insulin release can be controlled as a function of the glucose concentration in the environment. Polysaccharides (e.g., polysucrose, dextran, glycogen) can also be used with Con A to make similar glucose-sensitive insulin delivery systems. The unmodified insulin is loaded into an aqueous or nonaqueous reservoir covered by the glucose-sensitive membrane. The nonaqueous system showed better results, possibly due to better gel stability.[60,61] Con A can also be introduced as an additional physical linker to a chemically cross-linked hydrogel to increase cross-linking density. The complexation between Con A and the poly(2-glucosyloxyethyl methacrylate) hydrogel decreases the swelling ratio. The swelling of the hydrogel increases in the presence of glucose due to the dissociation of the complex. Insulin release in this system is controlled by the reversible swelling–shrinking volume transition of the hydrogel instead of phase transition.[24,25] The same concept can be used to design hydrogel systems that can respond to specific molecules using antigen–antibody associations. Antigen and a corresponding antibody were grafted to different polymer chains to form reversible polymer networks.[10] The hydrogel swelling was triggered by the presence of free antigen that competed with the polymer-bound antigen, leading to lowering of the hydrogel cross-linking density, as shown in Figure 10.8B.

Another type of modulated insulin delivery system utilizes the competitive desorption of glycosylated insulin from ConA conjugates by free glucose molecules.[22] Insulin molecules are usually glycosylated by introducing glucose, which can form a complex with ConA. The complementary and competitive binding behavior of Con A with glucose and glycosylated insulin is used as a modulator. The insulin then undergoes exchange-controlled release as shown in Figure 10.5. When the glucose concentration is high, the free glucose molecules compete with glucose–insulin conjugates at the ConA binding sites, and thus, the initially bounded glycosylated insulin is desorbed from the ConA in the presence of free glucose. The desorbed glucose–insulin conjugates are released to the surrounding tissue, and the studies have shown that they are bioactive. Various glycosylated insulins having different binding affinities to Con A have been synthesized to manipulate displacement of immobilized insulin from Con A at different glucose levels.[23,62-64]

The use of a protein such as ConA as a glucose-sensitive unit is not ideal for long-term applications. Proteins may denature during the lifetime of the device or may not function as intended upon slight changes in environmental conditions including pH and concentrations of specific salts. Many attempts have been made to utilize synthetic molecules for glucose sensing. One example is gel formation between polymers containing pendant phenylboronic groups (e.g., poly[3-(acrylamido) phenyl-boronic acid] and its copolymers) and polyol polymers (e.g., poly(vinyl alcohol) or PVA). They can form a gel through reversible complex formation between the coplanar phenylborate and hydroxyl groups, as described in Figure 10.9.[27,65] Glucose, having pendant hydroxyl groups, competes with polyol polymers for the borate groups. Terpolymers made of m-acrylamidophenylboronic acid, *N,N'*-dimethylaminopropyl-acrylamide (DMAPAA), and *N,N'*-dimethylacryl-amide allowed high glucose sensitivity at physiological pH through the interaction of phenylborate with amino groups. DMAPAA was introduced to stabilize the phenylborate–polyol complex at physiological pH. The glucose sensitivity of the system was greatly improved as compared with the previous systems without DMAPAA. This type of system will be highly useful if the polymers prove to be biocompatible and can be removed from the body.

A

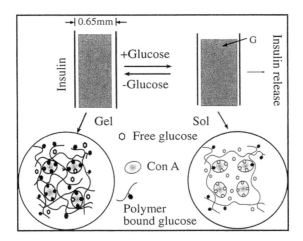

B.

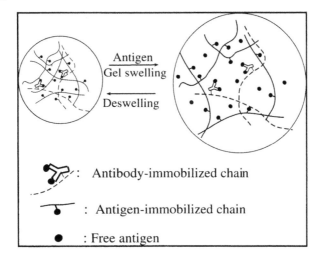

FIGURE 10.8 Examples of sol-gel phase-reversible hydrogel systems sensitive to glucose (A) and an antigen (B). (Redrawn from Kim, J.J., in *Industrial and Physical Pharmacy*, Purdue University, West Lafayette, IN, 1999, p. 162. With permission.)

10.3.4 ENZYME-SENSITIVE POLYMERS AND HYDROGELS

The presence of specific enzymes in different parts of the body makes it possible to utilize enzymatically degradable polymers and hydrogels for modulated drug delivery.[34] This approach has been used extensively for colon-specific drug delivery

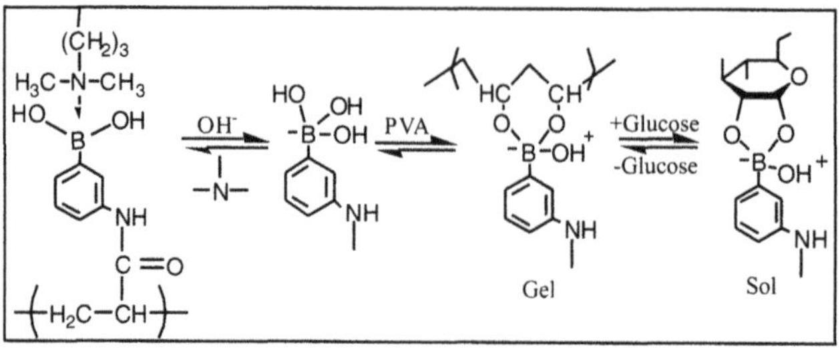

FIGURE 10.9 Sol–gel phase transistion of a polymer complex of polyphenylborate and poly(vinyl alcohol).

systems. Azoreductase produced by the microbial flora of the colon[66,67] degrades azoaromatic cross-linkers of hydrogels. Anionic polymers cross-linked with azoaromatic cross-linkers will swell in the intestine and release drugs when the hydrogel chains are degraded in the colon. The swelling kinetics and degradation kinetics can be controlled by the polymer composition[67] and the cross-linking density.[66]

10.3.5 PHOTOSENSITIVE POLYMERS AND HYDROGELS

The photosensitive polymers and hydrogels can be synthesized to possess sensitivity to UV,[68,69] visible light,[70-72] and infrared light.[73] Phase transitions of most of the photosensitive polymers and hydrogels are known to be due to the increase in local temperature upon exposure to light. Therefore, the system includes light-sensitive chromophores, such as the trisodium salt of copper chlorophyllin[70] or gold–gold sulfide nanoshells[74] which can absorb light and dissipate it locally as heat.

To be used as photo-modulated drug delivery systems, drug molecules are loaded into the light-sensitive hydrogel matrices. One visible light-modulated system was prepared by dispersing drug microreservoirs (lipid microspheres) into degradable matrices of cross-linked hyaluronic acid hydrogels. Methylene blue was incorporated in the hydrogel as a photosensitizer. The lipid microspheres were released in response to visible light-induced gel degradation.[72] UV irradiation modulated drug delivery was also investigated using poly(NIPAAm) hydrogels with photoreactive azobenzene groups.[69] Drug release increased upon UV irradiation when azobenzene was used as a pendant group of hydrogels. On the other hand, irradiation of hydrogels with azobenzene as a cross-linker caused a decrease in release. In another study, photothermally modulated drug delivery system was formed by incorporating gold–gold sulfide nanoshells into poly(NIPAAm-co-AAm) hydrogels.[74] Copolymers of N-isopropylacrylamide (NIPAAm) and acrylamide (AAm) exhibited LCSTs slightly above body temperature.

Burst release of a drug loaded in the hydrogel matrix will occur when the temperature of the copolymer exceeds the LCST, which causes the hydrogel to collapse. The photosensor in this system is a new class of nanoparticles designed to strongly absorb near-infrared light. When incorporated into the poly(NIPAAm-co-AAm) hydrogel, the nanoparticles can initiate a local temperature change when they absorb light at wavelengths between 800 and 1200 nm; the light is transmitted through tissue with relatively little attenuation. At 1064 nm, drug release from composite hydrogels has been significantly enhanced in response to irradiation. Additionally, under repeated near-IR irradiation, the nanoshell-composite hydrogels were able to release multiple bursts of protein in response.[74]

Recent studies, however, showed that thermosensitive hydrogels, such as poly(NIPAAm-co-AAm), reacted to light in the absence of local heating.[75] Shrinking was observed when the poly(NIPAAm-co-AAm) hydrogels were immersed in heavy water (D_2O) instead of normal water (H_2O) and a 1064-nm laser was irradiated to the gel. Since lights of different wavelengths can easily penetrate skin, photosensitive polymers and hydrogels will be very useful for modulated drug delivery in the future.

10.4 SMART POLYMERS AND HYDROGELS FOR CLINICAL APPLICATIONS

The literature is full of examples of modulated drug delivery utilizing various smart polymers and hydrogels. New polymers and hydrogels have better properties. Despite all these advances, modulated drug delivery systems are still far from practical clinical applications. This is not due to the lack of good designs. The main difficulty of applying polymers and hydrogels clinically stems from the lack of biocompatibility. If the modulated systems are to deliver drugs orally so that the unabsorbable polymers and hydrogels can be removed from the body, they will present little difficulty for clinical applications. Most applications of modulated drug delivery systems, however, are designed to be injected or implanted. Removal of the devices after use is not easy. Thus, biodegradable and biocompatible polymers are preferred, and yet the majority of smart polymers and hydrogels are not really biodegradable and their biocompatibilities have not been dealt with in depth.

Another important property to be improved in modulated drug delivery systems is the kinetics of drug delivery. Modulated delivery works best when the drug is delivered as fast as possible upon receiving signals. All the smart polymers and hydrogels described in this chapter work as intended, but in many situations their action (swelling or shrinking) is too slow. Miniaturization of the devices would shorten the response time, and microfabrication of the modulated delivery systems would present a new hope for effective clinical applications. The slow response is usually accompanied by slow turn-off of the release system. For modulated drug delivery to be truly successful, it is necessary to shorten the time for drug release and the time to shut off after a suitable amount of drug is released. Finally, the release profiles of modulated delivery systems should be predictable and reproducible. To achieve that, the hydrogel components forming the modulated delivery device should have good long-term stability. Maintaining long-term stability in the presence of abundant water at 37°C is a challenge for both polymers and proteins. Devising modulated delivery systems that meet all the challenges is, of course, difficult, but considering the advances made in the last few decades, we can be confident that such systems can be realized in the near future. Until a few years ago, we never worried about these problems, since all the efforts went into designing modulated drug delivery. Knowing what problems to solve is half way to solving the problems.

REFERENCES

1. Levi, F. et al. A chronopharmacologic phase II clinical trial with 5-fluorouracil, folinic acid, and oxaliplatin using an ambulatory multichannel programmable pump. High antitumor effectiveness against metastatic colorectal cancer, *Cancer*, 69, 893, 1992.
2. Falcone, A. et al. Infusions of fluorouracil and leucovorin: effects of the timing and semi-intermittency of drug delivery, *Oncology*, 57, 195, 1999.
3. Heller, J., Modulated release from drug delivery devices, *Crit. Rev. Ther. Drug Carrier Syst.*, 10, 253, 1993.
4. Heller, J., Feedback-controlled drug delivery, in *Controlled Drug Delivery: Challenge and Strategies*, Park, K., Ed., American Chemical Society, Washington, 1997, p. 127.
5. Park, K. and Park, H., Smart hydrogels, in *Concise Polymeric Materials Encyclopedia*, Salamone, J.C., Ed., CRC Press, Boca Raton, FL, 1999, p. 1476.
6. Takagi, T., A perspective of the intelligent materials, in *Proceedings of the First International Conference on Intelligent Materials*, Takagi, T. et al., Eds., Technomic, Lancaster, PA, 1993, p. 3.
7. Liang, C., Rogers, C.A.. and Malafeew, E., Preliminary investigation of shape memory polymers and their hybrid composites, presented at 1991 Annual Meeting of the American Society of Mechanical Engineers, Atlanta.
8. Lendlein, A., Schmidt, A.M., and Langer, R., AB polymer networks based on oligo (ε-caprolactone segments showing shape-memory properties. *PNAS*, 98, 842, 2001.
9. Lee, S.J. and Park, K., Synthesis and characterization of sol–gel phase-reversible hydrogels sensitive to glucose, *J. Molecular Recognition*, 9, 549, 1996.
10. Miyata, T., Asami, N., and Uragami, T., A reversibly antigen-responsive hydrogel, *Nature*, 399, 766, 1999.
11. Heller, J., Polymers for controlled parenteral delivery of peptides and proteins, *Adv. Drug Delivery Rev.*, 10, 163, 1993.
12. Kwon, I.C. et al., Drug release from electric current sensitive polymers. *J. Controlled Release*, 17, 149, 1991.
13. Sawahata, K. et al., Electrically controlled drug delivery system using polyelectrolyte gels, *J. Controlled Release*, 14, 253, 1990.
14. Yuk, S.H., Cho, S.H., and Lee, H.B, Electric current-sensitive drug delivery systems using sodium alginate/polyacrylic acid composites., *Pharm. Res.*, 9, 955, 1992.
15. Kwon, I.C., Bae, Y.H., and Kim, S.W., Electrically erodible polymer gel for controlled release of drugs, *Nature*, 354, 291, 1991.
16. Santini, J.T.J., Cima, M.J., and Langer, R., A controlled-release microchip, *Nature*, 397, 335, 1999.
17. Heller, M., Forster, A., and Tu, E., Active microeletronic chip devices which utilize controlled electrophoretic fields for multiplex DNA hybridization and other genomic applications, *Electrophoresis*, 21, 157, 2000.
18. Hsu, C.S. and Block, L.H., Anionic gels as vehicles for electrically-modulated drug delivery I. Solvent and drug transport phenomena, *Pharm. Res.*, 13, 1865, 1996.
19. Siegel, R.A. et al., pH-controlled release from hydrophobic/polyelectrolyte copolymer hydrogels, *J. Controlled Release*, 8, 179, 1988.
20. Brannon-Peppas, L. and Peppas, N.A., Dynamic and equilibrium swelling behavior of pH-sensitive hydrogels containing 2-hydroxyethyl methacrylate, *Biomaterials*, 11, 635, 1990.
21. Cunderlikova, B. et al., Increased binding of chlorine to lipoproteins at low pH values,*Int. J. Biochem. Cell Biol.*, 32, 759, 2000.

22. Brownlee, M. and Cerami, A., A glucose-controlled insulin-delivery system: semi-synthetic insulin bound to lectin, *Science*, 206, 1190, 1979.

23. Jeong, S.Y. et al., Self-regulating insulin delivery systems III. *In vivo* studies, *J. Controlled Release*, 2, 143, 1985.

24. Nakamae, K. et al., Formation of poly(glycosyloxyethyl methacrylate)–Concanavalin A complex and its glucose sensitivity, *J. Biomater. Sci. Polym. Edn.*, 6, 79, 1994.

25. Miyata, T. et al., Preparation of poly(2-glucosyloxyethyl methacrylate)–Concanavalin A complex hydrogel and its glucose-sensitivity, *Macromol. Chem. Phys.*, 197, 1135, 1996.

26. Taylor, M.J. et al., Delivery of insulin from aqueous and nonaqueous reservoirs governed by a glucose sensitive gel membrane, *J. Drug Targeting*, 3, 209, 1995.

27. Kitano, S. et al., A novel drug delivery system utilizing a glucose-responsive polymer complex between poly(vinyl alcohol) and poly(N-vinyl-2-pyrrolidone) with a phenyl boronic acid moiety *J. Controlled Release*, 19, 162, 1992.

28. Ishihara, K., Kobayashi, M., and Shinohara, I., Insulin permeation through amphiphilic polymer membranes having 2-hydroxyethyl methacrylate moiety, *Polym. J.*, 16, 647, 1984.

29. Ishihara, K., Kobayashi, M., and Shinohara, I., Glucose-induced permeation control of insulin through a complex membrane consisting of immobilized glucose oxidase and a poly(amine), *Polym. J.*, 16, 625, 1984.

30. Ito, Y. et al., An insulin-releasing system that is responsive to glucose, *J. Controlled Release*, 10, 195, 1989.

31. Hassan, C.M., Doyle, F.J., III, and Peppas, N.A., Dynamic behavior of glucose-responsive poly(methacrylic acid-g-ethylene glycol) hydrogels, *Macromolecules*, 30, 6166, 1997.

32. Heller, J. et al., Release of insulin from pH-sensitive poly(ortho esters), *J. Controlled Release*, 13, 295, 1990.

33. Jung, D., Magda, J., and Han, I., Catalase effects on glucose-sensitive hydrogels, *Macromolecules*, 33, 3332, 2000.

34. Heller, J., Pangburn, S.H., and Roskos, K.V., Development of enzymatically degradable protective coatings for use in triggered drug delivery systems: derivatized starch hydrogels, *Biomaterials*, 11, 345, 1990.

35. Bae, Y.H., Kim, S.W., and Valuev, L.I., Pulsatile drug delivery device using stimuli sensitive hydrogel, U.S. Patent, 5,226,902, 1993.

36. Gutowska, A. et al., Squeezing hydrogels for controlled oral drug delivery, *J. Controlled Release*, 48, 141, 1997.

37. Albin, G., Horbett, T.A., and Ratner, B.D., Glucose-sensitive membranes for controlled delivery of insulin: insulin transport studies, *J. Controlled Release*, 2, 153, 1985.

38. Kost, J. et al., Glucose-sensitive membranes containing glucose oxidase: activity, swelling, and permeability studies, *J. Biomed. Materials Res.*, 19, 1177, 1985.

39. Hoffman, A.S., Applications of thermally reversible polymers and hydrogels in therapeutics and diagnostics, *J. Controlled Release*, 6, 297, 1987.

40. Okano, T. et al., Thermally on–off switching polymers for drug permeation and release, *J. Controlled Release*, 11, 255, 1990.

41. Schild, H.G., Poly(N-isopropylacrylamide): experiment, theory and application, *Prog. Polym. Sci.*, 17, 163, 1992.

42. Feil, H., Bae, Y.H., and Kim, S.W., Mutual influence of pH and temperature on the swelling of ionizable and thermosensitive hydrogels, *Macromolecules*, 25, 5528, 1992.

43. Hirotsu, S., Coexistence of phases and the nature of first-order phase transition in poly(N-isopropylacrylamide) gels, *Adv. Polym. Sci.*, 110, 1, 1993.

44. Irie, M., Stimuli-responsive poly(N-isopropylacrylamide). Photo- and chemical-induced phase transitions. *Adv. Polym. Sci.*, 110, 490, 1993.

45. Dong, L.C. and A.S. Hoffman, Synthesis and application of thermally reversible heterogels for drug delivery, *J. Controlled Release* 13, 21, 1990.

46. Bromberg, L.E. and Ron, E.S., Temperature-responsive gels and thermogelling polymer matrices for protein and peptide delivery, *Adv. Drug Del. Rev.*, 31, 197, 1998.

47. Yoshida, R. et al., Pulsatile drug delivery systems using hydrogels, *Adv. Drug Del. Rev.*, 11, 85, 1993.

48. Bae, Y.H., Okano, T., and Kim, S.W., On–off thermocontrol of solute transport 1. Temperature dependence of swelling of N-isopropylacrylamide networks modified with hydrophobic components in water, *Pharm. Res.*, 8, 531, 1991.

49. Bae, Y.H., Okano, T., and Kim, S.W., On–off thermocontrol of solute transport 2. Solute release from thermosensitive hydrogels, *Pharm. Res.*, 8, 624, 1991.

50. Okuyama, Y. et al., Swelling-controlled zero order and sigmoidal drug release from thermo-responsive poly(N-isopropylacrylamide-co-butyl methacrylate) hydrogel, *J. Biomaterials Sci., Polym. Ed.*, 4, 545, 1993.

51. Gutowska, A. et al., Heparin release from thermosensitive hydrogels, *J. Controlled Release*, 22, 95, 1992.

52. Yoshida, R. et al., Surface-modulated skin layers of thermal responsive hydrogels as on–off switches I. Drug release, *J. Biomaterials Sci., Polym. Ed.*, 3, 155, 1991.

53. Yoshida, M. et al., Thermo-responsive hydrogels based on acryloyl-L-proline methyl ester and their use as long-acting testosterone delivery systems, *Drug Design Delivery*, 7, 159, 1991.

54. Katono, H. et al., Thermo-responsive swelling and drug release switching of interpenetrating polymer networks composed of poly(acrylamide-co-butyl methacrylate) and poly(acrylic acid), *J. Controlled Release*, 16, 215, 1991.

55. Jeong, B. et al., Biodegradable block copolymers as injectable drug delivery systems, *Nature*, 388, 860, 1997.

56. Jeong, B. et al., New biodegradable polymers for injectable drug delivery systems, *J. Controlled Release*, 62, 198, 1999.

57. Jeong, B., Bae, Y.H., and Kim, S.W., Drug release from biodegradable injectable thermosensitive hydrogel of PEG–PLGA–PEG triblock copolymers, *J. Controlled Release*, 63, 155, 2000.

58. Obaidat, A.A. and Park, K., Characterization of protein release through glucose-sensitive hydrogel membranes, *Biomaterials*, 18, 801, 1997.

59. Kim, J.J., Phase-reversible glucose-sensitive hydrogels for modulated insulin delivery, in *Industrial and Physical Pharmacy*, Purdue University, West Lafayette, IN, 1999, p. 162.

60. Taylor, M.J. et al., A self-regulated delivery system using unmodified solutes in glucose-sensitive gel membranes, *J. Pharm. Pharmacol.*, 467, Suppl. 2, 1051a, 1994.

61. Tanna, S. and Taylor, M.J., Characterization of model solute and insulin delivery across covalently modified lectin–polysaccharide gels sensitive to glucose, *Pharm. Pharmacol. Comm.*, 4, 117, 1998.

62. Sato, S. et al., Self-regulating insulin delivery systems II. *In vitro* studies, *J. Controlled Release*, 1, 67, 1984.

63. Seminoff, L.A., Olsen, G.B., and Kim, S.W., A self-regulating insulin delivery system I. Characterization of a synthetic glycosylated insulin derivative, *Int. J. Pharm.*, 54, 241, 1989.

64. Seminoff, L.A. et al., A self-regulating insulin delivery system II. *In vivo* characteristics of a synthetic glycosylated insulin, *Int. J. Pharm.*, 54, 251, 1989.

65. Hisamitsu, I. et al., Glucose-responsive gel from phenylborate polymer and polyvinyl alcohol: prompt response at physiological pH through the interaction of borate with amino group in the gel, *Pharm. Res.*, 14, 289, 1997.

66. Ghandehari, H., Kopeckova, P., and Kopecek, J., *In vitro* degradation of pH-sensitive hydrogels containing aromatic azo bonds, *Biomaterials*, 18, 861, 1997.

67. Akala, E.O., Kopeckova, P., and Kopecek, J., Novel pH-sensitive hydrogels with adjustable swelling kinetics, *Biomaterials*, 19, 1037, 1998.

68. Mamada, A. et al., Photoinduced phase transition of gels, *Macromolecules*, 23, 1517, 1990.

69. Tomer, R. and Florence, A., Photo-responsive hydrogels for potential responsive release applications, *Int. J. Pharmaceutics*, 99, R5, 1993.

70. Suzuki, A. and Tanaka, T., Phase transition in polymer gels induced by visible light, *Nature*, 346, 345, 1990.

71. Suzuki, A., Ishii, T., and Maruyama, Y., Optical switching in polymer gels, *J. Appl. Phys.*, 80, 131, 1996.

72. Yui, N., Okano, T., and Sakurai, Y., Photo-responsive degradation of heterogeneous hydrogels comprising crosslinked hyaluronic acid and lipid microspheres for temporal drug delivery, *J. Controlled Release*, 26, 141, 1993.

73. Zhang, X. et al., Bending of N-isopropylacrylamide gel under the influence of infrared light, *J. Chem. Phys.*, 102, 551, 1995.

74. Sershen, S. et al., Temperature-sensitive polymer-nanoshell composites for photothermally modulated drug delivery, *J. Biomed. Materials Res.*, 51, 293, 2000.

75. Juodkazis, S. et al., Reversible phase transitions in polymer gels induced by radiation forces, *Nature*, 408, 178, 2000.

76. Kim, S.W. et al., Self-regulated glycosylated insulin delivery, *J. Controlled Release*, 11, 193, 1990.

77. Makino, K. et al., Self-regulated delivery of insulin from microcapsules, *Biomater. Artif. Cells Immobilization Biotechnol.*, 19, 219, 1991.

11 Drug Targeting with Polymeric Micelle Drug Carriers

Masayuki Yokoyama

CONTENTS

This chapter discusses supramolecular assembly of polymers for drug targeting with a focus on polymeric micelles. It will explain why polymeric micelle supramolecular design is suitable for drug targeting and discuss the advantages of polymeric micelle systems over conventional polymeric drug targeting systems.

11.1 DRUG TARGETING

11.1.1 SIGNIFICANCE OF DRUG TARGETING

Drug targeting is selective drug delivery to specific physiological sites, organs, tissues, or cells where drug pharmacological activities are required. In principle, a drug without a targeting methodology is considered uniformly distributed throughout the body, as illustrated in Figure 11.1(a). A drug distributed to sites other than the therapeutic sites may cause toxic side effects. By increasing delivery to the therapeutic

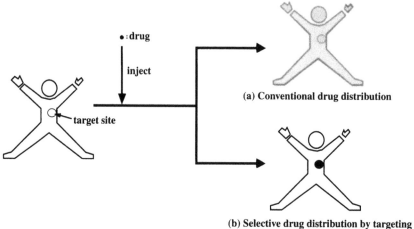

FIGURE 11.1 Concept of drug targeting.

sites and decreasing delivery to the unwanted sites, an improved therapeutic index can be obtained from enhanced drug action at the therapeutic sites and reduced drug action at the unwanted sites.

The first drug targeting idea was the "Magic Bullet" proposed by Paul Ehrlich in the 19th century (Figure 11.2). Ehrlich suggested that drug targeting could be achieved by a carrier that had a specific affinity to certain organs, tissues, or cells. This strategy was proposed even before the identification of antibodies, naturally occurring candidates to serve as carriers. Ehrlich's model assumed that a drug could exhibit its pharmacological activities only at the specific site to which it was delivered by the carrier. The essence of this concept is the separation of functions to achieve selective pharmacological action. The carrier handles delivery to the designated sites while the drug exerts pharmacological activity. Although this concept is very simple and requires only coupling of the drug with the carrier, drug targeting by the "Magic Bullet" alone has not been successful.

11.1.2 TARGETING METHODOLOGY

11.1.2.1 Classification of Drug Targeting Methodologies

Drug targeting may be classified as active or passive targeting.[1-3] Active targeting aims to increase the delivery of drug to the target by utilizing specific interactions at the target sites that require pharmacological activities. These interactions include antigen–antibody and ligand–receptor binding. Alternatively, physical signals such as magnetic field and temperature applied to the target sites externally can be utilized for active targeting. Carriers in this category include antibodies, transferrin, ferrite-containing liposomes, and thermoresponsive carriers.

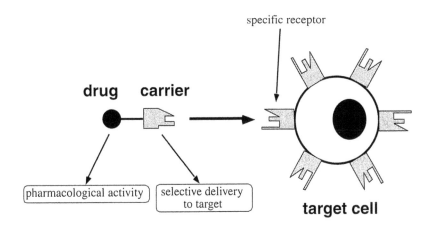

FIGURE 11.2 Ehrlich's "Magic Bullet."

Passive targeting is a methodology that increases the target/nontarget ratios of delivered drugs by adjusting the physical and chemical properties of the carriers to physiological and histological characteristics of the target and nontarget tissues, organs, and cells. This group of carriers includes synthetic polymers, natural polymers such as albumin, liposomes, microparticles (nanoparticle is a microparticle with a diameter smaller than 1 μm), and polymeric micelles. Influential characteristics for passive targeting are chemical factors such as hydrophilicity/hydrophobicity, positive/negative charges, and physical factors such as size and mass. Passive targeting can be achieved by minimizing nonspecific interactions with and delivery to nontarget organs, tissues, and cells as well as by maximizing delivery to the target.

11.1.2.2 Active Targeting vs. Passive Targeting?

Which targeting methodology — active or passive — is superior and more applicable to human use? The author believes both methodologies are important for drug targeting. Passive targeting methodology was underestimated in comparison with active targeting until about 10 years ago because of the very high specificity of monoclonal antibodies *in vitro*. It was speculated that this high specificity might provide highly selective *in vivo* delivery to targets when antibodies were simply conjugated with drugs. The general presumption was that passive targeting systems would never achieve such high selectivity.

Achievement of *in vivo* selective drug delivery with active targeting systems was not as easy as a simple extension of *in vitro* specificity to selective delivery *in vivo*. Consider a case of anticancer drug delivery by conjugation of the drug to an antibody possessing high binding specificity to surface antigens of tumor cells. Delivery of this conjugate is usually evaluated by the quantity accumulated at solid tumor sites.

The specificity of the antibody is not correlated with its accumulation phenomenon since transfer from the bloodstream to the interstitial spaces of tumor sites is made through the endothelial cells of blood vessels that do not express tumor-specific antigens. Several difficulties obstruct the success of *in vivo* delivery of the conjugate, including loss of antibody specificity by chemical conjugation of drugs and nonspecific uptake of drug–antibody conjugates due to physicochemical properties imported by the conjugated drugs. Passive targeting to solid tumors can be achieved by the EPR effect as described in the next section.

One correlation between active and passive targeting has often been recognized in a way shown in Figure 11.3(a). It shows active targeting as a different methodology from passive targeting. Some targeting systems such as immunoliposomes (antibody-binding liposomes) combine both methodologies. Passive targeting is as important as active targeting; the factors governing passive targeting are also important for active targeting systems. In this consideration, the correlation between both the targeting methodologies must be recognized as shown in Figure 11.3(b).[3] Passive targeting is a wider methodology that includes active targeting. The reasons for this are as follows:

1. The majority of a living body comprises nontarget sites. The liver, one of the largest targets of drugs, occupies only 2% of the weight of the entire body. That means, 98% of the body can be considered a nontarget site. Active targeting can be achieved within the small dose fraction remaining after nonspecific capture at nontarget sites throughout the entire body. Minimization of nonspecific capture at nontarget sites by passive targeting may therefore be important to maximize amounts delivered by the active targeting systems.
2. Passive targeting phenomena precede active targeting ones in most cases. The exceptions are intravascular targets such as lymphocytes and vascular endothelial cells. Most targets are located in the extravascular spaces. To reach these targets via the bloodstream, the first step must be extravasation through the vascular endothelia, followed by permeation through the interstitial spaces to the extravascular targets.

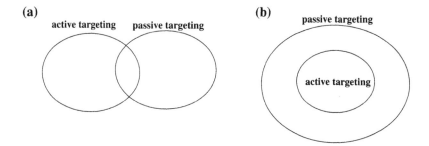

(a) active targeting   passive targeting

(b) passive targeting   active targeting

FIGURE 11.3 Correlation of active and passive targeting.

3. The passive aspects may become even more important as more drugs are introduced to the active targeting carriers. For antibody–drug conjugates, the physicochemical properties of the introduced drugs may reduce antibody specificity by steric hindrance and decrease the delivery to tumor sites by increasing nonspecific capture at nontarget tissues, particularly in the reticuloendothelial systems.

11.2   EPR EFFECT

Maeda et al. presented a new concept of targeting drugs to solid tumors by a passive targeting mechanism in 1986.[4] The concept is called the enhanced permeability and retention effect (EPR effect)[5] of polymers at solid tumor tissues. As illustrated in Figure 11.4, vascular permeability of tumor tissues is enhanced by the action of secreted chemical factors such as kinin. As a result of this increased vascular permeability, both polymers and low molecular weight compounds increase their transport from blood vessels to tumor tissues. However, low molecular weight compounds are more diffusible out of tumor tissues into blood circulation again than macromolecular compounds. Therefore, enhanced accumulation at tumor tissues is prominent only for macromolecules.

The lymphatic drainage system does not operate effectively in tumor tissues, and macromolecules are retained for prolonged periods in the tumor interstitium. As a consequence, polymers can accumulate efficiently in tumor sites. Maeda et al. first showed the EPR effect with Evans blue-modified albumin.[4] Intravenously injected Evans blue modified albumin was found in transplanted tumor S-180 tissue at higher concentrations than in normal muscle; the high concentration in the tumor was retained up to 6 days. They confirmed the EPR effect in a chemically induced tumor.[6]

In principle, the EPR effect should be seen in every solid tumor site for the following reasons. The first is the fact that the hyperpermeability of macromolecules at solid tumor sites has been known by many groups since the 1950.[7-9] Although opinions differ as to whether macromolecules translocate the vascular endothelial cells through intracellular channels such as vesiculovacuolar organelles (VVOs)[10] or through intercellular junctions,[11,12] the consensus is that macromolecules in solid tumor sites have 3 to 10 times as much permeability[13] as normal tissues.

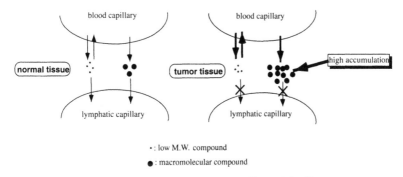

FIGURE 11.4 Enhanced permeability and retention effect (EPR effect).

The second reason to support the ubiquity of the EPR effect is a hypothesis presented by Dvorak et al.[14,15] It is widely accepted that angiogenesis[16,17] (new vasculature formation) is essential to tumor growth since tumor cells cannot obtain nutrients by diffusion from distant blood vessels beyond a certain limit of tumor volume. Dvorak et al. hypothesized that vascular hyperpermeability is required to achieve accumulation of plasma proteins in the interstitial spaces in order to form a new and provisional extravascular matrix that permits migration of endothelial cells and fibroblasts for new vascular formation.

One strong evidence for this hypothesis is the fact that vascular endothelial growth factor (VEGF) simultaneously possesses activity as vascular permeability factor (VPF). This very important and specific protein for angiogenesis was first discovered as VPF,[14,18] followed by the finding of VEGF.[19] These two activities indicate a tight connection between growth and hyperpermeability of vascular endothelial cells.

According to the EPR effect, specific targeting moieties such as antibodies are not necessary to obtain highly selective delivery to tumors. Any synthetic and natural macromolecules can selectively accumulate at solid tumor sites. However, carrier polymers must fulfill the following two requirements to avoid nonspecific capture at nontumor sites. First, they must possess appropriate size or molecular weight. Carrier diameters must be smaller than ca. 200 nm to allow them to evade reticuloendothelial system uptake.[20] Molecular weights above a critical value (ca. 40,000) are favorable for evading renal filtration. Second, carrier polymers should not allow strong interactions with or uptake by normal organs (especially the reticuloendothelial systems). This character is typically seen for cationic[21] and hydrophobic polymers.[22] Carrier polymers must be hydrophilic and neutral or weakly negative in their charge.[21] These requirements are effectively achieved in polymeric micelle carrier systems as described later in this chapter.

11.3   POLYMER–DRUG CONJUGATES

11.3.1 RINGSDORF'S MODEL

In 1975, Ringsdorf[23] presented a famous design for polymer–drug conjugates. As shown in Figure 11.5, his polymeric drug carrier system is composed of five components: polymer backbone, transport system, solubilizer, drug, and spacer. The spacer is an intermediate component between the polymer backbone and the drug, and it is expected to modulate drug release rate. The polymer backbone is made of a biodegradable or nonbiodegradable polymer. The transport system includes a homing device and a nonspecific resorption enhancer. Homing devices utilize specific interactions with the living system and are exemplified by antibodies and hormones. Nonspecific resorption enhancers contribute to efficient delivery of the drug by interactions with the living system based on their chemical and physical properties. Solubilizers are classified as lipid-soluble if they enhance adsorption of the drug to the lipid bilayers of cell membranes, and water-soluble if they maintain water solubility of the drug carrying system.

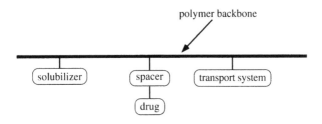

FIGURE 11.5 Ringsdorf's model for drug–polymer conjugates.

The solubilizing component is very important for two reasons. The low water solubility of drug–polymer conjugates often causes problems for *in vivo* injection. The solubilizer protects the conjugates from precipitation. Oil-solubles are considered to increase pharmacological activities by enhancing uptake of the conjugates by cells.

Although Ringsdorf's model was presented more than a quarter century ago, it retains its significance for macromolecular drug carrier design. One disadvantage is that one delivery property may be determined by plural components. Consider the need to increase the amount of conjugated drug per polymer chain in order to raise pharmacological activity. As the drug loading amount increases, other properties such as the water solubility of the conjugate, nonspecific interactions with cells, and drug release rate may change simultaneously since these properties are closely correlated with the hydrophobicity/hydrophilicity of the conjugate. It is not easy to control a property by changing the content of one component in Ringsdorf's design. This problem can be resolved by using a polymeric micelle carrier system because of its separated functionality.

11.3.2 PHPMA SYSTEM

The most advanced example of Ringsdorf's model in basic research and clinical application aspects is the carrier system based on poly[N-(2-hydroxypropyl)methacrylamide] (PHPMA) studied by Kopecek, Kopecekova, and Duncan et al.[24,25] The chemical structure of their system is shown in Figure 11.6. The biocompatibility of this polymer has been well characterized,[26] and it was found to have inert character when injected into the bloodstream.[27,28] They inserted a peptide spacer between the main polymer chain and the drug for selective drug release in cells. This tetrapeptide spacer was designed to ensure stability in the bloodstream during its delivery and to induce drug release inside lysosomes by enzymatic action; therefore, this system is also classified in the lysosomotropic agent that De Duve et al.[29] presented in 1974. With this peptide spacer, they succeeded in obtaining specific cytotoxicity at specific cells *in vivo* using cytotoxic agents as drugs and antibody[30,31] and sugar moiety[32] as a homing device. Even without specific targeting moieties, PHPMA–drug conjugates

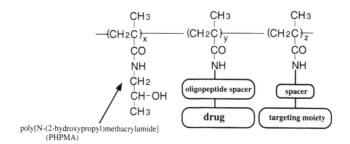

FIGURE 11.6 Kopecek's polymer–drug conjugates based on PHPMA.

were found to exert high *in vivo* antitumor activity.[38] They attributed this antitumor activity to the selective delivery of these conjugates by the EPR effect of solid tumor sites. Their system using adriamycin (doxorubicin) as the anticancer drug is named PK1 and its phase I clinical trials were completed in 1999. Phase II clinical trials in the United Kingdom were in progress in 2001.

The drug content of their drug–PHPMA conjugates was kept relatively low. Typically, 2 mol% (with respect to monomer units) of adriamycin was conjugated to the main chain PHPMA through the tetrapeptide spacer. The reason to maintain the low drug content is that the intact character of PHPMA may appear in the drug–polymer conjugates only within low drug substitution. If the drug content is high, distribution of the conjugates may be determined by the characters of the substituted drugs, not by the polymer. The hydrophobicity introduced by the drug may enhance nonspecific interactions with normal cells, especially the reticuloendothelial system. These interactions cause nonselective and unwanted capture at nontarget sites to a significant degree. The other reason to maintain low drug content is inhibition of association of the polymer chains of the conjugates. If hydrophobic drugs such as adriamycin were introduced at high levels, the substituted drug molecules would associate with each other to form heavy intrapolymer and interpolymer aggregates as was reported with model drugs.[34] The hydrophobic environment of these aggregates may make it difficult for hydrolytic enzymes to have access to the oligopeptide spacers. Therefore, the low drug content is preferable to obtain effective lysosomotropic release of drug based on the oligopeptide spacers.

11.4 POLYMERIC MICELLES

11.4.1 Use of Polymeric Micelles for Drug Targeting

A polymeric micelle is a supramolecular assembly of polymers with a spherical inner core and an outer shell, typically formed from block or graft copolymers. [35] The diameters of polymeric micelles range from 10 to 100 nm. Random and alternating copolymers can also form assemblies. They are not called polymeric micelles in general because they are much less discrete than polymeric micelles in terms of structure and assembling behavior. This is due to the larger entropy loss for the micellar structure formation from random and alternating copolymers than from graft and block copolymers.

As shown in Figure 11.7 using an AB type block copolymer, a micellar structure forms if one segment of the block copolymer can provide enough interchain cohesive interactions in a certain solvent. Most basic and applied studies of polymeric micelles have been done with AB or ABA type block copolymers because the close relationship between micelle-forming behavior and structures of polymers can be more easily evaluated with AB or ABA type block copolymers than with graft or multisegmented block copolymers.

Drugs can be incorporated into polymeric micelles both by chemical conjugation and physical entrapment. They can be incorporated into both the inner core and the outer shell, but the inner core is considered a more appropriate site for drug incorporation because possible interactions between the incorporated drug molecules or between the drug and the outer shell segment of the block copolymer may lead to intermicellar aggregation. The presence of drugs in the outer shell inhibits the separation of functionality that will be described later in this section.

Attractive interactions in the inner core utilized as the driving force of micelle formation are hydrophobic, electrostatic, π-π interactions, and hydrogen bonding. Most commonly, hydrophobic drugs are incorporated to the micelle inner core by hydrophobic interactions, since most drug molecules contain hydrophobic moieties in their structures even if they are water-soluble. Most polymeric micelle drug carrier systems were studied using hydrophobic interactions for drug incorporation. A few studies involved electrostatic interactions for DNA or protein incorporation.[36,37]

Polymeric micelles possess several advantages as drug carrier systems. Table 11.1 summarizes them. Polymeric micelles are of suitable size for drug targeting. Their diameters range from 10 to 100 nm. This range is suitable for long-term circulation in the blood. The large diameter allows them to escape from renal filtration. Even if the molecular weight of the constituting chains is lower than the molecular weight critical for renal filtration, these polymer chains can escape from the renal excretion by forming micellar structures that have diameters larger than the critical size for renal filtration.

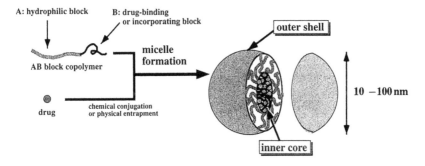

FIGURE 11.7 Polymeric micelle drug carrier system.

TABLE 11.1

Benefits of Polymeric Micelles as Drug Carriers for Drug Targeting

Appropriate size: 10 nm < diameter < 200 nm
Excretion as single polymer chain
Stable micelle formation in physiological environments
Separated functionality:

⎧ inner core   ⟶   drug incorporation ⟶   pharmacological activitiy
⎩ outer shell ⟶   interactions with biocomponents ⟶   delivery to target

Polymeric micelles are formed by intermolecular noncovalent interactions in an equilibrium with a single polymer chain form. All the polymer chains can be released as single polymer chains from the micelles over a long period to result in complete excretion from the renal route if the polymer chains have molecular weights lower than the critical values for renal filtration. This is an advantage of polymeric micelles over conventional PHPMA systems that required small molecular weights to ensure excretion from the renal route because PHPMA is not biodegradable, even though larger molecular weight PHPMA showed higher accumulation[38] at tumors by evading renal excretion.

Polymeric micelles are very stable molecular assemblies. This stability has static and dynamic aspects.[39-41] Static stability is described as an equilibrium constant between a single polymer chain and the micelle structure, or more conveniently by critical micelle concentration (cmc). Generally, polymeric micelles show very low cmc values,[42] these values are much smaller than typical cmc values of micelles formed from low molecular weight surfactants. Dynamic stability is characterized by low dissociation rates of micelles, and may be more important than static stability for *in vivo* drug delivery in physiological environments where metabolism, excretion, and interactions with biological factors (e.g., cells, proteins, and lipids) can destroy micellar structures. Low dissociation rates allow polymeric micelles to maintain their structures long enough to accomplish delivery to targets. The structural stability of polymeric micelles stated above is an important key for *in vivo* delivery in micellar form while eliminating the possible contributions of single polymer chains to drug delivery.

Many factors must be favorably incorporated in highly effective drug delivery systems. In the conventional polymer–drug conjugate systems, monomer units interfere with the functions of other monomer units in random copolymers. In contrast, with polymeric micelles, the required functions for drug delivery can be distinctly shared by the structurally separated segments of the block copolymer. The outer shell is responsible for interactions with biocomponents such as proteins and cells. These interactions may determine pharmacokinetic behavior and biodistribution of drugs. Therefore, *in vivo* delivery of drugs may be controlled by the outer shell segment independently of the inner core that expresses pharmacological activities. This heterogeneous structure is more effective for highly functionalized carrier systems than conventional polymeric carrier systems.

The differences between polymeric micelles and macromolecular assemblies made from random copolymers are worth mentioning. Sunamoto and Akiyoshi et al.[43-45] reported macromolecular assemblies made from pullulan randomly substituted with hydrophobic cholesterol moieties. Their system was made from random copolymers. They called these assemblies *nanoassociates*. The utility of these nano-associates for drug delivery was also examined. Akiyoshi et al. showed formation of associates from ca. polymer chains with diameters of 20 to 30 nm and incorporated a hydrophobic drug and several proteins.[43,44] *In vivo* delivery data have not yet been reported.

Nanoassociates differ from polymeric micelles in architecture of assembly. Nanoassociates were found to contain multiple (from 10 to 14) hydrophobic domains (cores) per particle,[45] while polymeric micelles have only one core per particle. Little is known about the advantages and disadvantages of nanoassociates as compared with polymeric micelles for drug delivery.

Ringsdorf et al.[46,47] reported the first application of polymeric micelles to drug carrier systems in 1984. A sulfidoderivative of cyclophosphamide (an anticancer drug analogue) was conjugated to lysine residues of poly(ethylene glycol)–poly(L-lysine) block copolymer. Since the sulfidoderivative of cyclophosphamide was hydrophilic, palmitic acid was also introduced as a hydrophobic component to the lysine residues of the block copolymer. Although micelle formation of this polymer–drug conjugate was suggested from data of dye solubilization experiments, formation of micellar structures was not confirmed by more direct methods such as laser light scattering or gel permeation chromatography. Ringsdorf et al. reported sustained release of the conjugated drug from the block copolymer, and attributed the decrease in the release rate to a depot effect of the hydrophobic micelle inner core. While they suggested polymeric micelle might serve as drug carriers from the viewpoint of mimicking functions of natural lipoproteins, their study was limited to the *in vitro* stage.

Kabanov et al.[48] reported an increase in activity *in vivo* of a neuroleptic drug (haloperidol) physically associated with a polymeric amphiphile (Pluronic® P-85, a poly(propylene oxide)–poly(ethylene oxide) block copolymer) coupled to a specific antibody. This is the first example of enhancement of drug activity *in vivo* by polymeric micelles. The reason for this enhancement of efficacy may be an increase in the amount of drug delivered to targets due to drug targeting or an increase in permeability of the drug through biological membranes produced by the polymeric amphiphile. Uptake of a model drug by brain microvessel endothelial cells increased in the presence of Pluronic P-85 at concentrations lower than its critical micelle concentration.[49] This indicates that Pluronic may increase the permeability of biological membranes by working as single chain (non-micelle-forming) surfactant. They also reported[50] that Pluronic circumvented multidrug resistance against anticancer drugs *in vitro* by changing uptake amounts and subcellular distribution of drug inside the resistant cells or inhibiting cellular functions for multidrug resistance expression. They also reported[51] that Pluronic enhanced *in vivo* anticancer activity of anthracycline drugs (adriamycin and epirubicin) against solid tumors. This is an innovative application of synthetic polymers for chemotherapy other than selective drug delivery to the target.

Yokoyama, Okano, and Kataoka et al. designed polymeric micelle systems using poly(ethylene glycol)–poly(amino acid) block copolymers in the late 1980s with a clear focus on selective delivery to the target by the carrier system. Thereafter, Yokoyama and Okano et al. developed thermoresponsive polymeric micelle systems. These are briefly explained in the following sections.

In the 1980s, studies of polymeric micelle drug carrier systems were done only by the three research groups named above. In the 1990s, a substantial increase in research activity by many research groups was reported in a large number of publications.[52-61] In some papers,[62-64] polymeric micelles were studied as nanospheres, nanoparticles, or nanoparticulates. The two-phase structure of the inner core and the outer shell formed from block or graft copolymers must be classified as a polymeric micelle even though the kinetic constant from the micellar structure into the single polymer chain is zero due to a kinetically frozen inner core.[65]

11.4.2 TARGETING OF AN ANTITUMOR DRUG TO SOLID TUMOR

Yokoyama, Okano, Kataoka et al.[66-75] studied passive targeting of an anticancer drug, adriamycin (doxorubicin), to solid tumors with a polymeric micelle system. The molecular design of their system is shown in Figure 11.8. Adriamycin (ADR) was chemically conjugated to aspartic acid residues of poly(ethylene glycol)–poly(aspartic acid) block copolymer by amide bond formation. The poly(ethylene glycol) (PEG) segment is hydrophilic, while the ADR-substituted poly(aspartic acid) chain is hydrophobic. Therefore, the obtained drug–block copolymer conjugate (PEG–P(Asp(ADR))) formed micellar structures due to its amphiphilic character with the ADR-substituted poly(aspartic acid) segment as the inner core and the PEG segment as the outer shell of the micelle. In the second step, ADR was incorporated into the inner core by physical entrapment utilizing hydrophobic and π-π interactions with the chemically conjugated ADR molecules. As a result, polymeric micelles containing the chemically conjugated and physically entrapped ADR in the inner core were obtained with the PEG outer shell phase.

Dramatic enhancement of antitumor activity was obtained by incorporation of ADR into a polymeric micelle system.[75] Figure 11.9 shows *in vivo* antitumor activity of the polymeric micelles containing both the chemically conjugated ADR and the physically conjugated ADR against murine colon adenocarcinoma.[26] For free ADR, only the maximum tolerated dose (10 mg/kg body weight) provided considerable inhibition effects of tumor growth; however, a decrease of tumor volume was never seen. For the polymeric micelles, a rapid decrease in tumor volume was observed in two doses (20 and 10 mg physically entrapped ADR/kg of body weight), and the tumors completely disappeared in all treated mice after day 21. All the treated mice survived over 60 days, while control mice were dead on around day 20. A subsequent dose (5 mg/kg) also produced considerable inhibition of tumor growth. Such great enhancement of antitumor activity is rarely seen in studies using various types of drug carriers. All these results clearly show that polymeric micelles appear promising for anticancer drug targeting.

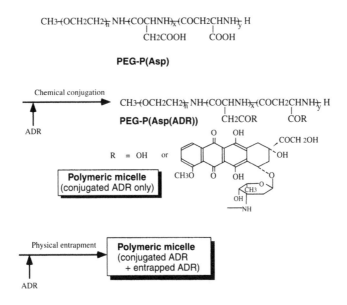

FIGURE 11.8 Chemical structure of polymeric micelle containing adriamycin (ADR).

Physically entrapped ADR played a major role in antitumor activity.[74] Little inhibition of tumor growth was observed with the polymeric micelle containing only the chemically conjugated ADR without the physically entrapped ADR. The antitumor activity of the polymeric micelles is considered to result from highly selective delivery of the physically entrapped ADR to tumors since the polymeric micelles accumulate selectively at tumor sites by ^{14}C-benzylamine labeling on PEG-P(Asp(ADR)) block copolymer. As shown in Figure 11.10, the physically entrapped ADR was delivered to the solid tumor site at much higher concentrations than free

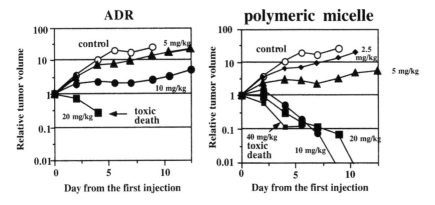

FIGURE 11.9 *In vivo* antitumor activity of free adriamycin (ADR) and polymeric micelle containing ADR.

ADR. Furthermore, the observed time profile with the peak concentration 24 h after intravenous injection and retention of this high concentration for longer periods post-injection indicates passive delivery by the EPR effect.

On the other hand, accumulation of the physically entrapped ADR in the polymeric micelle was the same as or lower than free ADR in normal organs and tissues. As a result of this contrast of accumulation between tumors and normal organs, highly selective delivery to the tumor with the polymeric micelle was obtained. Table 11.2 summarizes the biodistribution of polymeric micelles labeled by physically entrapped ADR. The physically entrapped ADR to accumulated at much higher levels than intact ADR. High accumulation ratios of tumor/heart and tumor/muscle were also obtained from this experiment using physical ADR labeling. These results clearly proved that the polymeric micelle carrier system selectively delivered anticancer drugs to solid tumor sites by utilizing the EPR effect and dramatically enhanced activity of the incorporated antitumor drug.

Although adriamycin shows some hydrophobic properties, it is still water-soluble. The demand for solubilization of water-insoluble drugs is strong for medical chemotherapy, particularly for cancer chemotherapy, since many new and potent anticancer drugs such as camptothecin and taxol are water insoluble or barely water-soluble. The incorporation of a water-insoluble anticancer agent, KRN-5500 (KRN), into polymeric micelles was studied.[76,77] Incorporation of water-insoluble drugs into polymeric micelles is considered more difficult than incorporating water-soluble drugs, because unentrapped water-insoluble drugs may co-precipitate with block copolymers. By choosing an appropriate structure of block copolymer, the water-insoluble KRN was successfully incorporated into polymeric micelles.[76] The polymeric micelle method showed higher antitumor activity than KRN injected in the conventional formulation. The polymeric micelle combination did not show toxic side effects,[77] while KRN in the conventional formulation showed severe side effects probably due to toxicities of organic solvents and surfactants used to dissolve KRN for intravenous injection. This indicates that polymeric micelle carrier systems are strong possibilities for drug targeting and are very effective for dissolving water-

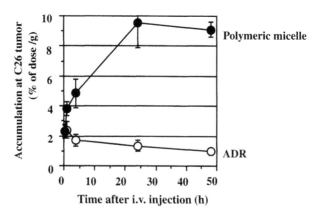

FIGURE 11.10 Enhanced accumulation of polymeric micelle at solid tumor.

TABLE 11.2
Enhanced Accumulation of Ratios Between Tumor and Normal Organs

Sample	Accumulation Ratio [a]	
	Tumor Muscle	Tumor Heart
Polymeric micelle	13.0 ± 7.1	6.2 ± 1.1
	19.0 ± 5.1	9.0 ± 0.6
ADR	1.4 ± 0.3	1.3 ± 0.2
	1.8 ± 0.4	2.0 ± 0.4

[a] Upper values, 24 h; lower values, 48 h after i.v. injection.
Values are shown by mean ± S.D., n = 3 or 4.

insoluble drugs for intravenous injection without causing toxic side effects. This success will expand the applications of polymeric micelle drug carrier systems to a variety of drugs, especially water-insoluble or barely water-soluble drugs.

11.4.3 THERMORESPONSIVE POLYMERIC MICELLES

In the previous section I explained a successful example of a polymeric micelle system containing the anticancer drug, adriamycin. Selective cytotoxic activity of the drug to tumor cells was obtained by a slow drug release rate that matched well to the time period required for delivery to solid tumor sites through the bloodstream. This drug release rate from the polymeric micelle achieved selective delivery to the target by avoiding a considerable amount of drug release during circulation in the bloodstream. This drug release, however, was not site-specific at solid tumor sites.

If the anticancer drug is released selectively at solid tumor sites from the polymeric micelle carriers, the therapeutic index must be raised by decreasing drug release in the bloodstream and by increasing delivery amounts of anticancer drug to tumors. From this perspective, Yokoyama and Okano et al.[78-83] designed a multitargeting anticancer drug system using thermoresponsive polymeric micelles. Multitargeting is the combination of two or more targeting methodologies to increase targeting selectivity. The drug targeting methodologies include selective delivery to therapeutic sites and selective drug release and/or activation at the therapeutic sites. By multiplying selectivities of each targeting methodology, spatial targeting selectivity can be raised. Furthermore, the timing and duration of drug action can be controlled. To design a multitargeting system to deliver anticancer drugs, we have chosen a combination of thermoresponsive polymeric micelles and local hyperthermia. After the polymeric micelles are delivered to tumor sites, local hyperthermia is applied. At the elevated temperature, the anticancer drug retained in the polymeric micelles is released by this temperature stimulus to express cytotoxic action to tumor cells. Furthermore, tumor cells are damaged more than normal cells by the elevated temperature. Thus, tumors are attacked by the selective cytotoxic activity of drugs and selective hyperthermia.

A thermoresponsive polymeric micelle is formed from block copolymers composed of a thermoresponsive block and a hydrophobic block. The thermoresponsive block forms the outer shell, while the hydrophobic block forms the inner core that incorporates drugs. A thermoresponsive polymer poly(N-isopropylacrylamide) chain is used a block for the outer shell, as illustrated in Figure 11.11. Poly(N-isopropylacrylamide) (PIPAAm) is known to exhibit phase transition at 32°C, and has been utilized for controlled release and intelligent materials. The phase transition temperature can be adjusted to an appropriate temperature (around 39°C) for this multitargeting system by introduction of hydrophilic comonomer, N,N-dimethylacrylamide. The inner core of the polymeric micelle is made of hydrophobic polymer blocks. Poly(butyl methacrylate) is used[78,79] for the inner core hydrophobic block because this polymer is considered to possess enough hydrophobicity to incorporate the hydrophobic drug and enough chain flexibility to exhibit substantial structural change when the outer thermoresponsive block shows phase transition. Alternatively, biodegradable poly(DL-lactide) is used[80,82] as the hydrophobic block for the inner core.

When temperature is raised above the transition temperature of the outer shell block, the outer shell is dehydrated, as illustrated in Figure 11.11(a). Drug is considered to be released upon heating above the transition temperature by two possible mechanisms, as illustrated in Figure 11(b).

The inner hydrophobic core phase is separated from the outer PIPAAm phase below the transition temperature. Upon heating above the transition temperature, the outer shell becomes hydrophobic and miscible with the inner core. The dehydrated outer shell polymer block is still lower in hydrophobicity than the inner core polymer block. The hydrophobicity of the inner core is lowered by this phase mixing with the less hydrophobic PIPAAm block, and accordingly hydrophobic drug molecules are located in a less hydrophobic atmosphere above the phase transition temperature than the inner core below the phase transition temperature. In general, drug release rates from polymeric materials are determined by diffusion coefficient of drug molecules in the polymeric materials and partition coefficient of drug molecules between the polymeric materials and aqueous phase outside the materials. The less hydrophobic atmosphere around drug molecules increases drug release rates by increasing drug partition in the aqueous phase. Therefore, the less hydrophobic polymeric materials incorporating hydrophobic drugs release drugs at higher rates. Thus, drug release can be enhanced by the lowered hydrophobicity around drug molecules above the transition temperature.

The second possible mechanism is illustrated in Figure 11.11(b)(2). Upon heating above the transition temperature, the outer shell aggregates. The inner core undergoes structural distortion upon this aggregation since the inner core polymer blocks are chemically connected to the aggregated outer shell polymer blocks. Due to the distortion, water enters the inner core and produces water channels for drug

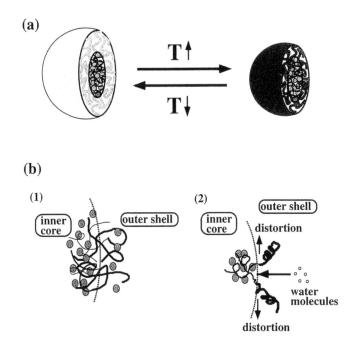

FIGURE 11.11 Thermoresponsive polymeric micelles for drug targeting. (a) Structure with drug-incorporating inner core and thermoresponsive outer shell. (b) Two possible mechanisms for enhanced drug release above transition temperature. (1) Phase mixing between inner core and outer shell. Drugs are located in a more hydrophilic atmosphere and/or moved to outer shell. (2) Aggregation of outer shell polymer segment induces mechanical distortion on inner core polymer segment. Water molecules move into inner core through the channel made by this distortion.

release. We have not determined experimentally which mechanism enhances drug release upon heating above the transition temperature.

The thermoresponsive drug delivery of the polymeric micelle formed from poly(butylmethacrylate)-poly(N-isopropylacrylamide) (PBMA–PIPAAm) block copolymer was examined.[81-83] First, hydrophobicity (polarity) of the inner core was measured using pyrene as a fluorescence probe. Upon heating above the phase transition temperature (32°C), the inner core was found to decrease its hydrophobicity. This decrease can be explained by both the mechanisms described above. Above the transition temperature, drug release was induced, as shown in Figure 11.12. Below the phase transition temperature, no drug release was observed after the initial burst up to 10% of incorporated adriamycin. In contrast, drug was rapidly released above the transition temperature. This polymeric micelle showed lower *in vitro* cytotoxic activity below the transition temperature and higher activity than adriamycin above the transition temperature. Another thermoresponsive polymeric micelle

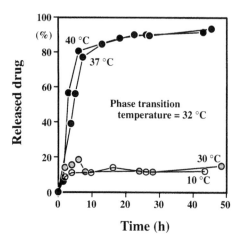

FIGURE 11.12 Thermoresponsive drug release from polymeric micelles.

incorporating adriamycin was obtained from biodegradable poly(IPAAm-*co*-DMAAm)–block–poly(DL-lactide) showing phase transition at 40°C that is preferable for multitargeting systems. This polymeric micelle[82] also showed enhanced drug release and cytotoxic activity at 42.5°C as compared with those at 37°C. These results indicate effective multitargeting systems with thermoresponsive polymeric micelles are very promising.

REFERENCES

1. Yokoyama, M. and Okano, T., Targetable drug carriers: present status and a future perspective, *Adv. Drug Delivery Rev.*, 21, 77, 1996.
2. Sugiyama Y., Importance of pharmacokinetic considerations in the development of drug delivery systems, *Adv. Drug. Delivery Rev.*, 19, 333, 1996.
3. Takakura, Y., Maruyama, K., and Yokoyama, M., Passive targeting of drug (in Japanese), *Drug Delivery Sys.*, 14, 425, 1999.
4. Matsumura, Y. and Maeda, H., A new concept for macromolecular therapeutics in cancer chemotherapy: mechanism of tumoritropic accumulation of proteins and the antitumor agent SMANCS, *Cancer Res.*, 46, 6387, 1986.
5. Maeda, H., Seymour, L. W., and Miyamoto, Y., Conjugates of anticancer agents and polymers: advantages of macromolecular therapeutics *in vivo*, *Bioconjugate Chem.*, 3, 351, 1992.
6. Maeda, H. et al., Antitumor effect of SMANCS on rat mammary tumor induced by 7,12 dimethylbenz[a]anthracene, *Cancer Res.*, 52, 1013, 1992.
7. Dvorak, H.F., Nagy, J.A., and Dvorak, A.M., Structure of solid tumors and their vasculature: implications for therapy with monoclonal antibodies, *Cancer Cells*, 3, 77, 1991.
8. Jain, R.K., Delivery of novel therapeutic agents in tumors: physiological barriers and strategies, *J. Natl. Cancer Inst.*, 81, 570, 1989.
9. Jain, R.K., Transport of molecules in the tumor interstitium: a review, *Cancer Res.*, 47, 3039, 1987.

10. Dvorak, H.F. et al., Pathways of macromolecular tracer transport across venules and small veins, *Lab. Invest.*, 47, 596, 1992.

11. Jain, R.K., Vascular permeability in a human tumor xenograft: molecular weight dependence and cutoff size, *Cancer Res.*, 55, 3752, 1995.

12. Jain, R.K., Microvascular permeability and interstitial penetration of sterically stabilized (stealth) liposomes in a human tumor xenograft, *Cancer Res.*, 54, 3352, 1994.

13. Jain, R.K., Transport of molecules across tumor vasculature, *Cancer Metastasis Rev.*, 6, 559, 1987.

14. Dvorak, H.F. et al., Vascular permeability factor/vascular endothelial growth factor, microvascular hyperpermeability, and angiogenesis, *Am. J. Pathol.*, 146, 1029, 1995.

15. Dvorak, H.F. et al., Vascular permeability factor, fibrin, and the pathogenesis of tumor stroma formation, *Ann. NY Acad. of Sci.*, 4, 667, 101, 1992.

16. Folkman, J., Clinical applications of research on angiogenesis, *New Engl. J. Med.*, 333, 1757, 1995.

17. Folkman, J., Angiogenesis in cancer, vascular, rheumatoid and other disease, *Nature Med.*, 1, 27, 1995.

18. Dvorak, H.F. et al., Tumor cells secrete a vascular permeability factor that promotes accumulation of ascites fluid, *Science*, 219, 983, 1983.

19. Ferrara, N. and Henzel, W.J., Pituitary follicular cells secrete a novel heparin-binding growth factor specific for vascular endothelial cells, *Biochem. Biophys. Res. Commun.*, 161, 851, 1989.

20. Huang, L. et al., Effect of liposome size on the circulation time and intraorgan distribution of amphipathic poly(ethylene glycol)-containing liposomes, *Biochim. Biophys. Acta*, 1190, 99,1994.

21. Takakura, Y. and Hashida, M., Macromolecular carrier systems for targeted drug delivery: pharmacokinetic consideration on biodistribution, *Pharm. Res.*, 13, 820, 1996.

22. Davis, S.S., The organ distribution and circulation time of intravenously injected colloidal carriers sterically stabilized with a block copolymer — Poloxamine 908. *Life Sci.*, 40, 367, 1987.

23. Ringsdorf, H., Structure and properties of pharmacologically active polymers., *J. Polym. Sci. Symp.*, 51, 135, 1975.

24. Putnam, D. and Kopecek, J., Polymer conjugates with anticancer activity, *Adv. Polymer Sci.*, 122, 55- (1995)

25. Duncan, R., Dimitrijevic, S., and Evagorou, E.G., The role of polymer conjugates in the diagnosis and treatment of cancer, *S.T.P. Pharma Sci.*, 6, 237, 1996.

26. Rihova, B., et al., Biocompatibility of N-(2-hydroxypropyl) methacrylamide copolymers containing adriamycin, *Biomaterials*, 10, 335, 1989.

27. Duncan, R. et al., Soluble, crosslinked N-(2-hydroxypropyl) methacrylamide copolymers as potential drug carriers. 2. Effect of molecular weight on blood clearance and body distribution in the rat after intravenous administration. Distribution of unfractionated copolymer after intraperitoneal, subcutaneous or oral administration, *J. Controlled Release*, 4, 253, 1987.

28. Seymour, L. W. et al., Effect of molecular weight of N-(2-hydroxypropyl)methacrylamide copolymers on body distribution and rate of excretion after subcutaneous, intraperitoneal, and intravenous administration to rats, *J. Biomed. Mater. Res.*, 21, 1341, 1987.

29. De Duve, C., Commentary: lysosomotropic agents, *Biochem. Pharmacol.*, 23, 2495, 1974.

30. Rihova, B. and Kopecek, J., Biological properties of targetable poly[N-(2-hydroxypropyl)methacrylamide] antibody conjugates, *J. Controlled Release*, 2, 289, 1985.

31. Duncan, R. et al., Evaluation of protein-N-(2-hydroxypropyl) methacrylamide copolymer conjugates as targetable drug carriers 2. Body distribution of conjugates containing transferrin, anti-transferrin receptor antibody or anti-Thy 1.2 antibody and effectiveness of transferrin-containing daunomycin conjugates against mouse L 1210 leukaemia *in vivo*, *J. Controlled Release*, 18, 25, 1992.

32. Duncan, R. et al., Fate of N-(2-hydroxypropyl)methacrylamide copolymers with pendant galactosamine residues after intravenous administration to rats, *Biochim. Biophys. Acta*, 880, 62, 1986.

33. Duncan, R. et al., Macromolecular prodrugs for use in targeted cancer chemotherapy: melpharan covalently coupled to N-(2-hydroxypropyl)methacrylamide copolymers., *J. Controlled Release*, 16, 121, 1991.

34. Ulbrich, K. et al., Solution properties of drug carriers based on poly[N-(2-hydroxypropyl)methacrylamide] containing biodegradable bonds, *Makromol. Chem.*, 188, 1261, 1987.

35. Tuzar, Z. and Kratochvil, P., Block and graft copolymer micelles in solution, *Adv. Colloid Interfacial Sci.*, 6, 201, 1976.

36. Katayose, S. and Kataoka. K., Remarkable increase in nuclease resistance of plasmid DNA through supramolecular assembly with poly(ethylene glycol) poly(L9lysine) block copolymer, *J. Pharm. Sci.*, 87, 160, 1998.

37. Harada, A. and Kataoka, K., Novel polyion complex micelles entrapping enzyme molecules in the core preparation of narrowly distributed micelles from lysozyme and poly(ethylene glycol)-poly(aspartic acid) block copolymer in aqueous medium, *Macromolecules*, 31, 288, 1998.

38. Seymour, L.W. et al., Influence of molecular weight on passive tumour accumulation of a soluble macromolecular drug, *Eur. J. Cancer*, 31A, 766, 1995.

39. Riess, G. et al., Investigation of polystyrene-poly(ethylene oxide) block copolymer micelle formation in organic and aqueous solutions by nonradiative energy transfer experiments, *Macromolecules*, 27, 1210 1994.

40. Wang, Y. et al., Exchange of chains between micelles of labeled polystyrene-block-poly(oxyethylene) as monitored by nonradiative singlet energy transfer, *Macromolecules*, 28, 904, 1995.

41. Desjardins, A. and Eisenberg, A., Colloidal properties of block ionomers. 1. Characterization of reverse micelles of styrene-b-methacrylate diblocks by size-exclusion chromatography, *Macromolecules*, 24, 5779, 1991.

42. Winnik, M. A. et al., Poly(styrene-ethylene oxide) block copolymer micelle formation in water: a fluorescence probe study, *Macromolecules*, 24, 1033, 1991.

43. Akiyoshi, K. et al., Self-assembled hydrogel nanoparticle of hydrophobized polysaccharide: complexation and stabilization of soluble proteins, in *Biomedical Functions and Biotechnology of Natural and Artificial Polymers*, Yalpani, M., Ed., ATL Press, Shrewsbury, MA, 1996, p. 115.

44. Nishikawa, T., Akiyoshi, K., and Sunamoto, J., Macromolecular complexation between bovine serum albumin and the self-assembled hydrogel nanoparticle of hydrophobized polysaccharides, *J. Am. Chem. Soc.*, 118, 6110, 1996.

45. Akiyoshi, K. and Sunamoto, J., Supramolecular assembly of hydrophobized polysaccharides, *Supramolecular Sci.*, 3, 157, 1996.

46. Bader, H., Ringsdorf, H., and Schmidt, B., Water soluble polymers in medicine, *Angew. Chem.*, 123/124, 457, 1984.

47. Ringsdorf, H. et al., Micelle-forming block copolymers: pinocytosis by macrophages and interaction with model membranes, *Makromol. Chem.*, 186, 725, 1985.

48. Kabanov, A.V. et al., The neuroleptic activity of haloperidol increases after its solubilization in surfactant micelles: micelles as microcontainers for drug targeting, *FEBS Lett.*, 258, 343, 1989.

49. Kabanov, A.V. and Alakhov, V.Y., Micelles of amphiphilic block copolymers as vehicles for drug delivery, in *Amphiphilic Block Copolymers: Self Assembly and Applications*, Alexandridis, P. and Lindman, B., Eds., Elsevier, Amsterdam, 1997, p. 1.

50. Kabanov, A. et al., Hypersensitizing effect of Pluronic L61 on cytotoxic activity, transport, and subcellular distribution of doxorubicin in multiple drug-resistant cells, *Cancer Res.*, 56, 3626, 1996.

51. Kabanov, A.V., Anthracycline antibiotics non-covalently incorporated into the block copolymer micelles: *in vivo* evaluation of anti-cancer activity, *Br. J. Cancer*, 74, 1545, 1996.

52. Newman, K.D., Samuel, J., and Kwon, G., Ovalbumin peptide encapsulated in poly(d,l lactic-co-glycolic acid) microspheres is capable of inducing a T helper type 1 immune response, *J. Controlled Release*, 54, 49, 1998.

53. Kwon, G. et al., Polymeric micelles for drug delivery: solubilization and haemolytic activity of amphotericin B, *J. Controlled Release*, 53, 131, 1998.

54. Kwon, G.S. et al., *In vitro* dissociation of antifungal efficacy and toxicity for amphotericin B-loaded poly(ethylene oxide)-block-poly(β-benzyl-L-aspartate) micelles, *J. Controlled Release*, 56, 285, 1998.

55. Rolland, A. et al., New macromolecular carriers for drugs. 1. Preparation and characterization of poly(oxyethylene-b-isoprene-b-oxyethylene) block copolymer aggregates, *J. Appl. Polym. Sci.*, 44, 1195, 1992.

56. Shin, I.L. et al., Methoxy poly(ethylene glycol)/e-caprolactone amphiphilic block copolymeric micelle containing indomethacin 1. Preparation and characterization, *J. Controlled Release*, 51, 1-11, 1998.

57. Feijen, J. et al., A controlled release system for proteins based on poly(ether ester)block copolymers: polymer network characterization, *J. Controlled Release*, 393, 1999.

58. Hoffman, A.S., A hydrophobically-modified bioadhesive polyelectrolyte hydrogel for drug delivery, *J. Controlled Release*, 49, 167, 1997.

59. Davies, S.S., Polylactide-poly(ethylene glycol) copolymers as drug delivery systems 1. Characterization of water dispersible micelle-forming systems, *Langmuir*, 12, 2153, 1996.

60. Trubetskoy, V.S. et al., Block-copolymer of polyethylene glycol and polylysine as a carrier of organic iodine: design of long-circulating particulate contrast medium for x-ray computed tomography, *J. Drug Targeting*, 4, 381, 1997.

61. Piskin, E. et al., Novel PDLLA/PEG copolymer micelles as drug carriers, *J. Biomater. Sci. Polymer Edn.*, 7, 359, 1995.

62. Langer, R. et al., Biodegradable long-circulating nanospheres, *Science*, 28, 1600, 1994.

63. Ha, J.C., Kim, S.Y., and Lee, Y.M., Poly(ethylene oxide)-poly(propylene oxide)–poly(ethylene oxide) ((pluoronic)/poly(ϵ-caprolactone) (PCL) amphiphilic block copolymeric nanospheres I. Preparation and characterization, *J. Controlled Release,* 62, 381, 1995.

64. Verrecchia, T. et al., Non-stealth (poly(lactic acid/albumin)) and stealth (poly(lactic acid-polyethylene glycol)) nanoparticles as injectable drug carriers, *J. Controlled Release*, 36, 49, 1995.

65. Prochazka, K. et al., Time-resolved fluorescence studies on the chain dynamics of naphthalene-labeled polystyrene-block-poly(methacrylic acid) micelles in aqueous media, *Macromolecules*, 25, 454, 1992.

66. Yokoyama, M. et al., Preparation of adriamycin-conjugated poly(ethylene glycol)-poly(aspartic acid) block copolymer. A new type of polymeric anticancer agent, *Die Makromol. Chem. Rapid Commun.*, 8, 431, 1987.

67. Yokoyama, M. et al., Molecular design for missile drug: synthesis of adriamycin conjugated with IgG using poly(ethylene glycol)-poly(aspartic acid) block copolymer as intermediate carrier, *Die Makromol. Chem.*, 190, 2041, 1989.

68. Yokoyama, M. et al., Characterization and anti-cancer activity of micelle-forming polymeric anti-cancer drug, adriamycin-conjugated poly(ethylene glycol)-poly(aspartic acid) block copolymer, *Cancer Res.*, 50, 1693, 1990.

69. Yokoyama, M. et al., Toxicity and antitumor activity against solid tumors of micelle-forming polymeric drug and its extremely long circulation in blood, *Cancer Res.*, 51, 3229, 1991.

70. Kwon, G.S. et al., Enhanced tumor accumulation and prolonged circulation times of micelle-forming poly(ethylene oxide–aspartate) block copolymer–adriamycin conjugates, *J. Controlled Release*, 29, 17, 1994.

71. Kwon, G.S. et al., Block copolymer micelles as vehicles for hydrophobic drugs, *Colloids Surfaces B Biointerfaces*, 2, 429, 1994.

72. Yokoyama, M., et al., Improved synthesis of adriamycin-conjugated poly(ethylene oxide)-poly(aspartic acid) block copolymer and formation of unimodal micellar structure with controlled amount of physically entrapped adriamycin, *J. Controlled Release*, 32, 269, 1994.

73. Kwon, G.S. et al., Physical entrapment of adriamycin in AB block copolymer micelles, *Pharm. Res.*, 12, 192, 1995.

74. Yokoyama, M. et al., Characterization of physical entrapment and chemical conjugation of adriamycin in polymeric micelles and their design for *in vivo* delivery to a solid tumor, *J. Controlled Release*, 50, 79, 1997.

75. Yokoyama, M. et al., Selective delivery of adriamycin to a solid tumor using a polymeric micelle carrier system, *J. Drug Targeting*, 7, 171, 1999.

76. Yokoyama, M. et al., Incorporation of water-insoluble anticancer drug into polymeric micelles and control of their particle size, *J. Controlled Release*, 55, 219, 1998.

77. Matsumura, Y. et al., Reduction of the adverse effects of an antitumor agent, KRN 5500 by incorporation of the drug into polymeric micelles, *Jpn. J. Cancer Res.*, 90, 122, 1999.

78. Chung, J.E. et al., Reversibly thermo-responsive alkyl-terminated poly(N-isopropylacrylamide) core-shell micellar structures, *Colloids Surfaces B Biointerfaces*, 9, 37, 1997.

79. Chung, J.E. et al., Effect of molecular architecture of hydrophobically modified poly(N-isopropylacrylamide) on the formation of thermo-responsive core-shell micellar drug carriers, *J. Controlled Release*, 53, 119, 1998.

80. Kohori, F., Preparation and characterization of thermally responsive block copolymer micelles comprising poly(N-isopropylacrylamide-b-DL-lactide), *J. Controlled Release*, 55, 87, 1998.

81. Chung, J.E. et al., Thermo-responsive drug delivery from polymeric micelles constructed using block copolymers of poly(N-isopropylacrylamide) and poly(butylmethacrylate), *J. Controlled Release*, 62, 115, 1999.

82. Kohori, F. et al., Control of adriamycin cytotoxic activity using thermally responsive polymeric micelles composed of poly(N-isopropylacrylamide-co-N,N-dimethylacrylamide)-b-poly(DL-lactide), *Colloids Surfaces B Biointerfaces*, 16, 195, 1999.

83. Chung, J.E., Yokoyama, M., and Okano, T., Inner core segment design for drug delivery control of thermo-responsive polymeric micelles, *J. Controlled Release*, 65, 93, 2000.

12 Gene Delivery

Tetsuji Yamaoka

CONTENTS

12.1 INTRODUCTION

Transfection of foreign genes into mammalian cells *in vitro* and *in vivo* is the most important technique of gene therapy.[1] More than 75% of the clinical protocols involving gene therapy to date employed viral vectors, such as retroviruses (about 50%), adenoviruses (about 20%), adenoassociated viruses, or pox viruses because of their excellent transgene expression. However, despite their high efficiency *in vitro,* their successful use *in vivo* is often limited by toxicity, immunogenicity, inflammatory properties, limited DNA size, and reproduction problems of the viruses.[1]

    Various nonviral gene carriers are attracting great attention because they are biologically safe and their chemical structures can be designed.[2-4] These nonviral gene carriers possess positively charged groups, and this permits complex formation with DNA and condensation of the DNA coils into globules.

    The most widely studied nonviral gene carrier is the cationic liposome,[3] used in about 20% of clinical trials. The liposomes are accumulated undesirably into the reticuloendothelial systems after systemic injection, resulting in limited *in vivo* applications.[5-7] Polymeric gene carriers also possess cation charges at the side and/or main chains and can condense DNA coils into 10^{-3} to 10^{-4} of their original volume[8] by forming polyion complexes that are conventionally advocated in the field of polymer science.[9-11] In contrast, transgene expression greatly depends on chemical structure and shape, such as the linear or branched structures of the polycations used, suggesting that the formed polyion complex should possess special characteristics for improved gene transfer.

Gene delivery involves control of more complicated factors than the conventional drug delivery system. The introduced gene should pass various barriers before being expressed: passing through the plasma membrane, internalization into cells, inhibited intracellular hydrolysis, controlled intracellular trafficking, and recognition by the transcription factors. Wu et al. reported the pioneering work in *in vitro* gene delivery through receptor-mediated endocytosis, using polycations having targeting ligands against hepatocytes, resulting in the improved uptake of the complexes. This approach was based on a similar strategy established in conventional drug delivery systems. However, base carrier materials with poor efficiency cannot lead to sufficient transgene expression even when the DNA molecules are delivered into the cells. This suggests the importance of the nonviral carrier materials. The interaction of DNA and histone, which is based on a similar mechanism, is a biologically active event and many researchers pay much attention to its function. In contrast, the characteristics of gene carrier/DNA complexes affecting the expression of the transgene have not been studied although the characteristic/function correlation in the complexes is apparently important.

Effective nonviral gene carrier/DNA complexes should achieve well controlled intracellular trafficking and be recognized by transcription factors after entering into the cells; in other words, the complexes should possess supramolecular structures which are biologically active. Recently, it has become clear that the physicochemical characteristics of the DNA/carrier complex functions through these various steps. The well controlled and specialized supramolecular structures of the complexes must be the key factors for gene delivery. Detailed information on the structure/function correlation of the supramolecular complexes would permit further molecular design of novel and effective gene carriers. In this chapter, various gene carriers are reviewed and the effects of the characteristics of supramolecular complexes on gene delivery efficiency will be discussed, with a focus on polymeric gene carriers.

12.2 NONVIRAL GENE CARRIERS

12.2.1 CATIONIC LIPOSOMES

Cationic liposomes are the most widely used nonviral vectors *in vitro* and *in vivo*.[12] A cationic liposome complex with DNA is known as a lipoplex while the complex of a cationic polymer is known as a polyplex. Among cationic compounds with different chemical structures shown in Figure 12.1, 1,2-dioleyloxypropyl-3-trimethylammonium bromide (DOTMA) is the most widely used because of its effective gene expression even *in vivo*.[2,3,13] The size[14] and the hydrophilicity[15] of the lipoplex are important factors for effective gene delivery as well as for the linear polycations described later. In spite of their high efficacy, they exhibit poor biocompatibility, unexpected accumulation into the liver or spleen, and rapid degradation of DNA when injected *in vivo*.

Lew et al. reported the pharmacokinetic analysis of plasmid DNA/cationic lipid complexes injected intravenously in mice by Southern blot analyses and showed that the DNA was rapidly degraded in the bloodstream with a half-life of less than 5 min; the intact DNA was no longer detectable at 1 h post-injection.[16] Serum proteins strongly inhibit the transfer efficiency of the transgene *in vitro* when cationic liposomes are used as carriers, maybe because of the degradation of DNA which is not encapsulated in the liposome membrane by nuclease contained in the serum. In addition, since many lipoplexes are polydisperse in size, charge, and stoichiometry,[17] the effective application *in vivo* is limited to local delivery such as inhalation[5,6] or injection directly into a tumor or tumor-feeding arteries.[7]

Various cationic liposomes with bioderived active ligands on their surfaces were also proposed. For example, fusogenic liposome, which is prepared by fusing

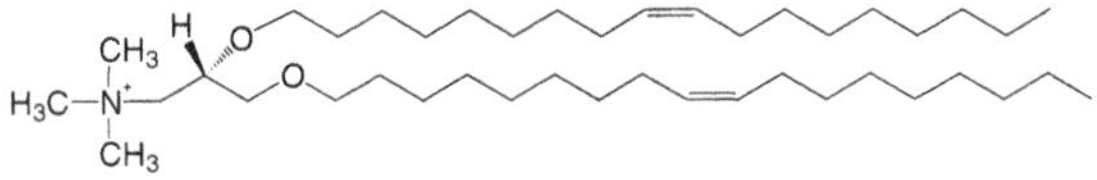

DOTMA [1,2-Dioleyloxypropyl-3-trimethyl ammonium bromide]

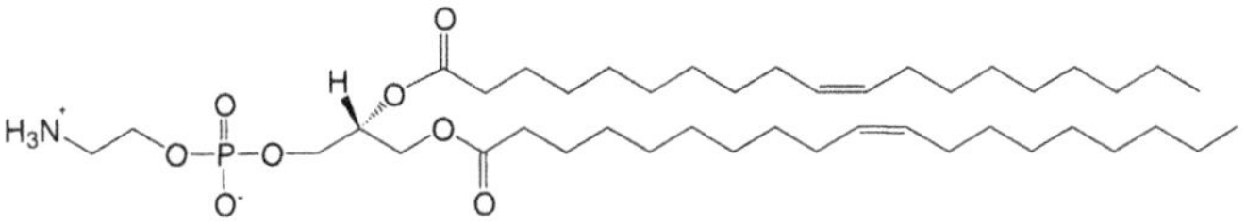

DOPE [Dioleoylphosphatidylethanolamine]

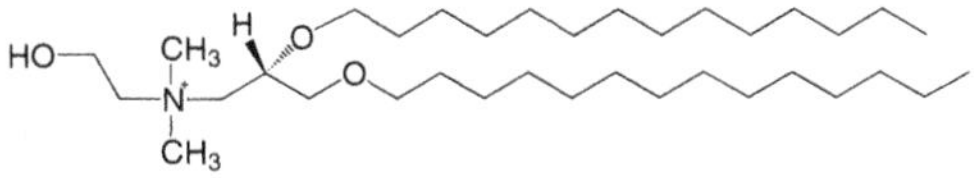

DMRIE [1,2-Dimyristyloxypropyl-3-dimethyl-hydroxyethyl ammonium bromide]

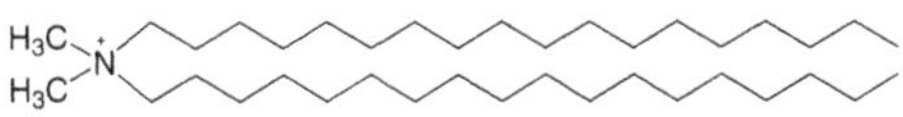

DDAB [Dimethyldioctadecyl ammonium bromide]

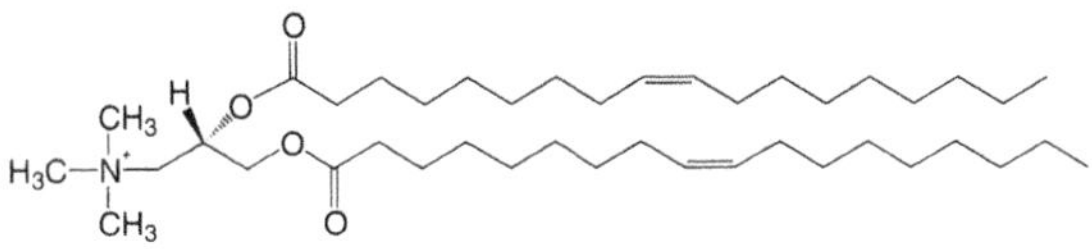

DOTAP [1,2-Dioleoyloxy-3-(trimethylammonio)propane]

FIGURE 12.1 Chemical structures of the compounds used for cationic liposomes.

unilamellar liposomes with UV-inactivated Sendai virus, produces high gene expression with low cytotoxicity *in vitro* even in the presence of 40% FCS in the medium.[18] The DNA encapsulated in the membranous structure of the liposome is strongly protected from the digestion by the nuclease, resulting in excellent expression even in *in vivo* gene transfer.[19]

12.2.2 LINEAR POLYCATIONS

Over the past decade, various cationic polymers have been proposed to act as effective gene carriers *in vitro*. Among them, poly(L-lysine) (PLL) is among the most widely studied polycations because those with various molecular weights are commercially available.[20] Cationic polysaccharides such as diethylaminoethyl–dextran (DEAE–dextran)[21,22] have been utilized in the field of molecular biology. Chitosan[23] was found to be much more effective than DEAE–dextran, and various synthetic polycations such as polyethyleneimine (PEI),[9,11,24-26] polybrene,[27,28] and cationic polymethacrylate derivatives[29,30] were also proposed. Since these polycations have been evaluated separately, little information on the effects of their chemical structures on gene-introducing efficiency has been offered, resulting in difficulty in designing novel carrier polycations.

In our group, various polycations with different chemical structures as shown in Figure 12.2 have been subjected to transfection experiments to determine the required chemical structures of effective polymeric gene carriers. Plasmid DNAs containing functional *lacZ* gene, EGFP gene, or luciferase gene were selected as reporter DNAs and transferred to various types of cells by the osmotic shock procedure reported by Takai et al. (Figure 12.3).[31] The osmotic shock procedure enabled us to analyze only the events following the release of the complexes from the endocytotic vesicles into the cytosols (details will be discussed later).

Agarose gel electrophoresis revealed that every polycation form complexes in a similar fashion, depending on the mixing ratio of polycation and DNA. The sizes of the complexes or their zeta potentials evaluated by dynamic light scattering are also similar, irrespective of polycations used. Despite these similarities, the expression of the transgene greatly depended on the chemical structures of the polycations. For all polycations, no gene expression was observed at the C/A ratio (the ratio of cationic groups of polycations to anionic phosphate groups of DNA) less than 1.0, suggesting the importance of the positively charged complexes that would interact effectively with the negatively charged cell surfaces. The qualitative results in gene expression by the polycations and their characteristic structures are summarized in Table 12.1. These results suggest that polycations having tertiary or quaternary ammonium groups led to high gene expression and those with primary ammonium groups were less efficient, indicating that the dissociation behavior of the cationic groups makes an important contribution to the high levels of gene expression. Only polycations with hydroxyl groups led to effective gene expression. According to these results, highly efficient water-soluble gene carriers would seem to have both dissociated cationic groups and sufficient hydroxyl groups. Although the role of the hydroxyl groups is still uncertain, we are focusing on the fact that the hydrophilic groups of

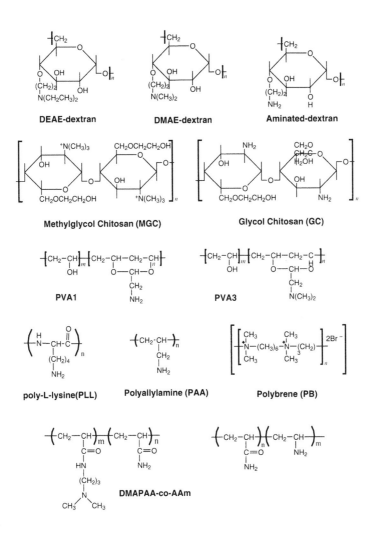

FIGURE 12.2 Chemical structures of polycations used by our group.

polycations strongly maintain the hydrophilic nature of the formed complexes, effectively prevent compaction of the complexes, and allow their disassembling discussed below.

Among the polycations evaluated, PLL and polybrene (PB), the most widely investigated as base polymers for gene carriers, were found to be the least effective. We have attempted to improve the capacity of PLL. Poly(lysine-co-serine), a random copolymer of L-lysine and serine with the unit composition of 3/1 (PLS), was employed as the polycation with hydroxyl groups. The ε-ammonium groups of PLL and PLS were converted into quaternary ammonium groups by their methylation, yielding Poly(N^{ε}-trimethyl-L-lysine) (PtmL) and Poly(N^{ε}-trimethyl-L-lysine-*co*-serine)

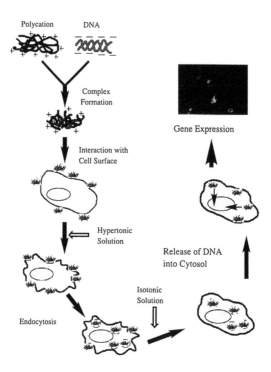

FIGURE 12.3 Mechanism of the osmotic shock procedure for *in vitro* gene transfer.

(PtmLS), respectively.[32] These polycations have similar molecular weights around 20,000 (Figure 12.4). pEGFP-N1 plasmid was transfected into COS-1 cells and the percentage of the cells expressing the EGFP gene was evaluated under a fluorescent microscope. The dependence of the transient expression of the introduced gene using the polypeptides on the C/A ratio is shown in Figure 12.4. PL and PtmL showed no transient expression irrespective of the C/A ratio, suggesting that the imparting of high basicity only to PL is not effective in enhancing transfection efficacy. Slightly enhanced expression was observed in the case of PLS with a C/A ratio around 10; PtmLS induced much higher transgene expression. The percent transient expression was rapidly increased at a C/A ratio of 3.0 which is in a good agreement with the fact that the total charge of the PtmLS/DNA complex became positive at C/A > 3.0.

The big difference in the efficacy of PLS and PtmLS indicates an important role of the quaternary ammonium groups in the presence of the hydrophilic residues. The amount of FITC-labeled DNA taken up by cells was in the range of 0.6 to 1.9 ng/10⁴ cells irrespective of the used polypeptides, suggesting that the difference in transient expression was determined at some point following the internalization of the complexes into the cells. When these complexes are subjected to *in vitro* transcription/translation using rabbit reticulocyte lysate, the amount of expressed luciferase for PLS and PtmLS were 3.48 and 2.31 times larger than PL and PtmL, re-

TABLE 12.1
Transient Expression of pCH110 Plasmid DNA Introduced into COS-1 Cells Using Various Polycations

Polycation	Main Chain	Hydrophilic Group	Cationic Group	Expression
DEAE-dextran			$-N(C_2H_5)_2$	Excellent
DMAE-dextran			$-N(CH_3)_2$	High
Aminated-dextran	Polysaccharide	-OH	$-NH_2$	Slight
MGC			$-N(CH_3)_2$	High
GC			$-NH_2$	Slight
PLL		—	$-NH_2$	None
DMAPAA-AAm		$-CONH_2$	$-N(CH_3)_2$	Low
AAm-NH₂	CH_2-CH_n	$-CONH_2$	$-NH_2$	None
PAA	$\mid$ x or $(CH_2-CXH)_n$	—	$-NH_2$	None
PVA-1		$-OH$	$-NH_2$	None
PVA-3		$-OH$	$-N(CH_3)_2$	Excellent
PB	$R-N(CH_3)_{2n}$	—	$-N(CH_3)_2$	None

spectively, indicating that the serine residues improve the transcription of the complexes, possibly because of their hydrophilic nature. Erbacher et al. also described the low efficiency of the PLL and the increased efficiency of gluconoylated PLL, and concluded that the decreased strength of the electrostatic interaction between DNA and gluconoylated PLL is a crucial factor in inducing high gene expression.

12.2.3 BRANCHED POLYCATIONS

The branched structures of gene carriers are considered to affect gene expression.[9,11,24-26] Plank et al. showed the efficacy of the branched structure,[33] while Ohashi et al. reported more efficient *in vivo* gene transfer using linear PEI than transfer using branched polyethyleneimine.[34] These results conflict with the viewpoint of the importance of the branched structure, and further research is necessary.

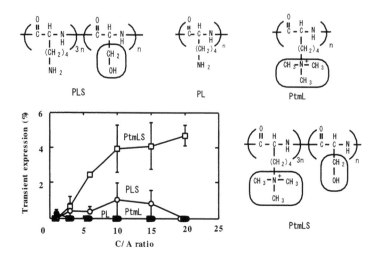

FIGURE 12.4 Transient expression of pEGFP gene introduced into COS-1 cells by the osmotic shock procedure using (●) PL, (○) PLS, (■) PtmL, and (□) PtmLS.

In 1993, Szoka and his coworkers proposed hyperbranched polyamidoamine (PAMAM) cascade polymers, a well-defined class of dendritic polymers from methyl acrylate and ethylenediamine, as novel gene carrier.[10] They successfully achieved very high levels of gene expression using "fractured dendrimers" that were significantly degraded by heat treatment at the amide linkage compared to the expression of intact dendrimers.[35] The great efficiency seems to be based on their high buffering capacity, which results in the rupture of the endocytotic vesicles and accelerates the DNA release from the endosome to the cytosol.[36]

12.2.4 SELF-ASSEMBLY OF BLOCK COPOLYMER/DNA COMPLEXES

Wolfert et al. reported transgene expression using AB type hydrophilic-cationic block copolymers such as poly(ethylene glycol)-poly(L-lysine) and poly-*N*-(2-hydroxypropyl) methacrylamide-poly(trimethylammonioethyl methacrylate chloride) block copolymers.[37] These copolymers spontaneously form a complex with DNA via the cationic segment resulting in small aggregates with sizes around 100 nm, which are stabilized by the hydrophilic segments poly(ethylene glycol) (PEG) or poly-*N*-(2-hydroxypropyl) methacrylamide, covering their surfaces. The extended structures of the complexes formed revealed high gene expression. Other characteristics of the PEG-PLL/DNA complexes, such as diameter, interexchange reaction with other polyanions, and stability of the DNA structure were also reported.[38,39]

12.3 FATE OF INTRODUCED GENES

The mechanism of gene transfer is thought to follow the general endocytotic process shown in Figure 12.5. A variety of polycations and other carriers condense DNA through electrostatic interaction. The interactions between the complexes and the cells are normally based on the electrostatic attractive forces between the positive charges of the complexes and the negative charges of the sialic acid at the cell surface. The attached complexes are internalized into the cells and usually localized in the endocytotic vesicles.

The vesicles are then transported in the cells as the internal pH of the vesicles gradually decreases to about 5.5 and fuse with the lysosomes, resulting in secondary lysosomes at which the incorporated DNA is hydrolyzed by the lysosomal enzymes. Even in the case of receptor-mediated endocytosis, the internalized DNA molecules are encapsulated in the endocytotic vesicles.[40] Therefore, the release of the DNA from the vesicle to the cytoplasm during this process is important for preventing DNA from hydrolysis. Next, the released DNA must be transported to the nucleus by some means and recognized by the transcript factors. This recognition may require the disassembly of the complex to release naked DNAs or somewhat specialized structures of the complexes by which the transcription of the DNA in the complexes is allowed. This transcription is the most important step for gene delivery, which is definitely different from conventional DDS for low molecular weight drugs such as antibiotics or antitumor agents. In the case of conventional DDSs, controlling the drug release rate based on the hydrolysis rate of the covalent bonding is effective and

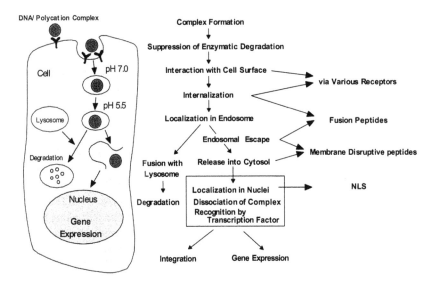

FIGURE 12.5 Proposed mechanisms of gene transfer by nonviral gene carriers.

the released drugs can diffuse to the site of action, while the DNA/carrier complexes should be controlled in the adequate structures for effective gene expression. Several research groups are investigating the characteristics of the complexes, the releasing mechanism of the naked DNA, and intracellular trafficking.

12.3.1 PHYSICOCHEMICAL PROPERTIES OF COMPLEXES

Although histones, spermidine, and spermine condense DNA molecules in cells and play an important role in gene transcription,[41,42] they do not necessarily improve the transfection efficiency when used as gene carriers perhaps because of the lower zeta-potentials of the complexes.[36] Polyplexes composed of polycations with sufficient molecular weights exhibit higher zeta potential, which facilitates the internalization of the complexes into the cells.[43] The physicochemical features of the polyplexes such as size, shape, aggregation properties, thermostability, surface charge, conformational change of DNA, and the ease of interexchange reactions with the other polyanions of transgene expression have attracted great attention.[36,44,45]

Various polycations have been found to form complexes of similar shape and size. Tang et al. studied the correlation of these factors and transfection efficiency using linear PLL, intact PAMAM dendrimers, fractured dendrimers, and branched PEI. These polycations formed similar complexes in terms of size and zeta potential, but exhibited different aggregation properties, suggesting the high gene expression induced by fractured dendrimers and branched PEI results from the stable complexes that do not aggregate over time.[36]

12.3.2 INTERACTION WITH CELL SURFACES

The complexes, which contain excessive polycation, have positive charges as a whole and then interact with cell surfaces by an electrostatic interaction. This interaction between the complex and the cell surface is not merely the starting stage for the internalization. The negative charges of the cell surface originate from the polysaccharides existing at the cell surface. Recently, Mislick et al. reported an important role of the proteoglycan other than the electrostatic interaction between the complexes and cell surface. DNA molecules in the complexes are replaced by the proteoglycan and released from the complex by interacting with proteoglycan at the surface.[46]

Some other noncovalent bondings are proposed for improving the complex/cell interaction. PEG is one of the candidates for improving cell/complex interaction because it is able to promote cell fusion through the perturbation of the plasma membrane. However, PEG may reduce the interaction because it is also the stabilizing agent for protein or other drugs in preventing endocytosis by the reticuloendothelial system.[47] These two conflicting effects must be carefully considered when designing gene carriers. Zhou et al. reported high gene expression using phosphatidylethanolamine, which has chemical features similar to cell surfaces, as a modification agent for low molecular weight PLL. This carrier also reduces the interaction of the complexes with serum proteins, resulting in effective gene expression *in vitro* even in the presence of 10% FCS.[48]

Some reports deal with the fusion of liposome to the plasma membrane, resulting in the direct gene delivery of DNA into the cytosol. However, DNA that forms complexes with cationic liposomes is not encapsulated in the liposomes but attaches outsides of liposomes. Thus we have no clear proof of the direct delivery of the DNA to the cytoplasm. Even when targeting moieties such as sugar or transferrin that can interact with cell surfaces are used, the complexes follow a similar trafficking pathway after the internalization.

12.3.3 INTRACELLULAR TRAFFICKING

Although the efficiency of gene delivery is known to depend greatly on the chemical structures of the gene carriers, the reason for the dependency is unclear. Because the big difference in the gene expression that depends on the carrier molecules used is observed even when the amount of the internalized DNA is taken into consideration, this difference must occur in some steps between the internalization into cells and the recognition by the transcript factors. One possible step is the release of the complexes or free DNA from the endocytotic vesicles to the cytoplasm. Gene delivery using various carriers should be analyzed separately before and after the release. For *in vitro* gene delivery, various introduction methods such as chloroquine treatment,[49] microinjection, and osmotic shock procedure have been employed.

The most widely selected method to enhance transfection efficacy is *in vitro* chloroquine treatment. The detailed mechanism of the chloroquine treatment is still unclear, but chloroquine seems to neutralize the acidic pH of endocytotic vesicles because of their weak acidity, resulting in the inactivation of lysosomal enzymes and inhibition of the fusion of endocytotic vesicles with lysosomes.[50] On the other hand, chloroquine is also known to form a complex with DNA, thus creating some difficulty for analyzing its mechanism.[51] DNA molecules transferred by the osmotic shock procedure were released into the cytosol by osmotic rupture of the endocytotic vesicle. Since the introduced gene should be traced and analyzed in a step-by-step manner in order to evaluate the roles of the carrier polycations, the osmotic shock procedure is a very useful method to deliver DNA into the cytosol more easily than microinjection. The osmotic shock procedure enables us to analyze the events following the release of the complexes from the endocytotic vesicle into the cytosol.

These treatments can be utilized only in *in vitro* experiments and are not applicable for clinical trials. The promising methods for *in vivo* treatment are raising osmotic pressure in the endosome by the action of the carrier polycations and fusion or rupture of the endosomal membrane by the actions of oligopeptides or polypeptides. Godby et al. showed that PEI internalized by the cells undergoes nuclear localization whether administered with or without DNA.[9] They suggested that the polyplexes come into contact with phospholipids of endosomes and the membranes are permeabilized and burst because of osmotic swelling, resulting in the coating of the polyplexes with the phospholipids. The coated complexes may enter the nucleus via fusion with the nuclear envelope.

The types and arrangements of cationic groups of the carriers are also reported to effect the endosomal escape of the internalized DNA. Cationic species partially protonated at physiological pH may act as proton sponges in the endocytotic vesicles and may result in disruption of the vesicle.[52] For example, dimethylaminoethyl groups improve endosomal escape much more effectively than trimethylaminoethyl groups based on their large buffering capacity.[47] The pKa of the cationic groups is also influenced by their arrangement, based on the polymer effect of the adjacent charged groups, resulting in large buffering capacity. This seems to be the reason for the high efficacy of dendrimers and PEI.

Another approach is enhanced endosomal release by use of a peptide that mimics the fusogenic activity of the virus[50] and membrane disruptive peptides.[53] This technique may be effective for improving the transgene expression. Midow et al. reported the efficacy of an addition of a 22-residue peptide derived from the influenza viral hemagglutinin HA2N-terminal polypeptide in the culture medium for gene transfection.

DNA molecules released from endocytotic vesicles into the cytosols may be delivered to the nuclei, but the mechanisms are unclear. One possibility is transportation through the nuclear membrane pore but this does not allow the complex, whose size is usually around 100 nm, to pass through. Another possibility is the accumulation during the mitotic event accompanying the nuclear membrane disappearance. To enhance trafficking through the nucleus pore, several nuclear localization signals (NLSs) were utilized.[54,55] NLSs are oligopeptides composed mainly of cationic residues. They are 5 to 20 amino acids long and have different sequences in many species.

NLS bound to PLL was evaluated by many researchers as a gene carrier and shown to be effective.[56] The importance of the disappearance of the nuclear membrane during the mitotic event is still being debated. The mitotic event was reported to be important for *in vitro* gene transfer in the case of lipoplexes.[57] Pollard et al. studied the nuclear localization of polyplexes and lipoplexes microinjected into the cells and indicated that polycations but not cationic lipids promote gene delivery from the cytoplasm to the nucleus. Moreover, when lipoplexes are injected into the nuclei of oocytes or mammalian cells, gene expression in the nucleus is prevented by the cationic lipids, while lipoplexes injected into the nuclei produce high gene expression.[11] Zauner et al. compared the role of mitosis in the transfection of confluent, contact-inhibited primary human cells using polyplexes and lipoplexes. The lipoplex cannot produce high gene expression at the confluent stage but polyplex can do so.[58] These results indicate that the intracellular trafficking and gene expression mechanisms for polyplex and lipoplex differ.

12.3.4 DISSOCIATION OF COMPLEXES

For transcription of the DNA molecules delivered into the cells, it is considered that the complexes (1) should be disassembled to release the free DNA or (2) should have somewhat well controlled structures that allow the transcription of DNA in the complexes without the disassembling.[59]

The ease of the dissociation of DNA/carrier complexes greatly depends on the strength of the electrostatic interaction between the plasmid and the polycations, which is quite important for the subsequent transcription of the transgene. In our experiment using polycations (Figure 12.2), only polycations having hydroxyl groups revealed higher gene expression. These hydroxyl groups seemed to impart hydrophilic nature to the complexes, resulting in the easy disassembling of the complexes and in releasing naked DNA in the cells. Indeed, adding other polyanions such as heparan sulfate or heparin, which are reported to play an important role of complex/cell surface interaction, easily disassembles the complexes. We then examined gene expression from the complexes by *in vitro* transcription/translation experiments. The complexes composed of the polycations having abundant hydroxyl groups showed higher gene expression even in this system. We confirmed that the hydroxyl groups and the amide groups may act similarly as nonionic hydrophilic groups.

Polycations carrying various saccharides were suggested to produce high gene expression due to the enhanced amounts of the internalized complexes and the decreased electrostatic interactions of the complexes based on weakened cationicity.[60,61] Chloroquine, which is known to form complexes with DNA, was also reported to enhance the dissociation of the complexes in addition to the neutralization and vacuolization of the endosomal and lysosomal vesicles. Erbacher et al. studied the efficacy of chloroquine and some other weak bases which can neutralize the pH inside the endocytotic vesicle and found that only chloroquine enhances transgene expression. They concluded that the strong effect of chloroquine on the gene transfer efficiency is not mainly related to the neutralization of the vesicles, but to the dissociation of the complexes.[62]

Heparan sulfate, which plays the main role in the interaction of the polyplexes with the cell surfaces, has been reported to take part in the disassembly of the polyplexes.[46] When polyanions such as heparan sulfate or heparin are added to the DNA/polycation complex solution, free DNA is released by the interexchange reaction. We recently clarified that this interexchange reaction was strongly improved by the nonionic–hydrophilic groups of carrier polycations such as hydroxyl or amide groups as mentioned above. Toncheva et al. studied gene transfer using PLL with a molecular weight of 1000 or 22,000 and its derivatives grafted with various hydrophilic polymers, including PEG, dextran, and poly [*N*-(hydroxypropyl)methacrylamide] (pHPMA). By analyzing the size, surface zeta potential, and aggregation properties of the complexes, they confirmed the efficacy of PEG–PLL and pHPMA–PLL.[63] Kabanov et al. reported that polyion interexchange reaction occurred when an adequate amount of polyanion was added to the polycation/DNA complex suspensions. The interexchange reaction of the complexes depended on the kind of polyanion added such as poly(vinyl sulfonate)[39] or poly(aspartic acid).[38] They also reported that the topology of the DNA (linear or super-coiled DNA) affects the stability of the polyplexes based on the phosphate group density of DNA.[45]

The fact that the carrier polycations that improve the interexchange reaction produce effective gene expression does not necessarily suggest the disassembling of the complexes in the cells before the transcription event. Since a weak complex with high hydrophilicity is thought to depress gene expression from the viewpoint of nuclease digestion of DNA, the ease of disassembling is not necessarily an advantage for gene expression. Indeed, the inverse effects of the nuclease resistance and the rate of interexchange reaction of polyplexes were pointed out.[64]

12.4 BIODERIVED MOLECULES AS TARGETING MOIETIES

Site-specific gene delivery is attracting great attention, especially for direct *in vivo* gene transfer using various biologically active moieties such as transferrin[20,65] and sugar.[50,60-62,66-68] These modifications bring DNA/carrier complexes to the target cells or organs and also enhance the internalization of complexes into the cells in a receptor-specific manner, which results in high gene expression.

In 1988, Wu et al. developed a system for targeting foreign genes to hepatocytes through receptor-mediated endocytosis for the internalization of DNA/carrier complexes. Hepatocytes possess unique receptors that bind and internalize galactose-terminal asialo glycoproteins. The asialo glycoproteins are internalized by their receptors and delivered into the lysosomes via membrane-limited vesicles.[19] Asialoorosomucoid-PLL carriers delivered pSV2-CAT plasmid DNA specifically to HepG2 hepatoma cells but not to the other receptor (-) cell lines.[67,68] The advantage of the use of the receptor-mediated endocytosis is not only the cell-type specificity of the gene transfer. Some types of cells, such as nonadherent primary hemopoietic cells, are well known to be difficult or almost impossible to transfect with foreign genes by conventional carriers because their endocytotic activity is quite low. Birnstiel and coworkers developed a system in which transferrin was selected as the ligand and named their system "transferrinfection."[69] They synthesized transferrin–PLL conjugates with various molecular weights of PLL and various transferrin ratios to PLL molecules. They found a strong correlation between DNA condensation evaluated under the electron microscope and cellular DNA uptake. One of the key factors for the high gene expression seems to be the sufficient condensing of DNA into a toroid structure, which may facilitate the endocytotic event.[40]

Other candidates for receptor-mediated gene delivery are the receptors for integlin,[70] insulin,[71] and some growth factors.[72] Interestingly, polycations bound to VEGF (vascular endothelial growth factor) could not deliver DNA into nucleus but bFGF (basic fibroblast growth factor) could. The PEI derivatives conjugated to the integrin-binding peptide CYGGRGDTP via a disulfide bridge produced transgene expression in integrin-expression epithelial (HeLa) cells and fibroblasts (MRC5) at the expression level of 10 to 100-fold as compared with PEI.

These studies used poly-L-lysine (PLL) as a carrier polymer and revealed improved endocytosis and excellent expression. However, the high gene expression did not necessarily result from improved endocytosis because the extent of improved transgene expression is often much larger than that which can be explained only by the enhanced amount of DNA ingested. Even in these cases, the physicochemical changes of the complexes play an important role in enhanced transgene expression.

12.5 CONCLUSIONS

Gene delivery is a biological and extremely complicated event. It might be reasonable and clever to use the functional ligands of the living body such as a cell surface receptor, nuclear localization signals, fusogenic peptides, and viral proteins. In contrast, the physicochemical character of the well controlled supramolecular complex of polyanionic DNA and polycation has great influence on transgene expression. Interestingly, the factor by which the transcription of DNAs, the final event in gene expression, can be promoted is not a biological one, but the physicochemical behavior of the supramolecular complexes. Development of safer and effective nonviral gene carriers through the cooperative effects of these factors can be expected in the near future.

REFERENCES

1. Smith, A.E, Viral vectors in gene therapy, *Annu. Rev. Microbiol.*, 49, 807-837, 1995.
2. Ledley, F.D., Nonviral gene therapy: the promise of genes as pharmaceutical products, *Hum. Gene Ther.*, 6, 1129-1144, 1995.
3. Behr, J.P., Gene transfer with synthetic cationic amphiphiles: prospects for gene therapy, *Bioconj. Chem.*, 5, 382-389, 1994.
4. Luo, D. and Saltzman, W.M., Synthetic DNA delivery systems, *Nat. Biotechnol.*, 18, 33-37, 2000.
5. Canonico, A.E. et al., Aerosol and intravenous transfection of human alpha 1-anti-trypsin gene to lungs of rabbits, *Am. J. Respir. Cell Mol. Biol.*, 10, 24-29, 1994.
6. Caplen, N.J. et al,, Liposome-mediated CFTR gene transfer to the nasal epithelium of patients with cystic fibrosis, *Nat. Med.*, 1, 39-46, 1995.
7. Nabel, E.G. et al., Safety and toxicity of catheter gene delivery to the pulmonary vasculature in a patient with metastatic melanoma, *Hum. Gene Ther.*, 5, 1089-1094, 1994.
8. De Smedt, S.C., Demeester, J., and Hennink, E., Cationic polymer based gene delivery system, *Pharm. Res.*, 17, 113-126, 2000.
9. Godbey, W.T., Wu, K.K., and Mikos, A.G., Tracking the intracellular path of poly(ethylenimine)/DNA complexes for gene delivery, *Proc. Natl. Acad. Sci. U.S.A.*, 96, 5177-5181, 1999.
10. Haensler, J. and Szoka, F.C., Polyamidoamine cascade polymers mediate efficient transfection of cells in culture, *Bioconj. Chem.*, 4, 372-379, 1993.
11. Pollard, H. et al., Polyethylenimine but not cationic lipids promotes transgene delivery to the nucleus in mammalian cells, *J. Biol. Chem.*, 273, 7507-7511, 1998.
12. Fraley, R. et al., Introduction of liposome-encapsulated SV40 DNA into cells, *J. Niol. Chem.*, 255, 10431-10435, 1980.
13. Felgner, P.L. et al., Lipofection: a highly efficient, lipid-mediated DNA-tranfection procedure, *Proc. Natl. Acad. Sci. U.S.A.*, 84, 7413-7417, 1987.
14. Ross, P.C. and Hui, S.W., Lipoplex size is a major determinant of *in vitro* lipofection efficiency, *Gene Ther.*, 6, 651-659, 1999.
15. Ross, P.C., and Hui, S.W., Polyethylene glycol enhances lipoplex-cell association and lipofection, *Biochim. Biophys. Acta*, 1421, 273-283, 1999.
16. Lew, D. et al., Cancer gene therapy using plasmid DNA: pharmacokinetic study of DNA following injection in mice, *Hum. Gene Ther.*, 6, 553-564, 1995.

17. Kabanov, A.V., Taking polycation gene delivery systems from *in vitro* to *in vivo*, Pharm. *Sci. Technol. Today*, 2, 365-372, 1999.

18. Mizuguchi, H. et al., Efficient gene transfer into mammalian cells using fusogenic liposome, *Biochem. Biophys. Res. Commun.*, 218, 402-407, 1996.

19. Kato, K. et al., Expression of hepatitis B virus surface antigen in adult rat liver. Co-introduction of DNA and nuclear protein by a simplified liposome method, *J. Biol. Chem.*, 266, 3361-3364, 1991.

20. Wagner, E. et al., Transferrin–polycation conjugates as carriers for DNA uptake into cells, *Proc. Natl. Acad. Sci. U.S.A.*, 87, 3410-3414 1990.

21. Sheldrick, P. et al., Infectious DNA from herpes simplex virus: infectivity of double-strand and single-strand molucules, *Proc. Natl. Acad. Sci. U.S.A.*, 70, 3621-3625, 1973.

22. Yamaoka, T. et al., Effect of cation content of polycation-tupe gene carriers on in vitro gene transfer, *Chem. Lett.*, 1998, 1171-1172, 1998.

23. Lee, K.Y. et al., Preparation of chitisan self aggregates as a gene delivery system, *J. Controlled Release*, 51, 213-220, 1998.

24. Boussif, O. et al., A versatile vector for gene and oligonucleotide transfer into cells in culture and *in vivo*: polyethyleneimine, *Proc. Natl. Acad. Sci. U.S.A.*, 92, 7297-7301, 1995

25. Remy, J.S. et al., Gene transfer with lipospermines and polyethylenimines, *Adv. Drug Deliv. Rev.*, 30, 85-95, 1998.

26. Ferrari, S. et al., ExGen 500 is an effecient vector for gene delivery to lung epithelial cells *in vitro* and *in vivo*, *Gene Ther.*, 4, 1100-1006, 1997.

27. Aubin, R.A. et al., Polybrene/DMSO-assisted gene transfer, *Mol. Biotechnol.*, 1, 29-48, 1994.

28. Mita, K., Zama, M., and Ichmura, S., Effect of charge density of cationic polyelectrolytes on complex formation with DNA, *Biopolymers*, 16, 1993-2004, 1977.

29. van de Wetering, P. et al., 2-(Dimethylamino.ethyl mathacrylate based copolymers as gene transfer agents, *J. Controlled Release*, 53, 145-153, 1998.

30. Cherng, J.Y. et al., Effect of size and serum proteins on transfection efficiency of poly ((2-dimethylamino)ethyl methacrylate)-plasmid nanoparticles, *Pharm. Res.*, 13, 1038-1042, 1996.

31. Takai, T. and Ohmori, H., DNA transfection of mouse lymphoid cells by the combination of DEAE-dextran-mediated DNA uptake and osmotic shock procedure, *Biochim. Biophys. Acta*, 1048, 105-109, 1991.

32. Yamaoka, T. et al., Enhanced expression of foreign gene transferred to mammalian cells *in vitro* using chemically modified poly(L-lysine) as gene carriers, *Chem. Lett.*, 118-119, 2000.

33. Plank, C. et al., Branched cationic peptides for gene delivery: role of type and number of cationic residues in formation and *in vitro* activity of DNA polyplex, *Human Gene Ther.*, 10, 319-332, 1999.

34. Ohashi, S. et al., Cationic polymer-mediated genetic transduction into cultured human chondrosarcoma-derived HCS-2/8 cells, *J. Orthop. Sci.*, 6, 75-81, 2001.

35. Tang, M.X., Redemann, C.T., and Szoka, F.C., *In vitro* gene delivery by degraded polyamidoamine dendrimers, *Bioconj. Chem.*, 7, 703-714, 1996.

36. Tang, M.X. and Szoka, F.C., The influence of polymer structure on the interactions of cationic polymers with DNA and morphology of the resulting complexes, *Gene Ther.*, 4, 823-932, 1997.

37. Wolfert, M.A. et al., Characterization of vectors for gene therapy formed by self-assembly of DNA with synthetic block co-polymers, *Hum. Gene. Ther.*, 7, 2123-2133, 1996.

38. Kabanov, A.V. and Kabanov, V.A., DNA complexes with polycations for the delivery of genetic material into cells, *Bioconj. Chem.*, 6, 7-20,1996.

39. Katayose, S. and Kataoka, K., Remarkable increase in nuclease resistance of plasmid DNA through supramoleclar assembly with poly(ethylene glycol)-poly(L-lysine) block copolymer, *J. Pharm. Sci.*, 87, 160-163, 1998.

40. Zenke, M. et al., Receptor-mediated endocytosis of transferin-polycation conjugates: an efficient way to introduce DNA into hematopoietic cells, *Proc. Natl. Acad. Sci. U.S.A.*, 88, 4255-4259, 1991.

41. Baeza, I. et al., Electron microscopy and biochemical properties of polyamine-compacted DNA, *Biochemistry*, 26, 6387-6392, 1987.

42. Peng, H.F. and Jackson, V., *In vitro* studies on the maintenance of transcription-induced stress by histones and polyamines, *J. Biol. Chem.*, 275, 657-668, 2000.

43. Wolfert, M.A. et al., Polyelectrolyte vectors for gene delivery: influence of cationic polymer on biophysical properties of complexes formed with DNA, *Bioconj. Chem.*, 10, 993-1004, 1999.

44. Ward, C.M., Fisher, K.D., and Seymour, L.W., Turbidometric analysis of polyelectrolyte complexes formed between poly(L-lysine) and DNA, *Colloid Surf. B: Biointerfaces*, 16, 253-260, 1999.

45. Bronich, T.K. et al., Recognition of DNA topology in reactions between plasmid DNA and cationic copolymers, *J. Am. Chem. Soc.*, 122, 8339-8443, 2000.

46. Mislick, K.A. and Baldeschwieler, J.D., Evidence for the role of proteoglycans in cation-mediated gene transfer, *Proc. Natl. Acad. Sci. U.S.A.*, 93, 12349-12354, 1996.

47. Zuidam, N.J. et al., Effects of physicochemical characteristics of poly(2-(dimethylamino)ethyl methacrylate)-based polyplexes on cellular association and internalization, *J. Drug Target.*, 8, 51-66, 2000.

48. Zhou, X., Klibanov, A.L., and Huang L., Lipophilic polylysines mediate efficient DNA transfection in mammalian cells, *Biochim. Biophys. Acta*, 1065, 8-14, 1991.

49. Yamaoka, T. et al., Transfection of foreign gene to mammalian cells using low-toxic cationic polymers, *Nucleic Acids Symp. Series*, 31, 229-230, 1994.

50. Midoux, P. et al., Specific gene transfer mediated by lactosylated poly-L-lysine into hepatoma cells, *Nucleic Acids Res.*, 21, 871-878, 1993.

51. Okada, C.Y. and Rechsteiner, M., Introduction of macromolecule into cultured mammalian cells by osmotic lysis of pinocytic vesicle, *Cell*, 23, 33-41, 1982.

52. Van de Wetering, P., Moret, E.E., and Schuurmans-Nieuwenbroek, N.M.E., Structure-activity relationships of water-soluble cationic methacrylate/methacrylamide polymers for nonviral gene delivery, *Bioconj. Chem.*, 10, 589-597, 1999.

53. Ohmori, N. et al., Importance of hydrophobic region in amphiphilic structures of α-helical peptides for their gene transferability into cells, *Biochem. Biophys. Res. Commun.*, 245, 259-265, 1998.

54. Garcia-Bustos, J., Heitman, J., and Hall, M.N., Nuclear protein localization, *Biochim. Biophys. Acta*, 1071, 83-101, 1991.

55. Yoneda, Y., How proteins are transported from cytoplasm to the nucleus, *J. Biol. Chem.*, 121, 811-817, 1997.

56. Chan, C.K. and Jans, D.A., Enhancement of polylysine-mediated transferrinfection by nuclear localization sequences: polylysine does not function as a nuclear localization sequence, *Hum. Gene Ther.*, 10, 319-332, 1999.

57. Mortimer, I. et al., Cationic lipid-mediated transfection of cells in culture requires mitotic activity, *Gene Ther.*, 6, 403-411, 1999.

58. Zauner, W. et al., Differential behaviour of lipid-based and polycation-based gene transfer systems in transfecting primary human fibroblasts: a potential role of polylysine in nuclear transport, *Biochim. Biophys. Acta*, 1428, 57-67, 1999.

59. Bielinska, A.U., Kukowska-Latallo, J.F., and Baker, J.R., The interaction of plasmid DNA with polyamidoamine dendrimers: mechanism of complex formation and analysis of alterations induced in nuclease sensitivity and transcriptional activity of the complexed DNA, *Biochim. Biophys. Acta*, 1353, 180-190, 1997.

60. Erbacher, P. et al., The reduction of the positive charges of polylysine by partial gluconoylation increases the transfection efficiency of polylysine/DNA complexes, *Biochim. Biophys. Acta*, 1324, 27-36, 1997.

61. Erbacher, P. et al., Glycosylated polylysine/DNA complexes: gene transfer efficiency in relation with the size and the sugar substitution level of glycosylated polylysine and with the plasmid size, *Bioconj. Chem.*, 6, 401-410, 1995.

62. Erbacher, P. et al., Putative role of chloroquine in gene transfer into a human hepatoma cell line by DNA/polylysine complexes, *Exp. Cell Res*, 225, 186-194, 1996.

63. Toncheva, V. et al., Novel vectors for gene delivery formed by self-assembly of DNA with poly(L-lysine) grafted with hydrophilic polymers, *Biochim. Biophys. Acta*, 1380, 354-368, 1998.

64. Dash, P.R. et al., Synthetic polymers for vectrial delivery of DNA: characterisation of polymer-DNA complexes by photon correlation spectroscopy and stability to nuclease degradation and disruption by polyanions *in vitro*, *J. Controlled Release*, 48, 269-276, 1997.

65. Wagner, E. et al., DNA-binding transferrin conjugates as functional gene-delivery agents: synthesis by linkage of polylysine of ethidium homodimer to the transferrin carbohydrate moiety, *Bioconj. Chem.*, 2, 226-231, 1991.

66. Wall, D.A., Wilson, G., and Hubbard A.L., The galactose-specific recognition system of mammalian liver: the route of ligand internalization in rat hepatocytes, *Cell*, 21, 79-93, 1980.

67. Wu, G.Y. and Wu, C.H., Evidence for targeted gene delivery to Hep G2 hepatoma cells *in vitro*, *Biochemistry*, 27, 887-892, 1988.

68. Wu, G.Y. and Wu, C.H., Receptor-mediated gene delivery and expression *in vivo*, *J. Biol. Chem.*, 263, 1, 4621-14624, 1988.

69. Wagner, E. et al., Transferrin-polycation-DNA complexes: the effect of polycations on the structure of the complex and DNA delivery to cells, *Proc. Natl. Acad. Sci. U.S.A.*, 88, 4255-4259, 1991.

70. Erbacher, P., Remy J.S., and Behr, J.P., Gene transfer with synthetic virus-like particles via the integrin-mediated endocytosis pathway, *Gene Ther.*, 6, 138-145, 1999.

71. Rosenkranz, A.A. et al., Receptor-mediated endocytosis and nuclear transport of a transfecting DNA construct, *Exp. Cell Res.*, 199, 323-329, 1992.

72. Fisher, K.D., et al., A versatile system for receptor-mediated gene delivery permits increased entry of DNA into target cells, enhanced delivery to the nucleus and elevated rates of transgene expression, *Gene Ther.*, 7, 1337-1343, 2000.

13 Sensing and Diagnosis

Mizuo Maeda

CONTENTS

13.1 INTRODUCTION

Recent developments in molecular biology make it possible to correlate small muta-tions of certain genes with heritable disorders and cancers. These findings promoted the study of gene mutation assays, especially in the fields of biomedical sensing and diagnosis. Various methods have been proposed to detect changes in DNA base se-quence.[1] One method relies on a sequence-specific enzymatic reaction and the other on an oligonucleotide probe. Enzyme-based methods may be more convenient and reliable in some cases, whereas the methods based on nucleic acid hybridization may be more general and widely applicable. Most of the latter methods take advantage of single-stranded DNA (ssDNA), which is immobilized on a solid surface such as polymer membrane, metal electrode, and latex particle.

A well known example of diagnostic methods that utilize supramolecular sys-tems is the latex agglutination immunoassay.[2] An antigen- or antibody-modified latex particle is cross-linked by the complementary antibody or antigen and the resulting particle assembly is detected by the increase in turbidity or light scattering intensity of the dispersion. Recently, the DNA diagnosis using the supramolecular assembling phenomenon of colloidal particles was reported by Mirkin et al.[3] Single-stranded DNA-modified gold nanoparticles were used as a detection probe; the particles were cross-linked by hybridization with the complementary DNA to form particle assem-blies. This aggregation behavior is easily detected by the color change of the disper-sion due to a red shift of the plasmon band.

In addition to Mirkin's study, single-stranded DNA-carrying colloidal particles have been recognized as useful tools in the field of molecular biology. Most of the particles are latex-based and are used for the sequence-specific separation of DNA[4] and RNA[5] and the detection of DNA[6] and RNA.[7] DNA-carrying colloidal particles reported thus far are commonly prepared by a two-step procedure: plain colloidal particle preparation followed by DNA immobilization to the particle.

The preparation of colloidal particles through the supramolecular assembly of amphiphilic copolymers has received much attention.[8a-8d] These particles are generally prepared by solvent exchange from nonselective solvent to selective solvent (water). As an alternative method, a lower critical solution temperature (LCST)-showing polymer, poly(N-isopropylacrylamide) (PNIPAAm), was used for the preparation of colloidal particles by simple heating above its LCST (~32°C).[9a-9c]

We developed a one-step method to preserve DNA-carrying colloidal particles through the self-organization of DNA-PNIPAAm graft copolymer (1). The copolymer is composed of a PNIPAAm main chain and a DNA (d(T)$_{12}$) graft chain, and forms a colloidal particle with a PNIPAAm core surrounded by hydrophilic DNA above the LCST. This particle aggregates in the presence of complementary DNA according to the cross-linking mechanism, and is observed as a turbidity increase of the dispersion.

We found another aggregation behavior of this DNA-containing colloidal particle. The mechanism is based on the stability change of the particle induced by the hybridization of the surface DNA with the complementary DNA. The DNA detection with selectivity in the sequence and also in the chain length (the number of nucleic bases) was achieved by the turbidimetric particle aggregation assay according to the supramolecular assembly mechanism.

In this chapter, two types of supramolecular assembling phenomena will be discussed in relation to gene mutation assay, which is one of the most important areas of biomedical sensing and diagnosis:

1. DNA-carrying colloidal nanoparticles prepared from DNA-PNIPAAm graft copolymer through supramolecular assembly
2. DNA-carrying nanoparticles assembled in the presence of complementary DNA to yield visibly detectable aggregates due to cross-linking or colloidal stability change.

13.2 DNA-CARRYING NANOPARTICLES

DNA graft copolymer (1) was prepared by copolymerization between N-isopropylacrylamide (NIPAAm) and DNA macromonomer (Figure 13.1). DNA macromonomer was synthesized by coupling reaction between methacryloyloxysuccinimide and amino-linked DNA having an aminohexyl linker at its 5'-terminus, as reported previously.[10] DNA macromonomer (0, 0.15, 0.30, and 0.60 μmol) was mixed with N-isopropylacrylamide (NIPAAm) (140 μmol) in buffer solution [10 mM Tris-HCl (pH 7.4)]. After flushing the solution with nitrogen, aqueous solutions of ammonium persulfate and N,N,N',N'-tetramethylethylenediamine were added. Polymerization was carried out at 25°C for 1 h. The unreacted NIPAAm monomer was removed by dialysis (Spectra/Por6, MWCO = 1000). The unreacted DNA

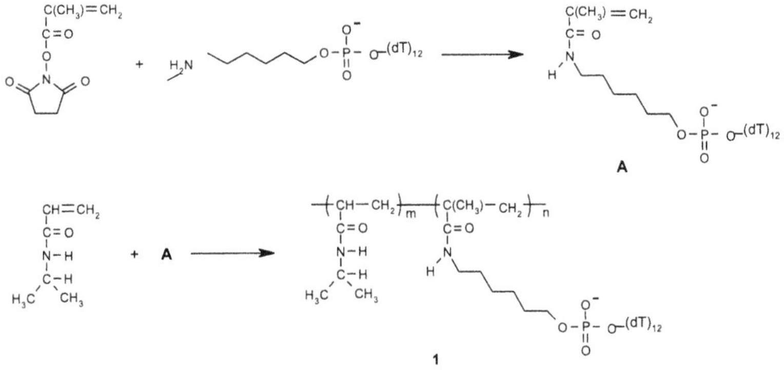

FIGURE 13.1 Synthetic route to DNA graft copolymer (**1**).

macromonomer was separated from **1** on a 1.5 × 10 cm Sephadex G-100 column. The composition of **1** was determined by dry weight and UV absorption at 260 nm due to DNA macromonomer unit using the molar extinction coefficient of 97,800 $M^{-1}cm^{-1}$.[13]

In order to obtain molecular data for graft copolymers, static light scattering (SLS) and dynamic light scattering (DLS) measurements were conducted with a DLS-7000 instrument (Otsuka Electronics) according to the literature.[12] The light source was an Ar ion laser (488 nm, 75 mW). The polymer solutions were filtered through 0.22-μm filters (Millipore) prior to measurements. For the determination of the Mw of each polymer, SLS measurement was carried out over the angular range from 30 to 140° and the concentration range from 0.5 to 2.3 mg/mL at 25°C in 10 mM Tris-HCl buffer (pH 7.4). The refractive index increment (dn/dC) of copolymer was calculated from the additive equation, dn/dC = $w_{PNIPAAm}$(dn/dC)$_{PNIPAAm}$ + w_{DNA}(dn/dC)$_{DNA}$, where w represents the weight fraction. The dn/dC of DNA macromonomer was measured by DRM-1021 (Otsuka Electronics) at 488 nm and determined to be 0.187 mL/g (25°C) and 0.192 mL/g (40°C). The literature values were used for the dn/dC of PNIPAAm.[13]

The properties of DNA graft copolymers are summarized in Table 13.1. The conversions of both monomers were about 70%. The molar ratios of DNA macromonomer units in the copolymers agreed with the feed ratios. The Mw values of the polymers were determined from Zimm plots and were almost constant ($\sim 2 \times 10^5$) irrespective of the DNA macromonomer fraction.

The polymer concentration for LCST measurement was 0.1 mg/mL in 10 mM Tris-HCl (pH 7.4)/5 mM MgCl$_2$. The solution turbidity was monitored at 500 nm by raising the solution temperature (0.5°C/min). LCST was defined as the temperature at which the turbidity began to increase. Only one transition was observed for all the polymers. As a result, the LCSTs of polymers increased with increasing DNA macromonomer fractions. Since this tendency is in line with the behavior of copolymers of NIPAAm and hydrophilic comonomers such as acrylamide and acrylic acid,[14] the DNA macromonomer was considered to act as a hydrophilic part in the copolymer.

TABLE 13.1

Molecular Parameters of Polymers

Sample	Mw	mol% DNA	DNA graft number	LCST[a] (°C)
D-0	2.1 x 10⁵	—	—	33.4
D-0.085	2.2 × 10⁵	0.085	1.6	34.5
D-0.17	2.3 × 10⁵	0.17	3.2	34.9
D-0.36	2.6 × 10⁵	0.36	7.3	35.8

[a] Determined by turbidity measurements as described in the text.

To form the colloidal particle from **1**, the temperature of the solution was raised to 40°C, which was higher than the phase transition temperature of the copolymer. The copolymer solution was 0.1 mg/mL in 10 mM Tris-HCl (pH 7.4)/5 mM MgCl$_2$. The colloidal particles were examined by DLS analysis conducted at a detection angle of 90°. Figure 13.2 shows the hydrodynamic radius (Rh) distributions of colloidal particles. The radii of colloidal particles increased as DNA macromonomer fractions in copolymers decreased. Table 13.2 summarizes the results of DLS analyses of colloidal particles. The association numbers (copolymers per particle) increased with decreasing fractions of DNA macromonomer in copolymers. The radius of each particle remained constant at least for several hours when heated to 40°C. When the particle dispersions were cooled to room temperature to dissociate the particles into the individual copolymers and the solutions were heated to 40°C again, particles of the same size were formed (relative difference was ±2%).

The ratios of radius of gyration (R_g) and (R_h) of colloidal particles (R_g/R_h) were calculated to range from 0.72 to 0.81, which is close to the theoretical value for a hard sphere (0.776).[15] The density of core of the colloidal particle (ρ) was calculated from the equation, $\rho = Mw/(4/3r_{core}^3 N_A)$. Assuming that $r_{core} \sim R_h$, the calculated ρ values roughly agreed with that reported for the collapsed PNIPAAm homopolymer (0.36 g/cm³)[16] as shown in Table 13.2. However, if the thickness of the DNA layer is assumed to be about 7.8 nm which is estimated from a polymer brush conformation of DNA on the core surface, the calculated values are about two times larger than that of collapsed PNIPAAm homopolymer. These results may indicate that the DNA layer was not detected by the light scattering method due to the low density of this layer or that the DNA existed as a flat conformation on the core surface.

The value of surface area per DNA (S_{DNA}) calculated from the assumption of $r_{core} \sim R_h$, was roughly constant for all the particles. This is very similar to the case of colloidal particles formed from poly(NIPAAm-co-acrylic acid)[13] and should be explained as follows. In the particle formation process, the association of copolymers stops when the surface area per DNA reaches a certain value and this value is constant irrespective of the copolymer composition. This is the reason why the copolymer with a smaller DNA fraction formed a larger particle.

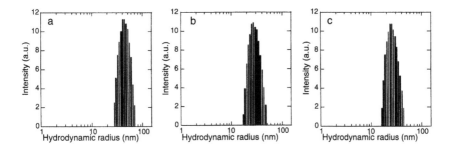

FIGURE 13.2 z-Weighted hydrodynamic radius distributions of colloidal particles formed from copolymers (1) at 40°C in 10 mM Tris-HCl (pH 7.4)/5 mM MgCl$_2$. (a) D-0.085, (b) D-0.17, (c) D-0.36. Copolymer concentration was 0.1 mg/mL.

TABLE 13.2
Results of Light Scattering Analysis of Colloidal Particles Formed from Copolymers at 40°C

Sample	Mw of particle	R_g (nm)	$R_h{}^a$ (nm)	Rg/Rh	Association number	S_{DNA} (nm^2/DNA)	ρ (g/cm^3)
D-0.085	7.6×10^7	35	43	0.81	350	40	0.38
D-0.17	2.0×10^7	21	29	0.72	87	36	0.33
D-0.36	8.6×10^6	18	25	0.72	33	31	0.22

^{a} Rh was calculated from Stokes-Einstein equation.[12]

13.3 DNA-DEPENDENT ASSEMBLY OF NANOPARTICLES

The complementary DNA recognition by the particle surface DNA (d(T)$_{12}$) was examined. The copolymer solution was 0.1 mg/mL in 10 mM Tris-HCl (pH 7.4)/5 mM MgCl$_2$. After the formation of colloidal particle from D-0.17 at 40°C, the cross-linking DNA [equimolar mixture of 3′-d(A)$_{12}$(TG)$_6$-5′ and 5′-d(AC)$_6$(A)$_{12}$-3′] having complementary d(A)$_{12}$ regions at both ends or noncross-linking DNA [equimolar mixture of 3′-d(A)$_{12}$(TG)$_6$-5′ and 5′-d(AC)$_6$-3′] having a d(A)$_{12}$ region at only one end was added to the particle dispersion and the turbidity change of the dispersion was monitored. As shown in Figure 13.2, the turbidity did not change by the addition of non-crosslinking DNA and increased steeply with cross-linking DNA. Moreover, when the temperature of the turbid dispersion with cross-linking DNA was raised, the turbidity began to decrease at 44°C and reached the same value before DNA addition. This phenomenon should be explained by assembly and dissociation between the particles according to the hybridization of cross-linking DNA (d(A)$_{12}$ regions) with the surface DNA (d(T)$_{12}$). In fact, the temperature range of this particle dissociation process was included in that of the melting of free DNA duplex formed from 5'-d(AC)$_6$(A)$_{12}$-3' and d(T)$_{12}$ (26 to 47°C).

The effect of DNA addition on the particle size was investigated for D-0.17 by light scattering measurements. On the addition of noncross-linking DNA to the colloidal particles at 40°C, R_h did not change for more than 3 h. Although the hybridization of noncross-linking DNA with the surface DNA would lead to the increase in overall hydrophilicity of the particle, the particle size remained constant. This indicates a relatively slow rate of copolymer exchange at 40°C. When the particle assembly formed by the addition of cross-linking DNA at 40°C was heated to 50°C, the dispersed colloidal particle was found to have R_h of 31 nm, which was very close to that of the original colloidal particle.

Thus we found that the DNA-carrying colloidal particles are easily prepared from PNIPAAm–graft-DNA by heating through supramolecular assembly. The particle surface DNA recognizes the complementary cross-linking DNA so that the

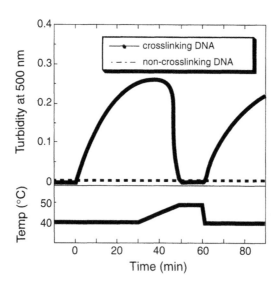

FIGURE 13.3 Turbidity change of colloidal dispersion induced by DNA addition at 40°C and the effect of temperature on dispersion turbidity. The dispersion (700 µL) contains 0.1 mg/mL of D-0.17 (1.0 nmol of d(T)$_{12}$ strand). At 0 min, 11 µL of cross-linking DNA (44 µM equimolar) mixture of 3'-d(A)$_{12}$(TG)$_6$-5' and 5'-d(AC)$_6$(A)$_{12}$-3') or non-cross-linking DNA (equimolar mixture of 3'-d(A)$_{12}$(TG)$_6$-5' and 5'-d(AC)$_6$-3') is added. The dispersion temperature is changed between 40 and 50°C periodically.

particle assembly formed shows easily detectable turbidity changes. These particles may be useful for turbidimetric DNA detection.

13.4   COLLOIDAL PROPERTIES OF DNA-CARRYING NANOPARTICLES

We studied in detail the stability of the DNA-carrying colloidal particles by changing the concentrations of coexisting salts ($MgCl_2$ and NaCl). Generally, colloidal particles in dispersion are known to aggregate at a certain salt concentration called the critical coagulation concentration. We prepared a graft copolymer having DNA branches of 5'-GCCACCAGC-3' in order to investigate more precisely DNA sequence recognition using a series of target DNAs (**I** through **V**) which are listed in Table 13.3.

Figure 13.4 shows the optical density of particle dispersion at 500 nm after the mixing with NaCl or $MgCl_2$ solution. The increase of optical density resulting from the aggregation of colloidal particle was observed at 20 mM of $MgCl_2$ but not for NaCl in the concentration range of 10 to 1400 mM. The stability of the colloidal particles was also examined in the presence of complementary DNA (**I**) or its one point-mismatching DNA (**II**). Surprisingly, the optical density of the particle dispersion in the presence of **I** increased steeply at 10 mM for $MgCl_2$ and at 400 mM for NaCl. No change was observed in the presence of **II**; the behavior with the one-point mutant was very similar to the DNA absence. These results suggest that the instability of the colloidal dispersion in the presence of **I** should be caused by the selective hybridization of the particle surface DNA with its complementary DNA (**I**).

To confirm this conjecture, we investigated the temperature effect on the particle aggregate formed in the presence of **I** at an NaCl concentration of 500 mM. As the temperature increased, the absorbance of the dispersion decreased steeply in the narrow temperature range and then reached almost zero, as shown in Figure 13.5 (bottom). The R_h of colloidal particles at 55°C was 22 nm, which agreed with that of the particles at that temperature without the addition of DNA, indicating that the aggregate dissociated into the individual particle. Since the temperature range of this

TABLE 13.3   Graft Copolymer

Code	Sequence (3'–5')	Description
I	CGGTGGTCG	Complementary
II	CGGT**A**GTCG	Point mutant
III	**TT**CGGTGGTCG	Different length (two bases longer)
IV	**TTTTT**CGGTGGTCG	Different length (five bases longer)
V	CGGTGGTCG**TT**	Different length (two bases longer)

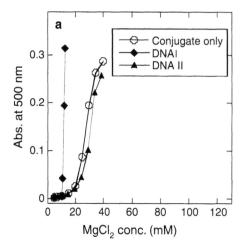

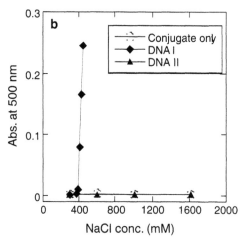

FIGURE 13.4 Absorbance of the colloidal particle dispersion as a function of concentration of (a) $MgCl_2$ and (b) NaCl in the absence and presence of complementary DNA (**I**) or one point-mismatching DNA (**II**) at 40°C. The colloidal particle concentration was 0.1 mg/mL, containing 2.8 µM of DNA unit. The target DNA concentration was 2.8 µM.

aggregate dissociation process was included in the temperature range of the dissociation of free duplex DNA (38 to 63°C), the aggregate dissociation should be attributed to the dissociation of DNA duplex on the particle. From these results, it can be concluded that the stability decrease of colloidal dispersion was induced by the duplex formation of the surface DNA. Generally, the binding of Mg^{2+} and Na^+ to the duplex of DNA or RNA is stronger than binding to single-stranded DNA or RNA, because of the higher anionic charge density of the duplex.[17] Thus, the absolute value of the electric potential of the particle surface should be smaller when the surface DNA was in duplex state, so that the particle became less stable.

It should be noted that the dissociation of aggregate took place at a very narrow temperature range in comparison with the melting of free duplex DNA (Figure 13.5). A similar phenomenon was reported for the aggregate from DNA modified-gold

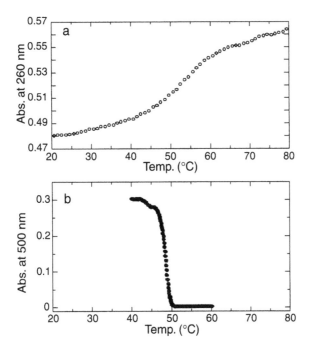

FIGURE 13.5 Temperature dependence of absorbance of the particle aggregate formed in the presence of **I** (b) and melting curve of free duplex DNA (a) in 500 mM NaCl/10 mM Tris-HCl buffer (pH 7.4). The concentrations of the colloidal particle and **I** were the same as those in Figure 13.4. The free duplex DNA concentration was 2.8 μM. Heating rate was 0.5°C/min.

nanoparticles cross-linked by the complementary DNA.[3] This property is important for the discriminative detection of DNA duplexes based on small differences in melting temperatures between probe DNA and the target DNAs.

We presumed that the discrimination of the target DNA in the chain length would also be possible according to the aggregation mechanism: the hybridization of particle surface DNA with the longer DNAs (**III** and **V**) should result in the protruding of a single-stranded region at the end of the duplex DNA, so that the colloidal particles would become more stable than when the particle hybridized with the same length DNA (**I**) to give a perfect duplex. Figure 13.6 shows the stability of the dispersion against NaCl. The particle was clearly more stable in the presence of **III** and **V** than in the presence of **I** as we expected. In the presence of **V**, having an additional T_2 at its 5′-terminus, the particle became more stable than in the presence of **III** or **IV**, having an additional T_2 or T_5 at its 3′-terminus, respectively. Since the hybridization of **V** with the particle shell DNA should result in the exposure of the protruding single-stranded region at the outer surface of colloidal particles, the property of the single-stranded region, namely the lower affinity to Na⁺, remarkably appeared in this

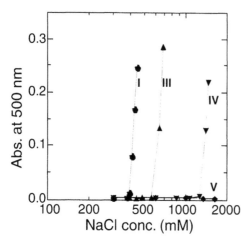

FIGURE 13.6 Absorbance of the colloidal particle dispersion as a function of NaCl concentration in the presence of complementary DNA (**I**) or complementary but longer DNAs (**III** through **V**) at 40°C. The concentrations of colloidal particle and the target DNA were the same as those in Figure 13.4.

case. The comparison between **III** and **IV** indicates that the particle is more stable in the presence of the longer DNA (**IV**). These results suggest that particle aggregation according to the proposed mechanism would be applicable to chain length-selective DNA detection. It was reported that a few base deletions in a certain region of the genome is closely related to a cancer,[18] and this method may be applicable as a diagnostic tool.

Finally, we demonstrated the turbidimetric detection of DNA with sequence and chain length selectivity. After the addition of DNA (**I** through **III** and **V**), the time-dependent absorbance change of the particle dispersion containing 500 m*M* NaCl was monitored. The absorbance did not change by the addition of either one point-mismatching DNA (**II**) or longer DNAs (**III** and **V**), while the absorbance increased steeply by the addition of complementary DNA **I** and was saturated within 5 min.

13.5 CONCLUSION

In this chapter, a typical example of supramolecular systems which are useful for biological sensing and diagnosis was explained. We proposed a novel aggregation mechanism of DNA-containing colloidal particles, which is based on the stability decrease of colloidal particles accompanied by the duplex formation of the shell DNA with the complementary DNA. Using the particle aggregation assay according to the above mechanism, sequence- and chain length-selective DNA detection was attained (Figure 13.7). However, further research must be carried out before it can be applied to biomedical gene diagnosis since the present results are limited to short oligonucleotides.

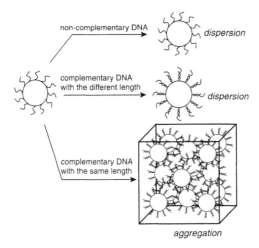

FIGURE 13.7 DNA sequence- and chain length-selective aggregations of the DNA-carrying colloidal particles.

REFERENCES

1.   Lyamichev, V.I. et al., *Biochemistry*, 39, 9523, 2000.
2.   Gella, F.J., Serra, J., and Gener, J., *Pure Appl. Chem.*, 63, 1131, 1991.
3a. Mirkin, C.A. et al., *Nature*, 382, 607, 1996.
3b. Elghanian, R. et al., *Science*, 277, 1078, 1997.
3c. Storhoff, J.J. et al., *J. Am. Chem. Soc.*, 120, 1959, 1998.
3d. Reynolds, R.A., III, Mirkin, C.A., and Letsinger, R.L., *J. Am. Chem. Soc.*, 122, 3795, 2000.
3e. Storhoff, J.J. et al., *J. Am. Chem. Soc.*, 122, 4640, 2000.
4.   Kuribayashi-Ohta, K. et al., *Biochim. Biophys. Acta*, 1156, 204, 1993.
5.   Imai, T. et al., *J Colloid Interface Sci.*, 177, 245, 1996.
6.   Hatakeyama, M. et al., *Colloids Surf. A Physicohem. Eng. Asp.*, 153, 445, 1999.
7.   Ihara, T., Kurohara, K., and Jyo, A., *Chem. Lett.*, 1999, 1041.
8a. Gao, Z. et al., *Macromolecules*, 27, 7923, 1994.
8b. Prochazka, K. et al., *Macromolecules*, 29, 6518, 1996.
8c. Li, M., Jiang, M., Zhu, L., Wu, C., *Macromolecules*, 30, 2201, 1997.
8d. Kataoka, K., Ishihara, A., Harada, A., Miyazaki, H., *Macromolecules*, 31, 6071, 1998.
9a. Topp, M.D.C. et al., *Macromolecules*, 30, 8518, 1997.
9b. Qiu, X. and Wu, C., *Macromolecules*, 30, 7921, 1997.
9c. Liang, D. et al., *Macromolecules*, 32, 6326, 1999.
10. Mori, T., Umeno, D., and Maeda, M., *Biotechnol. Bioeng.*, 72, 261, 2001.
11. Cantor, C.R., Warshaw, M.M., and Shapiro, H., *Biopolymers*, 9, 1059, 1970.
12. Harada, A. and Kataoka, K., *Macromolecules*, 31, 288, 1998.
13. Qiu, X., Kwan, C.M.S., and Wu, C., *Macromolecules*, 30, 6090, 1997.
14a. Taylor, L.D. and Cerankowski, L.D., *J. Polym. Sci., Polym. Chem. Ed.*, 13, 2551, 1975.
14b. Yoo, M.K. et al., *Polymer*, 39, 3703, 1998.

15. Douglas, J.F., Roovers, J., and Freed, K.F., *Macromolecules*, 23, 4168, 1990.
16. Meewes, M. et al., *Macromolecules*, 24, 5811, 1991.
17. Kankia, B.I. and Marky, L. A., *J. Phys. Chem. B*, 103, 8759, 1999.
18. Akiyama, Y et al., *Gastroenterology*, 112, 33, 1997.

14 Organic/Inorganic Supramolecular Assembly

Akio Kishida

CONTENTS

14.1 INTRODUCTION

Mineralized tissue, such as shell, pearl, bone, dentin, and cementum are indispensable to living organisms. Those naturally occurring mineralized tissues contain inorganic salts and organic substances. The organic materials occupy approximately 49% of the volume of human bone. The organic matter is mostly collagen (90%); the remainder consists of proteoglycans and other noncollagenous proteins. From these data, one can assume that organic substances might play some important role in mineralized tissues.

These mineralized tissues are not random aggregations of inorganic salts, and they have well-organized structures. Figure 14.1 is a group of scanning electron micrographs of the structure of pearl that illustrate the ordered structure of mineralized tissue. Microscale observation reveals that mineralized tissue is an organic/inorganic hybrid. The structures of the mineralized tissues are very sophisticated and have gathered the attention of inorganic material researchers for years.

What is the relation between biomineralization and organic/inorganic supramolecular assembly? The organized structure of mineralized tissue fits the definition of

0-8493-0965-4/02/$0.00+$1.50

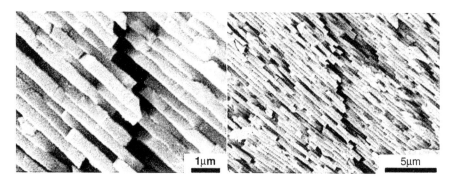

FIGURE 14.1 Scanning electron micrographs of the pearl.

supramolecular assembly well. Biomineralization is one example of the practical use of organic/inorganic supramolecular assemblies in biological applications.

Why did nature use supramolecular structured organic/inorganic assemblies such as bones and shells to protect organisms from enemies? One of the answers is their excellent physical properties. The incorporation of organic material into inorganic structures often leads to composites of great strength and toughness. For example, mother of pearl or nacre has a composition of 95% calcium carbonate but is 500 to 3000 times stronger than chalk. It is composed of layers of plates of aragonite (a form of calcium carbonate) separated by a thin layer of protein matrix.[4] Thus, naturally occurring organic/inorganic supramolecular assemblies represent an excellent balance of strength and toughness; synthetic materials often lack this balance.

To develop new materials that have the same mechanical character, it is essential to clarify the mechanisms of naturally occurring organic/inorganic supramolecular assembly formation and develop a new process for fabricating the assemblies. In the following sections, the principal phenomena of biomineralization and the process of organic/inorganic supramolecular assembly will be discussed.

14.2   BIOMINERALIZATION

Biomineralization, the biological formation of mineral deposits, is one of the most widespread processes in nature. The process of biomineralization is characterized by the close association of organic and inorganic materials to form biomaterials at organic interfaces during the stages of formation. Nature determines a crystal's size, shape, and crystallographic orientation, and the resulting materials have excellent properties such as high strength, resistance to fracture, and aesthetic value.

In eukaryotes, the process of mineral deposition at extracellular sites is mediated and regulated by the proteins and other components the cells secrete to form the matrix. The processes involved in the formation of biominerals can be summarized into five steps:

1. The cells first form the structural components of the extracellular matrix: an enclosed protein cage, a lipid vesicle, and a protein-polysaccharide complex.
2. The cells secrete the regulatory macromolecules that modify the properties of the matrix.
3. Transport of inorganic ions into the mineralization site and nucleation of ion clusters on functional groups on the site surface occur.
4. By changing the pH of surroundings, stereospecific nucleation of mineral crystal takes place.
5. Higher ordered small structures of biominerals are formed by transportation and assemblage of crystals.

These biomineralization processes are conducted by cells that take charge of preparing mineralized tissues; in animals, they are osteoblasts and odontoblasts. This growth process is mimicked to produce mineralized composites, but it is impossible to trace the full functions of those cells.

Because of the low solubility products of the carbonates, phosphates, and sulfates and the relatively high levels of calcium in extracellular fluids, calcium salts are usually present in biominerals. Calcium phosphates and carbonates are present in a variety of organisms and have a great number of functions.

14.3 PREPARATION OF ORGANIC/INORGANIC SUPRAMOLECULAR ASSEMBLY

For preparing organic/inorganic supramolecular assemblies, various biomimetic approaches were used. One approach was the use of an organic surface as a template. Langmuir–Blodgett (LB) film or other polymer films are used as templates for inorganic crystals of a specific polymorphism and orientation. Another technique is the use of solubilized ions or polymers that may interact with the growing crystal. The use of phase-separated microenvironments such as vesicles, foams, microemulsions, and hydrogels is the third approach.

14.3.1 THE USE OF ORGANIC SURFACES AS TEMPLATES

LB film is a typical supramolecular assembly. LB film is used because one can control the distribution, orientation, and density of the functional group with ease. The particular amphiphile headgroup, its spacing, and the condition of the subphase effect the orientation, morphology, and phase of the crystal nucleated from it.

For example, when a supersaturated calcium bicarbonate solution is allowed to stand, calcium carbonate crystals will precipitate. Normally, a polymorphic mixture largely composed of calcite rhombs will form. The crystals consisted of unusual pyramid–shaped calcite forms on the surface of the monolayer of n-eicosyl sulfate. It seems that the tridentate sulfate headgroup mimics the arrangement of carbonate groups of calcite crystal.[5]

Tanaka et al. prepared LB films with the same functional groups as collagen and used them as templates for hydroxyapatite (HAp: $Ca_{10}(PO_4)_6(OH)_2$) formation in a simulated body fluid (in mM: Na^+ 142, K^+ 5.0, Cl^- 148, HCO_3^- 4.2, HPO_4^{2-} 1.0, SO_4^{2-} 0.5).[6] Nucleation of HAp took place on the monolayers of the carboxyl groups, while no nucleation occurred on the monolayers of the amino groups. IR spectra analyses revealed that an interfacial interaction between carboxyl groups and Ca ions was important for HAp nucleation.

An apatite layer was also formed on polyethyleneterephthalate (PET) substrates by the following biomimetic process. PET substrates were placed on granular particles of a $CaO–SiO_2$-based glass in simulated body fluid (SBF) with ion concentrations nearly equal to those of human blood plasma to form apatite nuclei on their surfaces (first treatment). They then were soaked in modified SBFs, the ion concentrations of which were changed to give a variation in ionic activity product of apatite, in order to make the apatite nuclei grow (second treatment).[7]

Kato et al. succeeded in forming aragonite and vaterite selectively on chitosan films.[8] They used poly(aspartate) as a soluble additive.

14.3.2 The Use of Soluble Additives

The presence of soluble additives in solution from which the crystals nucleate and develop is also known to have significant effect on the morphologies and faces of the crystals. Water-soluble polymers bearing ionic groups act as a template for nucleation. Kato et al. reported that poly(acrylic acid) (PAAc) works as a precursor for nucleation and as a pH controller at the same time.[9] Some additives have an affinity for a particular face of a crystal and can inhibit its growth, leading to a departure from the normal morphology. This effect results in an increase in the relative area of that face as growth proceeds, compared to a control crystal. Normal crystallographic development can be markedly altered with additives present at only millimolar levels.

14.3.3 The Use of Microenvironments

Biomineralization processes often depend on the use of a shaped vesicle to guide nuclei formation and control crystal shape. The vesicle serves as a reaction site for nucleation. Another candidate is the hydrogel. The use of hydrogels is an up-to-date technique to develop a three-dimensional matrix of supramolecular architecture.

14.3.3.1 The Use of Surfactants and Lipid Vesicles

Supersaturated water-in-oil microemulsions have been used to synthesize microskeletal calcium phosphates by controlled nucleation and vectorial growth in constrained reaction environments. Walsh et al. reported the preparation of a porous micrometer-scale reticulated HAp structure using bicontinuous microemulsion, with a structure composed of a self-organized interconnected network of surfactant-bounded-water filled channels surrounded by oil. This is somewhat different from the natural mineralization processes; however, it is expected that highly ordered HAp crystal arrays will be obtained by improving the process.

14.3.3.2 The Use of Hydrogels as Microenvironments

The hydrogel is another candidate that can provide microenvironments for biomineralization. Hydrogels are currently used for biomedical applications; for instance, poly(2-hydroxyethyl methacrylate) (PHEMA) is used for contact lenses. However, the use of hydrogels is sometimes limited by calcification.

Calcification is a type of biomineralization but in most cases, it is considered a nonwilling reaction to biomaterials. The calcification of biomaterials is an important pathologic process observed in hydrogels and also in many kind of biomaterials,[11] for example, those observed in artificial blood pumps (artificial hearts),[12] heart valves,[13,14] and soft contact lenses.[15] Calcification has also been observed in polyurethane,[11] silicone rubber,[16] and PHEMA.[17] Calcification lowered the performance of the materials by changing their bulk properties or causing thrombosis, and a great deal of research has been done on calcification.[18-21]

Calcified material is important and useful for biomedical purposes. HAp, one of the main components of calcified material or bone, is a biofunctional inorganic material. In the hydrogel–HAp system, apatite crystals and polymer chains are entangled, and their mechanical properties and biological activities are unique.

The calcification mechanism has not yet been clarified. Many possible factors, such as animal species, age, hormone levels, types of materials, shear stress, surface defects, protein adsorption, hydrophilicity, and thrombus may contribute to the calcification of biomedical materials *in vivo*.[22,23] Most studies of calcification have been done *in vivo*[18,21] because it was assumed that devitalized cells and cellular debris were the keys to calcification. Recent research revealed that the physicochemical activity of materials is another essential factor for calcium phosphate deposition in the initial stage of calcification. In 1990, Kokubo et al. developed a biomimetic process that served as an *in vitro* calcification model.[24] The biomimetic process is as follows; SBF (1.0) and concentrated SBF (1.5) were prepared by dissolving inorganic salts. The biomimetic process has two steps: the first is nucleation, which uses $CaO–SiO_2$ based glass (nominal composition: MgO 4.6, CaO 44.7, SiO_2 34.0, P_2O_5 16.2, and CaF_2 0.5 wt%) and 1.0 SBF. The second is the HAp growing step which uses 1.5 SBF. Nucleation was performed at 37°C for 24 h for each substrate, then the substrates were transferred into the 1.5 SBF (2 ml/gel) and soaked for various periods in the 1.5 SBF, which was replaced every 2 days. Using this process, HAp formation on/in the hydrogels was studied. Nonionic hydrogels consisting of hydroxyl groups bearing polymers were used to clarify the effects of the surroundings near the hydroxyl groups. Figure 14.2 shows the cross-sectional views of (a) PVA, (b) agarose, and (c) polyacrylamide (PAAm) hydrogels after the biomimetic process. A thin, continuous white layer of crystals of HAp was observed on the PVA and PAAm hydrogels. No such white layer was observed on the agarose hydrogel.

Table 14.1 summarizes the amount of the deposited calcium on/in each hydrogel (second soaking for 7 days) in relation to the swelling ratios and the bound water content. The swelling ratios of agarose gels were very high and they only had small amounts of bound water. The PVA and PAAm gels showed a reverse correlation between the swelling ratio and the bound water content. The relationship of the amount

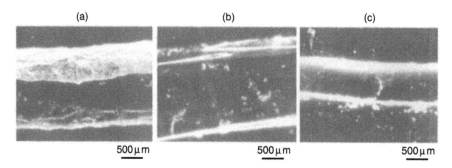

FIGURE 14.2 Cross-sectional views of hydrogels after biomimetic process.

of deposited calcium, the swelling ratio, and the bound water content varied. In this system, the swelling ratio and the bound water content were the essential physico-chemical factors that seemed to be related to HAp formation on/in hydrogels. The greater bound water content provides a large number of nucleation sites for HAp. The higher the swelling ratio, the larger the number of ions supplied into a hydrogel matrix from a solution (here 1.5 SBF) to grow HAp nuclei.

To prevent calcification, it is necessary to modify chemical structures, such as by introduction of sulfonate groups.[21] Considering the definitive characteristics of hydrogels for use as implants, the swelling ratio seems to be more important than the bound water content because, when hydrogels are implanted *in vivo*, their nucleation sites will be provided by cell debris, denatured proteins, and adsorbed lipids.

The biomimetic process can effectively prepare apatite composites on the surfaces of various kinds of materials; however, it takes a long time to form a large amount of apatite using this process. To overcome these obstacles, a novel apatite formation process was developed.[25] This process (alternate soaking process) is based on the widely known wet process of apatite preparation.[26] In the first step, hydrogel is soaked in a $CaCl_2$/Tris-HCl aqueous solution (pH 7.4); in the second, the gel is soaked in an Na_2HPO_4 aqueous solution. The apatite content in the PVA–apatite composites obtained by this method was increased by increasing the number of reaction cycles. After six reaction cycles, a PVA gel with a high swelling ratio contained approximately 70 wt% of apatite in the composite. A gel with a low swelling ratio contains about 15 wt% of formed apatite in the composite. Figure 14.3 shows cross-sectional views of the PVA gels after each cycle; apatite crystals were formed on the surfaces of the gels and inside the gels after 15 reaction cycles.

Bone contains about 70 to 80 wt% apatite in a collagen matrix. One goal of fabricating organic/inorganic supramolecular assemblies is to prepare a matrix that has the same apatite content and the same or better mechanical properties. Using a hydrogel as a template of the microenvironment for deposition of inorganic crystals is expected to yield the desired organic/inorganic supramolecular assembly.

TABLE 14.1
The Amounts of Deposited Calcium on/in Nonionic Hydrogels

Hydrogel		Swelling ratio	Bound water content [c] (%)	Ca deposited (mg/gel)
PVA	1.0[a]	18.0	13.3	103.0
	3.0[a]	5.6	27.6	7.2
	5.0[a]	1.5	68.1	0.6
Agarose	1.0[b]	8.8	1.0	152.4
	2.0[b]	45.3	0.0	153.1
	3.0[b]	32.8	1.2	161.6
PAAm	1.0[a]	31.9	5.4	45.4
	4.0[a]	16.9	6.8	130.2
	8.0[a]	12.7	7.8	138.8

[a] Cross-linker (mol%)
[b] Solution concentration (wt%).
[c] Determined by differential scanning calorimetry.

14.3.3.3 The Use of Grafted Surfaces as Microenvironments

One of the requirements of HAp coating onto organic polymer substrates is good adhesion to the substrates. In order to enhance the interaction between the inorganic apatite and the organic polymers, some studies introduced hydrophilic polar groups such as phosphate[27,28] carboxyls and hydroxyls[28-30] onto hydrophobic substrates

Another strategy is to create the microenvironment for biomineralization on the surface. Surface graft polymerization of hydrophilic polymers was adopted for this objective. Commonly used hydrophilic polymers, PAAm and PAAc, were grafted onto polyethylene (PE) film surfaces. Carboxyl groups can enhance apatite deposition on polymer substrates.[28-30] Using an alternate soaking process, the effect of PAAm and PAAc grafting densities on apatite formation was investigated. X-ray diffraction analysis indicated that HAP was coated on PAAm- or PAAc- grafted PE films. The amount of apatite coated on PAAm-grafted PE (PAAm-g-PE) films increased with an increase in the number of reaction cycles and the grafting density of the PAAm. Similar to PAAm-g-PE, the amount of apatite coated on PAAc-grafted PE (PAAc-g-PE) films increased linearly with an increase in the grafting density of the PAAc up to around 30 µg/cm.[2] No significant increase in the apatite coating on the

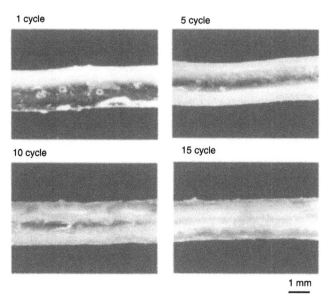

FIGURE 14.3 Cross-sectional views of PVA hydrogel after alternate soaking process.

PAAc-g-PE films was observed even after 50 reaction cycles when the grafting densities of PAAc were over 30 $\mu g/cm^2$. Apatite coating was not observed on the original PE films. As shown in Figure 14.4, scanning electron microscopic images reveal the aggregation of apatite crystals on all PAAm-g-PE films and PAAc-g-PE films with grafting densities from 10 to 30 $\mu g/cm^2$. On the other hand, a dense apatite layer with some cracks was coated when the grafting density of the PAAc chains was over 30 $\mu g/cm.^2$ These results indicate that it is possible to coat apatite on hydrophilic polymer–grafted PE films by an alternate soaking process and that apatite crystal morphology can be controlled as a function of polymer type and density.

Kato et al. grafted an organophosphate polymer onto a PE film by surface graft polymerization of a phosphate-containing monomer.[27,28] Apatite formation was done by immersing the grafted film into SBF. To distinguish the effect of phosphate groups on the deposition of the apatite layer from simple calcium absorption by the anion, a comparative study was done using a PE film with surface immobilized carboxylic groups. Calcium phosphate deposition was observed on all the materials investigated, but the kinetics, composition, deposit amount, and bonding strength of the new phase were found to be significantly different among the modified materials, depending on the density and chemical nature of the surface-immobilized ionic groups. The polymeric materials modified by surface graft polymerization of a phosphate-containing monomer produced a carbonated HAp layer firmly bonded with the material upon immersion in SBF.

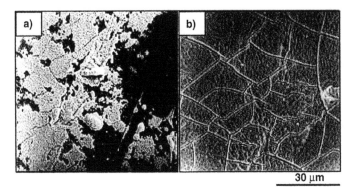

FIGURE 14.4 Scanning electron micrograph of poly(acrylic acid) (PAAc)-grafted poly(ethylene) film surface after 50 cycles of alternate soaking process: (a) $10\ \mu g/cm^2$, (b) $43\ \mu g/cm^2$.

14.4 SUMMARY

Much progress has been made in the understanding of mineralization processes and in the preparation of synthetic complex structures in recent years. Organic materials such as lipids, surfactants, and polymers play important roles as triggers for nucleation and as templates for arrangement of crystals. It is essential to control the three-dimensional positioning of organic materials and inorganic crystals. We can expect to achieve large-scale precision positioning of functional groups with nanometer-sized resolution. Supramolecular assembly is one of the possible techniques.

The ultimate goal of the study of organic/inorganic supramolecular assembly is to produce new materials that have far superior properties than present synthetic materials. The challenges are (1) the control of crystal growth by organic materials, (2) the alignment of the crystals on a two-dimensional surface, (3) accumulating two-dimensional order-structured hybrids, and (4) preparation of hierarchical structures organized on a wide scale. These problems will be conquered, and highly elaborated and finely controlled organic/inorganic supramolecular assemblies will be of great importance for our society.

ACKNOWLEDGMENTS

A part of this work was done in collaboration with Professor Akashi and Professor Serizawa of Kagoshima University. The author is grateful to Professor Kokubo and Doctor Tanahashi of Kyoto University for their advice and suggestions about the biomimetic process. The authors would also like to acknowledge Dr. Kamino of the Kagoshima Prefecture Institute of Industrial Technology, Professor Hirata, and Lecturer Fukushige of Kagoshima University for their help.

REFERENCES

1. Mann, S. et al., Crystal tectonics: chemical construction and self-organization, *Dalton*, 21, 3753, 2000.
2. Mann, S., The chemistry of form, *Angew. Chem. Int. Ed.*, 39, 3393, 2000.
3. Lowenstam, H.A. and Weiner, S., *On Biomineralization*, Oxford University Press, New York, 1989.
4. Jackson, A.P., Vincent, J.F.V., and Turner, R.M., A physical model of nacre, *Comos. Sci. Technol.*, 36, 255, 1989.
5. Mann S. et al., Crystallization at inorganic–organic interfaces: biominerals and biomimetic synthesis, *Science*, 261, 1286, 1993.
6. Sato, K., Kumagai, Y., and Tanaka, J., Apatite formation on organic monolayers in simulated body environment, *J. Biomed. Mater. Res.*, 50, 16, 2000.
7. Kim, H.M. et al., Composition and structure of the apatite formed on PET substrates in SBF modified with various ionic activity products, *J. Biomed. Mater. Res.*, 46, 228, 1999.
8. Sugawara, A. and Kato, T., Aragonite $CaCO_3$ thin-film formation by cooperation of Mg^{2+} and organic polymer matrices, *Chem. Commun.*, 6, 487, 2000.
9. Kamei, S. et al., Histologic and mechanical evaluation for bone bonding of polymer surfaces grafted with a phosphate-containing polymer, *J. Biomed. Mater. Res.*, 37, 384, 1997.
10. Walsh, D., Hopwood, J.D., and Mann, S., Crystal tectonic: construction of reticulated calcium phosphate frameworks in discontinuous reverse microemulsions, *Science*, 264, 1576, 1994.
11. Harasaki, H. et al., Calcification in blood pumps, *Trans. ASAIO*, 25, 305, 1979.
12. Thoma, R. J. and Phillips, R. E., The role of material surface chemistry in important device calcification: a hypothesis, *J. Heart Valve Dis.*, 4, 214, 1995.
13. Neethling, W.N. et al., Processing factors as determinants of tissue valve calcification, *J. Cardiovasc. Surg. Torino*, 33, 285, 1992.
14. Fisher, A.C. et al., Calcification modeling in artificial heart valves, *Int. J. Artif. Organs*, 15, 284, 1992.
15. Bucher, P.J., Buchi, E.R., and Daicker, B.C., Dystrophic calcification of an implanted hydroxyethylmethacrylate intraocular lens, *Arch. Ophthalmol.*, 113, 1431, 1995.
16. Brockhurst, R.J. et al., Dystrophic calcification of silicone scleral bucking implant materials, *Am. J. Ophthalmol.*, 115, 524, 1993.
17. Imai, Y. and Watanabe, A., Effect of hydrophilicity and chemical structure of hydrogels on calcification, in *Progress in Artificial Organs*, Nose, Y., Kjellstranc, C.M., and Ivanurich, P., Eds., ISAO Press, Cleveland, 994, 1985.
18. Girardot, J.M. and Girardot M.N., Amide cross-linking an alternative to glutaraldehyde fixation, *J. Heart Valve Dis.*, 5, 518, 1996.
19. Joshi, R.R. et al., Calcification of polyurethanes implanted subdermally in rats is enhanced by calciphylaxis, *J. Biomed. Mater. Res.*, 31, 201, 1996.
20. Golomb, G. et al., Mechanical properties and histology of charge modified bioprosthetic tissue resistant to calcification, *Biomaterials*, 13, 353, 1992.
21. Han, D.K. et al., *In vivo* biostability and calcification resistance of surface-modified PU-PEG-SO_3, *J. Biomed. Mater. Res.*, 27, 1063, 1993.
22. Coleman, D.L., Mineralization of blood pump bladders, *Trans. ASAIO*, 27, 708, 1981.
23. Nose, Y., Harasaki, H., and Murray, J., Mineralization of artificial surfaces that contact blood, *Trans ASAIO*, 27, 714, 1981.

24. Kokubo, T., Surface chemistry of bioactive glass-ceramics, *J. Non-Cryst. Sol.*, 120, 138, 1990.
25. Taguchi, T., Kishida, A., and Akashi, M., Hydroxyapatite formation on/in poly(vinyl alcohol) hydrogel matrices using a novel alternate soaking process, *Chem. Lett.,* 711, 1998.
26. Correia, R.N. et al., Wet synthesis and characterization of modified hydroxyapatite powders, *J. Mater. Sci. Mat. Med.*, 7, 501, 1996.
27. Kato, K., Eika, Y., and Ikada, Y., Deposition of a hydroxyapatite thin layer onto a polymer surface carrying grafted phosphate polymer chains, *J. Biomed. Mater. Res.*, 32, 687, 1996.
28. Tretinnikov, O.N., Kato, K., and Ikada, Y., *In vitro* hydroxyapatite deposition onto a film surface-grafted with organophosphate polymer, *J. Biomed. Mater. Res.*, 28, 1365, 1994.
29. Tanahashi, M. et al., Apatite coated on organic polymers by biomimetic process: improvement in its adhesion to substrate by NaOH treatment, *J. Appl. Biomater.*, 5, 339, 1994.
30. Tanahashi, M. et al., Apatite coated on organic polymers by biomimetic process: improvement in its adhesion to substrate by glow-discharge treatment, *J. Biomed. Mater. Res.*, 29, 349, 1995.

15 Biomimetic Function

Katsuhiko Ariga

CONTENTS

15.1 INTRODUCTION

In the biomimetic approach, we analyze biological functions and develop artificial systems that simulate or regenerate them. Most biological functions result from highly sophisticated sequential events where specific recognitions and reactions are driven by multiple weak dynamics such as electrostatic interaction, hydrogen bonding, and hydrophobic interaction. Supermolecules such as host–guest systems can sometimes be regarded as good models of biological receptor–substrate systems. A well designed host might induce the chemical reaction of a bound guest molecule and serve as an effective mimic of an enzyme function. The first part of this chapter discusses several examples of artificial receptors and artificial enzymes as individual biomimetic elements.

Many sophisticated functions are expressed at biological membranes where lipids, proteins, and sugars are organized in the required manner. Therefore, biomimetic membranes, which are mimics of biological membranes, are important parts of these functions. The biomimetic membranes provide a unique interfacial environment where molecular interactions are significantly modified. Different functional molecules can be co-immobilized on the biomimetic membranes where conjugation of the functions is highly possible. Later in this chapter, the functions expressed on the biomimetic membrane are described.

0-8493-0965-4/02/$0.00+$1.50
© 2002 by CRC Press LLC

15.2 INDIVIDUAL BIOMIMETIC ELEMENTS

15.2.1 ARTIFICIAL RECEPTORS

In biological systems, chemical reactions, energy conversions, and signal transmissions proceed in a well-organized way. Such organization heavily depends on the abilities of functional molecules to recognize their partner molecules. Molecular recognition of incredibly high specificity and efficiency is achieved by biological receptors. Therefore, the development of artificial receptors is a vital target in biomimetic chemistry, and host–guest chemistry plays a central role.

During the recognition process of biological receptors, the cooperative nature of interacting groups leads to incredibly high specificity and efficiency. In order to mimic such receptors by the supramolecular method, multiple recognition sites have to be assembled in their proper positions. However, an assembly of individual sites sometimes accompanies a serious entropy loss, resulting in less favorable guest binding. To avoid any entropic disadvantage, an artificial receptor must have recognition sites at the proper positions in a relatively rigid backbone. The recognition sites are preorganized, and any unnecessary entropy loss upon guest binding is suppressed. Preorganization is one of the most important keys in designing artificial receptors. Several examples of the artificial receptors are shown in Figure 15.1.

Many cyclic molecules have been used as artificial receptors,[1] because their limited conformational flexibility is advantageous for preorganization. Crown ether was the first artificial receptor. The crown ethers can recognize various cations through interaction with lone pairs on oxygen atoms, and recognition efficiency is determined by size matching between the guest ions and the inner diameter of the crown ether. It can be regarded as a mimic of biological ionophores such as valinomycin, which can bind and carry potassium ions. Cryptands have three-dimensionally linked cyclic structures and can more decisively recognize target guests than the crown ethers can. The rigid nature of the cryptand has a large effect of the preorganization.

Another well known artificial receptor is cyclodextrin, which is a cyclic oligomer of glucose, that provides a rigid hydrophobic core. Molecular recognition by cyclodextrin is mainly driven by the van der Waals contact, and thus cyclodextrin can recognize the sizes and shapes of guest molecules. The chemical modification of OH groups leads to an additional interaction between the cyclodextrin and the guest molecule. The introduction of the additional functional groups is useful for designing artificial enzymes as described later.

Other cyclic molecules have been synthesized as artificial receptors, some of which are called calixarenes, cyclophanes, and carcerands. In addition, acyclic molecules with many interacting groups on a rigid backbone have been developed as artificial receptors.[2,3] Some are called molecular clefts. Many kinds of receptor sites are organized on a cleft-like rigid backbone, and their cooperative interaction with a guest molecule leads to highly efficient recognition.

The organic syntheses of receptors with complicated structures are not always easy, and approaches based on organic chemistry are not always practical. Therefore, we need alternative methodologies that can be applied to many kinds of guest

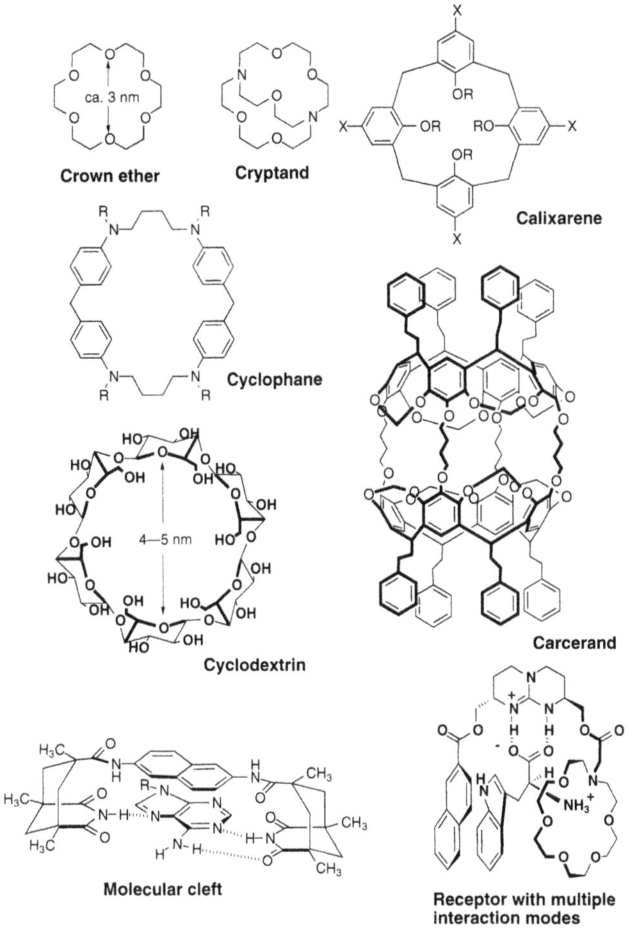

FIGURE 15.1 Artificial receptors.

molecules. One alternative is a molecular imprinting technique in which a guest molecule is used as a template and its surrounding is rigidified as a mold (Figure 15.2).[4] In the example shown in Figure 15.2, the guest molecule possesses three characteristic functional groups (A, B, and C), and these groups specifically interact with three different monomers (X, Y, and Z, respectively) (step I). The monomers were copolymerized with matrix monomers to immobilize the positions of recognition sites (X, Y, and Z) (step II). After the removal of the guest molecule, the remaining pores in the solid material can memorize sizes, shapes, and positions of the functional groups of the guest molecule (step III). Rebinding of the guest molecule to the pore then occurs efficiently (step IV). This methodology does not require complicated organic syntheses.

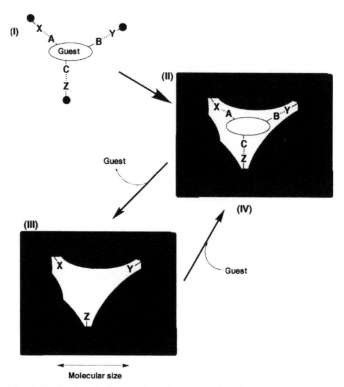

FIGURE 15.2 Molecular imprinting method. A guest molecule possesses three characteristic functional groups (A, B, and C) that can be recognized specifically by monomers X, Y, and Z, respectively. A formed pore can efficiently accommodate the guest molecule (step III to step IV).

If the most suitable receptor is selected from numerous candidates by a simple procedure, trial-and-error steps in molecular design can be eliminated. Combinatorial chemistry uses this concept.[5] We synthesized a group of receptor candidates called a library. After the library is prepared, a tag which identifies every receptor molecule is sometimes attached to each receptor candidate in a systematic way. Binding of the receptor candidates to a target guest is examined in one batch. The molecule having the greatest affinity to the guest molecule is selected from the library.

15.2.2 ARTIFICIAL ENZYMES

Enzymes are biological catalysts that can provide desirable reactions with high selectivity and efficiency. The utilization of naturally occurring enzymes under unnatural conditions can produce great benefits with current technology. However, enzymes do not always catalyze all the reactions desired. Conditions suitable for enzyme functions are usually limited and far from the conditions required for engineering processes. The amounts of naturally occurring enzymes is usually limited, and the extraction process is sometimes expensive and time consuming. Therefore, the development of enzyme mimics (artificial enzymes) that can overcome these disadvantages is desirable. Artificial enzymes in molecular devices would be useful for performing information conversion. The application of the artificial enzymes to a biological system also provides benefits. In this section, artificial enzymes for phosphodiester hydrolysis are described. Phosphodiester cleavage is important for nucleic acid modification, and thus, these kinds of artificial enzymes are important in gene technology.

Figure 15.3A shows the reaction mechanism of RNA hydrolysis by ribonuclease A. In the first step, the 2′-OH group of the RNA is activated through removal of the 2′-proton by histidine 12, and a P–O–C linkage is exchanged by the nucleophilic attack of the activated 2′-oxygen on the phosphorus atom, resulting in a cyclic phosphodiester (base 1 side) and a ribose terminal (base 2 side). Protonation of the phosphodiester by histidine 119 increases the electrophilicity of the phosphorus atom to help the nucleophilic attack by the 2′-oxygen. The histidines' catalytic roles are reversed in step II. Water is activated by the neutral histidine 119, and the activated water similarly attacks the cyclic phosphodiester. Cleavage of the cyclic ester is promoted through protonation by the other histidine (12). Cooperation of the neutral and protonated histidines is crucial in these reaction steps.

FIGURE 15.3 (A) Mechanism of RNA hydrolysis by nuclease. (B) Cyclodextrin-type artificial enzyme for cyclic phosphodiester hydrolysis. This enzyme mimics the second step of RNA cleavage. (C) Molecular cleft-type artificial enzyme for RNA hydrolysis.

This mechanism suggests that appropriate positioning of the two histidines would lead to efficient artificial ribonuclease under an optimized pH condition. Figure 15.3B shows an artificial ribonuclease that has a cyclodextrin core as the hydrophobic pocket with two histidine residues as catalytic sites.[6] This artificial enzyme catalyzed the second step of the phosphodiester cleavage. The hydrophobic part of the cyclic phosphodiester (substrate) was accommodated into the core of the cyclodextrin and the phosphodiester was exposed between the two histidines. The water molecule was activated through proton removal by the neutral histidine (left), and the activated water caused the nucleophilic attack on a phosphate atom. The protonated histidine (right) assisted this nucleophilic attack through protonation of the phosphodiester. Because cooperative function of the neutral and protonated histidines was important, the maximum activity of the artificial ribonuclease was obtained at around the pK_a of the histidines (ca. pH 7). However, this artificial enzyme cannot cleave RNA; it catalyzes only the second step.

RNA was cleaved by the artificial enzyme shown in Figure 15.3C. The enzyme is a mimic of staphylococcal nuclease.[7] It is a molecular-cleft-type of artificial enzyme in which guanidinium residues connected to a rigid backbone can immobilize an RNA phosphodiester moiety. Imidazole in solution activated 2'-OH and then nucleophilically attacked the phosphate. The transition state during the hydrolysis can be stabilized through electrostatic hydrogen bonding with the guanidiniums. This stabilization increased the reaction rate of the RNA cleavage.

To develop an artificial restriction enzyme that can cleave the desirable sequence, an oligonucleotide tag should be attached to the catalysis site. The artificial enzyme shown in Figure 15.4 has an oligonucleotide tag (rectangle) connected to a metal-chelate catalysis site (circle).[8] The catalytic site was fixed on the particular site of a substrate upon base pairing between the artificial enzyme and the substrate. The site-specific hydrolysis of RNA and DNA was achieved by the Ru–chelate and Ce–chelate enzymes, respectively.

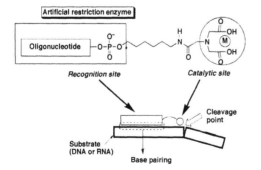

FIGURE 15.4 Artificial restriction enzyme. Oligonucleotide part (rectangle) in the artificial enzyme can recognize a substrate sequence and cleavage the substrate by the catalytic site (circle).

The supramolecular system described in Figure 15.5 was proposed to catalyze a self-replication process.[9] Condensation between the adenosine derivative (A) and Kemp's acid derivative (B) provides C. Compound C can bind A and B and catalyze the condensation between A and B, thus producing C. As a result, compound C was self-replicated. It is surprising that such a simple system can realize the self-replication process which is one of the key events of life.

Enzymes have precisely constructed active sites consisting of finely designed sequences of amino acids. Construction of such complicated structures by organic syntheses is energy- and time-consuming. The utilization of a biological system might overcome this problem. A biological immune system has an excellent ability to bind any type of outer substance (antigen), and a specific antibody is biologically produced for every antigen. This system would be useful for the construction of various enzyme-mimic sites, because the antibody for the transition state of the particular reaction could catalyze the corresponding reaction. This type of artificial enzyme is called a catalytic antibody. Because the transition state is usually unstable, the analog of the state is used for the preparation of the catalytic antibody.[10] Figure 15.6 shows the catalytic antibody for ester hydrolysis. The carboxylic acid ester hydrolysis proceeds via a tetrahedral transition state which is produced by nucleophilic attack of a hydroxide ion on a carbonyl carbon. Therefore, a phosphonic acid ester can be a good analog of the tetrehedral transition state. In this example, albumin-bound phosphonic acid ester was dosed to animals, and an antibody recognizing the analog was then immunologically obtained. The obtained antibody can stabilize the transition state and induce the rate enhancement of the carboxylic acid ester hydrolysis.

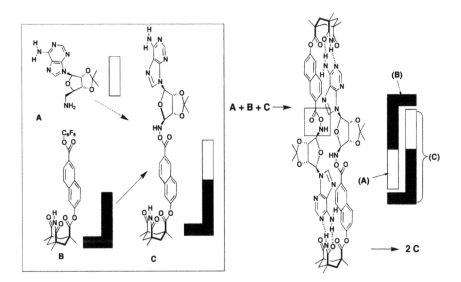

FIGURE 15.5 Self-replication based on molecular recognition. Compound C can bind A and B resulting in formation of C through condensation between A and B.

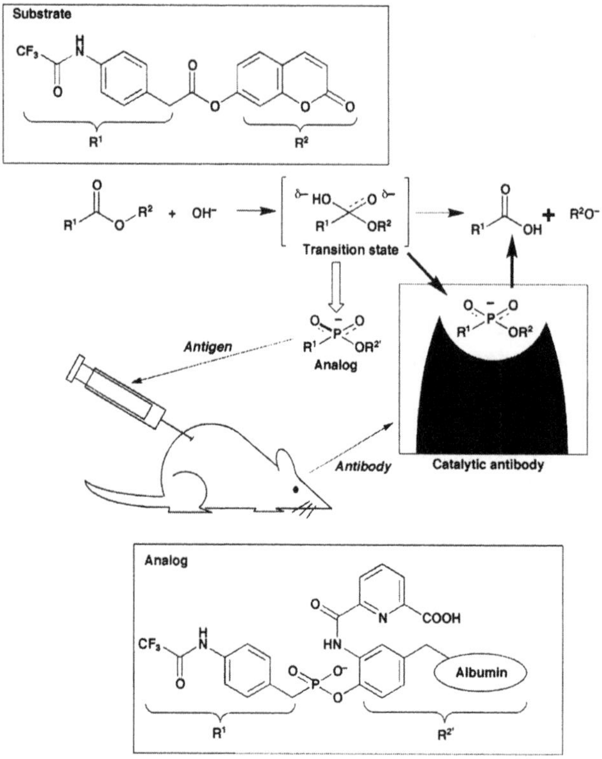

FIGURE 15.6 Catalytic antibody for ester hydrolysis. Albumin-bound phosphonic acid ester was used as an analog of a tetrahedron transition state of carboxylic acid ester hydrolysis. The antibody for the analog obtained from the animal can effectively catalyze carboxylic acid ester hydrolysis.

15.3 BIOMIMETIC FUNCTIONS AT MEMBRANE MEDIA

Biological systems are supported by various membrane structures, and many functions are expressed with the aid of the membranes. The development of membrane mimics and membrane-related artificial functions is one of key areas of biomimetic chemistry. This section discusses biomimetic approaches related to membrane structures.

15.3.1 PERMEABILITY CONTROL THROUGH BIOMIMETIC MEMBRANES

All biological membranes have a common general structure which is the assembly of lipids, proteins, and so on. The lipid molecules spontaneously form a continuous double layer structure (lipid bilayer) as a basic structure, and the proteins are accommodated in this structure. The most essential role of the membrane is defining the insides and outsides of the cell structures. The membranes are highly sensitive filters and allow active transport. The asymmetric distribution of ions is maintained across the membranes, and the gradient of the ion concentration can be regarded as one kind of energy that drives ATP synthesis and electrical signal transmission. Therefore, the primary target of the biomimetic function of the membrane structure should be permeability control.

Simple but useful models of cell membranes are liposomes and vesicles that have spherical shapes and lipid bilayer skins. The permeation control from the inside of these structures has been extensively researched with the aim of designing a drug delivery system (DDS). However, the structures are simple assemblies of lipids that are not strong enough for practical use. This disadvantage can be overcome through hybridization of the bilayer membrane with solid supports.

Figure 15.7A shows a bilayer-immobilized capsule.[11] The capsule as a solid support was prepared by interfacial condensation by dropping ethylendiamine alkaline solution into a cyclohexane/chloroform solution of 1,10-decyldicarbonyl chloride. The obtained capsule has a 2-mm diameter and was exposed to a hot dodecane solution of lipids. A large number of the lipid bilayer structures (multibilayers) were immobilized in the skin of the capsule by cooling the solution. Water-soluble substances were incorporated in the inner cell of the capsule by dialysis before the bilayer immobilization. The permeation of the trapped substance was controlled by a

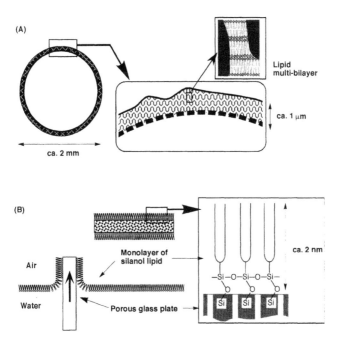

FIGURE 15.7 (A) Multiple layers of lipid bilayer structures are immobilized in a skin (1-µm thickness) of a nylon capsule (2-mm diameter). (B) Monolayer (2-nm thickness) is covalently immobilized on porous glass plate.

change in the physical state of the lipid bilayers. For example, the transition from the gel to the liquid crystalline state of the bilayer structure induced a drastic change in the permeability of small substances inside the capsule. Designing a lipid structure allows for other types of permeation controls that can be driven by pH change, the addition of calcium ion, and the application of an electric field.

Permeation control by a single lipid monolayer was also performed (Figure 15.7B).[12] A monolayer of a silanol lipid was covalently immobilized onto a porous glass plate. The monolayer structure was also stabilized through a siloxane-like linkage between the lipids. The permeability of aqueous substances through the glass plate was controlled by the transition from the gel to liquid crystalline state of the monolayer. Recently, a self-assembled vesicle of the silanol lipid was demonstrated. The obtained vesicle has a basic bilayer structure with a rigid ceramic-like shell. This sufficiently stable cell membrane mimic is called Cerasome.[13]

In biological membranes, some proteins form a channel structure in a cell membrane and achieve active transport of particular ions. Therefore, the development of an artificial ion channel is an attractive target in membrane-related biomimetic approaches. Several oligopeptides have been used as mimics of the channel proteins.[14] They form an amphiphilic α-helix having both hydrophilic and hydrophobic sides. Such helices spontaneously assemble to form hydrophilic channels for ions in the hydrophobic lipid membrane. The structure of the hydrophilic channel can be controlled through modification of the amino acid sequences, resulting in the control of ion permeability and selectivity. Stacking assemblies of cyclic peptides[15] or crown ethers[16] also provide channel structures in the lipid membrane. As shown in Figure 15.8, lipid mimics having various chain structures spontaneously formed hydrophilic channels in the lipid bilayers.[17] Such a supramolecular approach based on self-assembling properties seems to be more convenient than the construction of an entire channel structure.

15.3.2 MOLECULAR RECOGNITION OF MEMBRANES

Hydrogen bonding is highly directional compared with other noncovalent interactions such as electrostatic, van der Waals, and hydrophobic interactions. The directionality of the hydrogen bonding significantly contributes to the molecular recognition in biological systems, although an aqueous medium is not good for hydrogen bond formation. In order to mimic biological hydrogen bonding, molecular recognition sites were embedded in a hydrophobic environment dispersed in or located at aqueous interfaces. The aqueous phase contacting the organic phase displays unique properties different from those of bulk water. The creation of well organized hydrogen bonding sites in the interfacial environment may open the way to achieving molecular recognition through effective hydrogen bonding in aqueous media.[18]

The effect of the interfacial environment was examined using the guanidinium–phosphate system. The binding of nucleotides such as AMP to the aqueous micelles and bilayers of guanidiniums was studied and Langmuir analysis with varied guest concentrations gave AMP binding constants of 10^2 to 10^4 M^{-1}.[19] These values are significantly greater than that between molecularly dispersed guanidinium

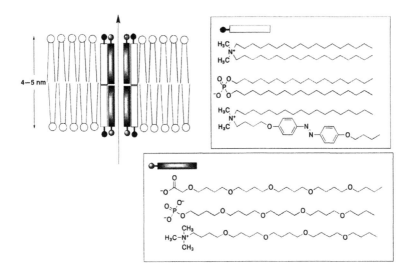

FIGURE 15.8 Self-assembled artificial channel.

and phosphate in water (1.4 M^{-1}). It can be concluded that the guest binding is enhanced at the aqueous mesoscopic interfaces. Molecular recognition at a macroscopic interface was also investigated at the air–water interface. A water-insoluble guanidinium amphiphile was spread on water, and the interaction of its monolayer with aqueous nucleotides such as AMP and ATP was investigated (Figure 15.9A). A significantly large binding constant (10^6 to 10^7 M^{-1}) was observed at the macroscopic interface.[20]

The molecular recognition abilitites of nucleotides and related compounds, sugars, nucleic acid bases, peptides, amino acids, and other compounds through complementary hydrogen bonding were investigated at the air–water interface.[18] Two examples of base pair mimics at the air–water interface are shown in Figure 15.9B. The binding of aqueous thymine to a receptor monolayer with the diaminotriazine function was investigated.[21] The FT–IR spectral changes are consistent with the guest binding via complementary hydrogen bonding. Elemental analyses by x-ray photoelectron spectroscopy (XPS) revealed equimolar binding stoichiometry. The mode of hydrogen bonding is altered in the binding of aqueous adenine to the orotate-type monolayer that possesses the cyclic imide function.[22] Conceivably, the stacking of bound adenine molecules accelerates the binding. A similar stacking interaction is well known in the double-helix formation of DNA.

Molecular recognition by mixed monolayers was also demonstrated. The recognition of aqueous flavin adenine dinucleotide (FAD) was investigated by using mixed monolayers of guanidinium, orotate, and diaminotriazine amphiphiles (Figure 15.9C).[23] Isoalloxazine, phosphates, and adenosine moieties in FAD were recognized through hydrogen bonding by diaminotriazine, guanidiniums, and orotate in the

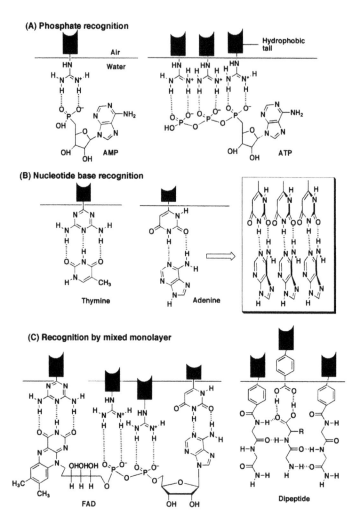

FIGURE 15.9 Molecular recognition at the air–water interface: (A) phosphate recognition; (B) nucleotide base; (C) recognition by mixed monolayer.

mixed monolayer, respectively. The XPS analyses of the mixed film transferred from aqueous FAD (0.01 mM) confirmed the binding stoichiometry proposed in Figure 15.9C.

In order to develop protein-like recognition sites by assembling rather simple amphiphiles, the recognition of aqueous dipeptides was investigated at the surface of the monolayer of the oligopeptide-functionalized amphiphile. Highly water-soluble dipeptides were bound from the aqueous subphase to monolayers of peptide-derivatized dialkyl amphiphiles.[24] The binding selectivity was essentially determined by the hydrogen bonding mode and the extent of the hydrophobic interaction when additional interaction at the guest terminal was absent. However, mixing of a second component to the monolayer would change the situation. Participation of the second amphiphile to the binding increased the binding efficiency and/or altered binding selectivity due to formation of additional hydrogen bonding (Figure 15.9C).

15.3.3 SIGNAL TRANSDUCTION AND ENERGY CONVERSION ON AN ARTIFICIAL MEMBRANE

A G-protein plays an important role in biological signal transduction, and its mechanism is shown in Figure 15.10A. The G-protein consists of three subunits (α, β, and γ) with GTP (or GDP) and couples the receptor function and enzyme (effector, adenylate cyclase) activation. The G-protein in its inactivated form exists as a trimer with GDP bound to the α subunit. When the first signal molecule (hormone, etc.) binds to a receptor, the G-protein is activated through binding to the receptor–signal complex. The guanyl–nucleotide-binding site on the α subunit is altered, allowing GTP to bind in place of GDP. The binding of GTP is thought to dissociate the α subunit from the β and γ subunits. The dissociated α subunit tightly binds to the enzyme (adenylate cyclase) which is activated to produce the cyclic AMP (second signal). Within less than a minute, the α subunit hydrolyzes its bound GTP to GDP, causing the α subunit to dissociate from the enzyme. Reassociation of the α subunit and β and γ subunits reforms the inactivated form of the G-protein.

Figure 15.10B shows a mimic of the signal transduction system[25] where lactate dehydrogenase (LDH, effector) immobilized on the bilayer vesicle is inhibited by Cu^{2+} (G-protein mimic) in the initial (off) state. When a suitable signal molecule

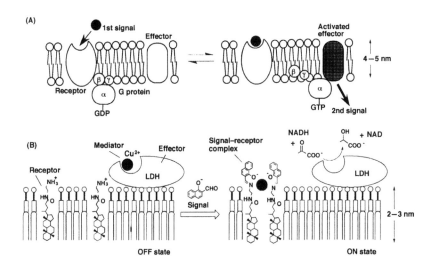

FIGURE 15.10 (A) G-protein-mediated signal transduction system found in naturally occurring systems. (B) Artificial signal transduction system. Addition of hydroxynaphthaldehyde (signal molecule) can activate LDH bound to a lipid membrane.

(hydroxynaphthaldehyde) is added to the system, a signal–receptor complex (Schiff's base) is formed through a reaction between the receptor amine and the signal aldehyde. Because the signal–receptor complex has a higher affinity for the metal ion than the enzyme, the metal ion is removed from the enzyme and the enzyme is activated (on state). In the on state, the system catalytically produced lactate and NAD. This system is driven by the difference in the binding affinity to the metal ion of the enzyme, the uncomplexed receptor, and the signal–receptor complex.

One of the most elegant examples of functional arrays seen in biological systems is dye/protein organization for a photosynthesis system. In a bacterial reaction center (Figure 15.11A), several dyes and proteins are systematically organized in a lipid bilayer membrane.[26] The absorption of photoenergy to a bacteriochlorophile special pair (BC–BC) induces electron transfer to a quinone (Q_A) via a bacteriopheophytin (BP). Another quinone (Q_B) accepts two electrons from the reaction center and two protons from the inner cell and turns into a hydroquinone (Q_BH_2). The trapped electrons and protons are carried to the outside of the cell by cytchrome b/c_1. The electrons are returned to the BC–BC special pair by cytochrome c_2. The protons are transported from the inside to the outside of the cell. ATP can be synthesized by ATPase with the proton gradient as a driving force.

The photoenergy-driven ATP synthesis was mimicked by the system shown in Figure 14.11B.[27] The triad carotene–porphyrin–quinone (C-P-Q) molecule was buried in a lipid bilayer membrane. Visible light irradiation induced charge separation in the triad, i.e., carotene and quinone became a cation radical and anion radical, respectively. Another hydrophobic quinone (Q_s) located in the membrane accepted an electron from the triad quinone and a proton from the outside, resulting in the semiquinone formation. The semiquinone diffused to the inside of the membrane where it donated the electron to the carotene and released the proton to the inside of the bilayer membrane. The ATPase immobilized in the lipid bilayer converted ADP to ATP using the resulting proton gradient.

15.4 THE FUTURE OF BIOMIMETIC CHEMISTRY

Recently, much attention has been paid to nanotechnology — a methodology that develops mechanical machines and information converters with nanometer-scale structural precision. However, the 1999 nanotechnology research direction of the U.S. pointed out that current artificial technologies are inferior to those found in natural systems. The efficiency of energy conversion in mitochondrial and photosynthetic systems significantly exceeds the efficiency of any artificial system. Dogs can smell and bats can hear more sensitively than most artificial sensors. Information conversions in the brain and nervous system are much more sophisticated than those of current computers. We must learn from biological systems, and biomimetic approaches in supramolecular chemistry are indispensable to the future of our technology.

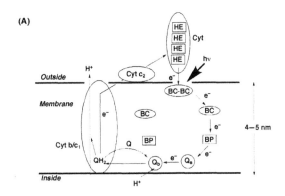

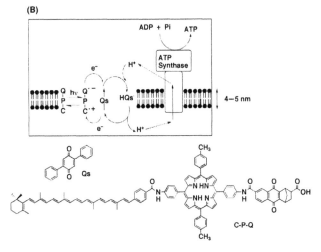

FIGURE 15.11 (A) Proton gradient formation at bacterial reaction center. (B) Photo-induced ATP synthesis as a photosynthesis mimic.

REFERENCES

1. Lehn, J.-M., *Supramolecular Chemistry — Concepts and Perspectives*, VCH Press, New York, 1995.
2. Rebek J., Jr., *Acc. Chem. Res.*, 23, 399, 1990.
3. Galan, A. et al., *Am. Chem. Soc.*, 114, 1511, 1992.
4. Wulff, G., *Angew. Chem, Int. Ed. Engl.*, 34, 1812, 1995.
5. Tarasow, T.M. et al., *Nature*, 389, 54, 1997.
6. Desper, J.M. and Breslow, R., *J. Am. Chem. Soc.,* 116, 12081, 1994.
7. Smith, J., Ariga, K., and Anslyn, E.V., *J. Am. Chem. Soc.*, 115, 362, 1993.
8. Komiyama, M. et al., *Methods Enzymol.*, 341, 455, 2001.
9. Tjivikua, T., Ballester, P., and Rebek, J., Jr., *J. Am. Chem. Soc.*, 112, 8200, 1990.

10. Tramontano, A., Janda, K.D., and Lerner, R.A., *Proc. Natl. Acad. Sci. U.S.A.*, 83, 6737, 1986.
11. Okahata, Y., Ariga, K., and Seki, T., *J. Am. Chem. Soc.*, 110, 2495, 1988.
12. Ariga, K. and Okahata, Y., *J. Am. Chem. Soc.*, 111, 5618, 1989.
13. Katagiri, K., Ariga, K., Kikuchi, J., *Chem. Lett.*, 661, 1999.
14. Åkerfeld, K.S. et al., *Acc. Chem. Res.*, 26, 191, 1993.
15. Ghadiri, M.R., Granja, J.R., and Buehler, L.K., *Nature*, 369, 301, 1994.
16. Voyer, N. and Robitaille, M., *J. Am. Chem. Soc.*, 117, 6599, 1995.
17. Kobuke, Y. Ueda, K., and Sokabe, M. *J. Am. Chem. Soc.*, 114, 7618, 1992.
18. Ariga, K. and Kunitake, T., *Acc. Chem. Res.*, 31, 371, 1998.
19. Onda, M. et al., *J. Am. Chem. Soc.*, 118, 8524, 1996.
20. Sasaki, D.Y., Kurihara, K., and Kunitake, T., *J. Am. Chem. Soc.*, 113, 9685, 1991.
21. Kurihara, K. et al., *J. Am. Chem. Soc.,* 113, 5077, 1991.
22. Kawahara, T., Kurihara, K., and Kunitake, T., *Chem. Lett.*, 1839, 1992.
23. Taguchi, K., Ariga, K., and Kunitake, T., *Chem. Lett.,* 701, 1995.
24. Cha, X., Ariga, K., and Kunitake, T., *J. Am. Chem. Soc.*, 118, 9545, 1996.
25. Kikuchi, J., Ariga, K., and Ikeda, K., *Chem. Commun.*, 547, 1999.
26. Deisenhofer, J. and Michel, H., Angew. *Chem. Int. Ed. Engl.*, 28, 829, 1989.
27. Steinberg-Yfrach, G. et al., *Nature*, 392, 479, 1998.

16 Supramolecular Surfaces

Kazuhiko Ishihara

CONTENTS

16.1 INTRODUCTION

The biomembrane is the medium through which all cells interact with their environment. Singer and Nicolson proposed the structure of the biomembrane as a fluid mosaic model.[1] Proteins, which generally comprise about half the total mass of biomembrane, determine the specific membrane functions. The chemical composition and physical properties of biomembrane phospholipids may modulate protein function and cell behavior.[2] The phospholipids provide the hydrophobic environment necessary for the functioning of intrinsic membrane proteins. Each phospholipid is characterized by a phase separation, above which the chains are in a more fluid state. Some intrinsic proteins require fluid environments for their activities, while others operate in fixed, immobilized conditions. Biomembanes appear to maintain a particular distribution of fatty acids that provide the fluidity appropriate for the function of the tissue.

The polar head groups are in contact with water and contribute largely to the interfacial properties of cell surfaces. The predominant head group is phosphorylcholine, which forms the polar group of sphingomyelin and phosphatidylcholine. Phosphorylcholine, an electrically neutral, Zwitter ionic head group, which presents on the external surfaces of cells, is inert in blood coagulation assays.[3] Indeed,

0-8493-0965-4/02/$0.00+$1.50
© 2002 by CRC Press LLC

327

Noishiki found a very important fact during evaluation of *in vivo* blood compatibility for a polyester vascular prosthesis.[4] The luminal surface of the implanted vascular graft was covered with a double membrane similar to a biomembrane. This result indicates the importance of considering phospholipid components in blood–material interactions. This chapter presents an overview of new biointerfaces with supramolecular structures by molecular assembly of phospholipids.

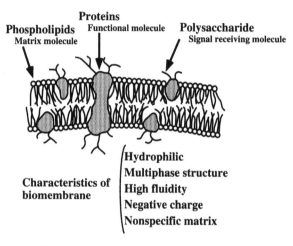

FIGURE 16.1 Structure and characteristics of biomembrane.

16.2 BIOMEMBRANE MIMICKING FOR SUPRAMOLECULAR SURFACES

The biomembrane has a supramolecular surface, constructed of three major chemical species: proteins, polysaccharides, and phospholipids (See Figure 16.1). These molecules form molecular assemblies and do not covalently bind each other. Therefore, fluidity of the biomembrane is very high and its surface is hydrophilic. These characteristics are important aspects of designing polymer biomaterials.

Figure 16.2, shows a molecular assembly with phospholipids and phospholipid polymers. Phospholipid molecules form assemblies in aqueous media, such as liposomes and lipid microspheres and can be injected directly into the bloodstream to function as drug carriers.[5] This characteristic is important. Thus, if the phospholipid molecules can immobilize in a highly organized manner, the surface has biocompatibility and blood compatibility that will weaken interactions between the biocomponents and materials surface.

Hall et al. used thromboelastography to investigate the effect of phospholipid adsorption on coagulation of blood exposed to the substrates, and found that coagulation on the surfaces coated with phospholipids.[6] Their attempts are not successful because of the unsuitability and very weak mechanical properties of phospholipid-

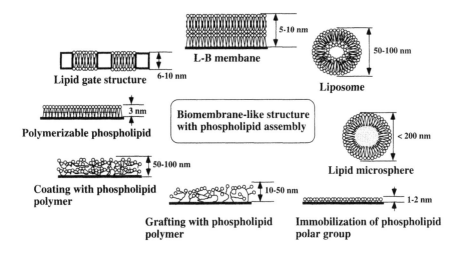

FIGURE 16.2 Various phospholipid assemblies.

coated surfaces. Kono et al. prepared porous polyamide microcapsules coated with phospholipid bilayer membrane like a phospholipid gate and investigated the interactions with platelets.[7] The phospholipid coating significantly suppressed the platelet adhesion onto the microcapsules.

16.3 PHOSPHOLIPID DERIVATIVE-ASSEMBLED SURFACES

Many researchers tried to prepare stable surfaces with phospholipids by polymerization of phospholipids and the chemical reaction between phospholipid and substrate as shown in Figure 16.3.

Coyle et al. reported that the cell adhesion properties of chemisorbed phospholipid monolayers on gold, prepared from phosphatidylcholine with thiol groups, have been defined.[8] In the presence of a nonadhesive protein, albumin, adhesion of cells to the surface was minimal; in the presence of fibronectin and vitronectin, substantial adhesion was observed. The ability of the phospholipid monolayer to support adhesion of cells was essentially independent of the molecular structures of the phosphatidylcholine derivatives employed. Kohler and coworkers developed a process of covalent grafting of modified phosphorylcholine molecules to substrate based on the premise of achieving blood compatibility through mimicking the chemical constituents of the biologically inert surfaces of inactivated platelet membranes.[9] The phosphatidylcholine-modified substrates were used in the platelet adhesion assay. These substrates reduced the number of adherent platelets over 80% compared with the original substrate.

Marra and coworkers reported that a stabilized phosphatidylcholine containing polymeric surfaces was produced by *in situ* polymerization of a self-assembled lipid monolayer on an alkylated substrate.[10] They introduced long alkyl groups on the glass

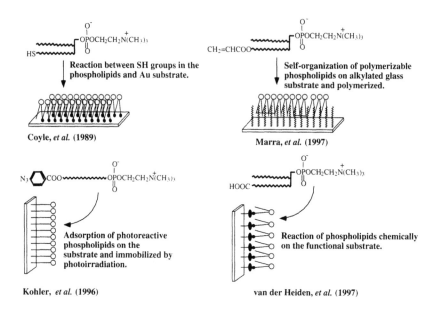

FIGURE 16.3 Methods of preparation of immobilization of phospholipid molecules.

surface and then unilamellar vesicles of phospholipid derivatives with polymerizable groups were fused on the substrate. Free radical polymerization with aqueous medium using water-soluble initiator was carried out to obtain a stabilized phospholipid surface. The surface analysis with contact angle measurement and x-ray photoelectron spectroscopic (XPS) analysis clearly indicated the formation of a closed packed phosphorylcholine surface.

van der Heiden and coworkers studied a photochemical modification using phospholipid analogue having an azide group.[11] They synthesized two compounds that had different types of spacers: tri(ethylene oxide) and hexamethylene chains. These compounds were physically adsorbed to the substrate surface. Upon UV irradiation, the azide group reacted to the substrate and the surface was covered with the compounds.

Blood compatibility *in vitro* was tested with thrombin generation assays and platelet adhesion tests. Clotting times were clearly prolonged for the modified surfaces. Platelet adhesion was observed on the original substrate surface, whereas it was suppressed on the modified surface. Liu et al. reported that a phosphorylcholine group was introduced onto the surface of substrate by a combination of graft polymerization of acrylic acid and subsequent chemical reactions.[12] The characterization of the modified surface revealed that a sufficient number of phosphorylcholine groups could be located at the surface. The platelet adhesion test indicated that the platelets hardly adhered on the modified surface in contrast to adherence to the original substrate, but it was affected by the existence of various functional groups generated during the first graft polymerization process on the surface.

16.4 POLYMERS WITH PHOSPHORYLCHOLINE GROUPS FOR SURFACE MODIFICATION

16.4.1 PHOSPHOLIPID POLYMERS

A polymer having phosphorylcholine in the side chain has been synthesized to make a preparation of phosphorylcholine-assembled surface much easier. The synthesis of a monomer with phosphorylcholine group may be excellent for this purpose.

A methacrylate monomer with a phospholipid polar group, 2-methacryloyloxyethyl phosphorylcholine (MPC, Figure 16.4) and its polymers were synthesized and the performance at their surfaces was evaluated.[13-14] MPC can be easily polymerized by a conventional radical polymerization technique. The solubility of the poly(MPC) is very unique, that is, it can be dissolved in water and alcohols such as methanol, ethanol, and 2-propanol, but it cannot be dissolved in a water–alcohol mixture in the range of 60 to 90 wt% of alcohol. MPC can be copolymerized with other vinyl compounds such as methacrylate, acrylate, and styrene derivatives through radical polymerization. It is possible to prepare MPC polymers with various architectures: random copolymer, block-type copolymer, and graft-type copolymer.[15-16] A reactive poly(MPC) with a reactive group in the one terminal of the polymer chain could be obtained.[17-19]

Monomers bearing phosphorylcholine groups shown in Figure 16.5 were synthesized with strong help from the structure and function of MPC and its polymers.[20-26] Changes were carried out with attention paid to the chemical structure of the polymerizable group, the length and mobility of the spacer portions between polymerizable groups and phosphorylcholine groups, and chemical structure of the phospholipid polar group.

The phosphorylcholine group was also introduced in the polyurethane and polycarbonate. Baumgartner et al. and Mathieu et al. prepared polyurethanes with phosphorylcholine groups to control protein adsorption and cell attachment.[27-28] Iwasaki et al. prepared polycarbonate as a new biodegradable polymer by polycondensation between 1,3-dicholoroisopropyl phosphorylcholine and 1,4-dibromobutane.[29]

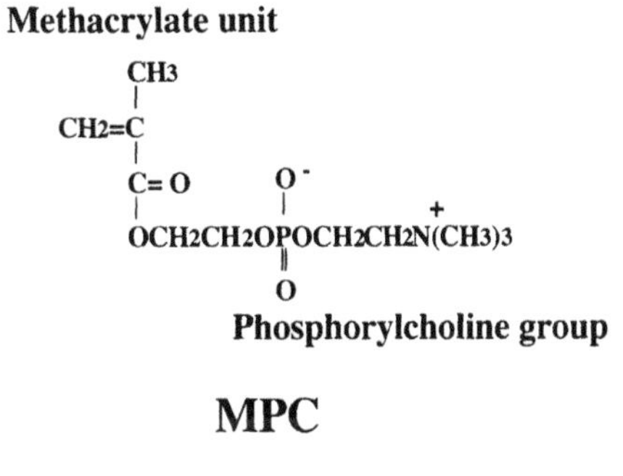

Methacrylate unit

$$CH_3$$
$$|$$
$$CH_2=C$$
$$|$$
$$C=O \qquad O^-$$
$$| \qquad |$$
$$OCH_2CH_2OPOCH_2CH_2N(CH_3)_3^+$$
$$||$$
$$O$$

Phosphorylcholine group

MPC

FIGURE 16.4 Chemical structure of 2-methacryloyloxyethyl phosphorylcholine (MPC).

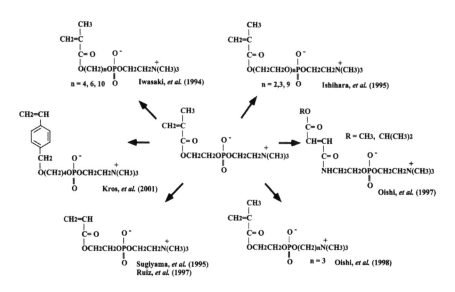

FIGURE 16.5 Chemical structures of MPC derivatives.

16.4.2 PREPARATION OF BIOMEMBRANE-LIKE SURFACES WITH PHOSPHOLIPID POLYMERS

Surface modification of a substrate with a phospholipid polymer is an effective technique for making phospholipid polar group-assembled surfaces; the surface becomes biomembrane-like. The surface modification of substrate polymers with the MPC polymer is carried out by various methods in the medical field. Simple coating easily improves surface properties. Surface grafting, cross-linking at the surface, and chemical reaction to the substrate are effective steps to stabilize the modification layer. The molecular structure of the MPC polymer can be regulated to adapt these modifications. Figure 16.6 is an XPS chart of a surface modified by simple dip coating with poly[MPC-co-n-butyl methacrylate(BMA)]. The XPS signals attributed to methacrylate and phosphorylcholine groups are observed. The surface concentration of the MPC units is about 30 mol%, which is almost the same as that of the polymer used for coating.[13-14]

The surface properties of the MPC polymer are summarized in Table 16.1.[30] Water contact angle is a good parameter for revealing the hydrophilic–hydrophobic nature and mobility of polymer chains at the surface.[31] The advancing and receding contact angles correspond to the surface hydrophilicity in the air and in water, respectively. The difference between these values reflects molecular mobility when the surface is in contact with aqueous media.

Surfaces of the MPC polymer in the air are hydrophobic, similarly to poly(BMA) and poly(ethylene terephthalate)(PET), but they become hydrophilic in water. A large hysteresis was observed when the MPC polymer was immersed in water.

That means the mobility of the polymer chains is very high. The surface ζ-potential of the PET became zero after modification with the MPC polymer. This indicates that the surface was covered completely with the phosphorylcholine group, because the

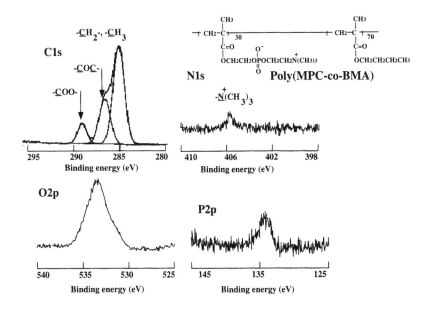

FIGURE 16.6 XPS chart of poly(MPC-co-BMA) surface.

TABLE 16.1
Surface Properties of Phospholipid Polymers

	Contact angle by water (deg)[a]		ζ-potential of polymer surface (mV)[b]
	Advancing	Receding	
Glass	<10	<10	−60
Poly(HEMA)	60	18	−15.8
Poly(BMA)	77	70	−38.5
Poly(MPC-co-BMA)[c]	81	33	−0.4
PET	83	45	−40.9
Poly(MPC)[d]	54	—	—
DDPC monolayer[e]	64	44	—

[a] K.M. DeFife et al., *J. Biomed. Mater. Res.*, 29, 431, 1995
[b] T. Ueda et al., *J. Biomed. Mater. Res.*, 29, 381, 1995, in PBX, pH 7.4, ionic strength, 0.15
[c] MPC unit mole composition: 30%
[d] K. Jinbo et al., *J. Soc. Cosmet. Chem. Japan*, 33, 147, 1999.
[e] Didodecanoyl phosphatidylcholine (DDPC) was arranged on alkylated glass to make monolayered membrane, K.G. Marra et al., *Macromolecules*, 30, 6483, 1997.

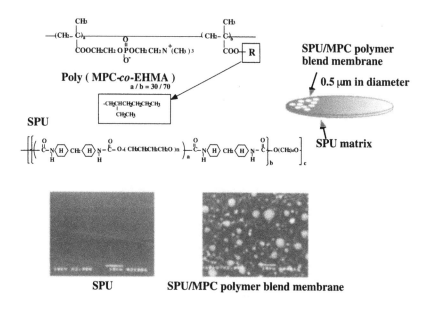

FIGURE 16.7 Surface modification of SPU by blending with the MPC polymer. White dots observed in the SPU/MPC polymer blend membrane are MPC polymer domain-stained with osmium tetraoxide.

MPC is electrically neutral through inner salt formation. Both surface characteristics indicate that the interaction between the MPC polymer surface and biocomponents, proteins, and cells is weakened.

Blending of the MPC polymer to other polymeric materials is another good method. Figure 16.7 is a scanning electron microscopic view of the MPC polymer blended to segmented polyurethane which is used as a medical implant elastomer.[32-34] The figure shows that the 10 wt% of the MPC polymer forms a domain in the segmented polyurethane matrix that is 0.5 μm in diameter and is distributed evenly. The MPC polymer in the blended membrane remained stable; it barely reached out from the membrane even when continuous stress is applied to the blend membrane.

A modification of the cellulose hemodialysis membrane with MPC polymers (Figure 16.8) required maintaining permeability of the solute.[35] However, cellulose is hydrophilic and swells in water, and it is difficult to coat the MPC polymer with cellulose. Thus, direct grafting of the MPC on the surface of cellulose, the chemical reaction of the carboxylic acid moiety in the MPC polymer, and the hydroxyl groups on the cellulose membrane were investigated. A much more effective modification was coating the surface with a water-soluble graft copolymer composed of cellulose backbone and poly (MPC) chains. An aqueous solution containing the graft polymer was used for coating and then drying the membrane; the graft polymer can bind

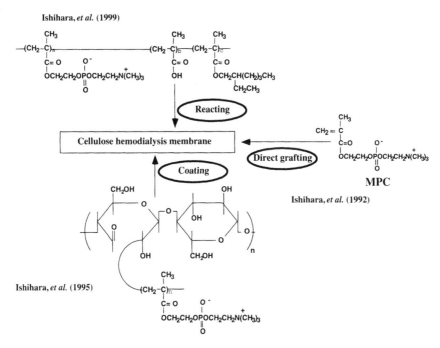

FIGURE 16.8 Surface modification of cellulose hemodialysis membrane with MPC and its polymers.

tightly through hydrogen bonding between cellulose chains. These modification methods indicate the applicability of the MPC polymers with various molecular structures.

Graft polymerization of MPC on the substrate initiated by irradiation of the corona, plasma, and light was also reported and the surface became hydrophilic and protein adsorption-resistible.[36-38]

The microspheres covered with the phosphorylcholine group have structures similar to those of cells. Sugiyama and Aoki prepared microspheres from emulsifier-free emulsion polymerization of MPC and alkyl methacrylate.[39] Uchida, Akashi, and coworkers synthesized an MPC macromonomer and used it as an emulsifier for polymerization of styrene in aqueous medium.[19] They obtained a very fine microsphere with a core-shell structure. Konno et al. prepared poly(L-lactic acid) (PLA) microspheres by solvent evaporation using the amphiphilic MPC polymer.[40] This method is good for preparing polymeric microspheres because it does not need any monomer and initiator during preparation. The MPC polymer chains were entangled with PLA chains and a stable surface was formed. These microspheres interact with proteins more mildly than conventional polystyrene microspheres.

16.5 BIOLOGICAL RESPONSE TO THE PHOSPHOLIPID POLYMERS

16.5.1 ADSORPTION AND ADHESION OF BLOOD COMPONENTS ON PHOSPHOLIPID POLYMERS

Protein adsorption is one of the most important phenomena in determining the bio-compatibility of materials.[41-42] In general, proteins are adsorbed on a surface within a few minutes when the material contacts body fluids such as blood, plasma, and tears. Protein adsorption on the MPC polymers from human plasma determined by ra-dioimmunoassay and an immunogold-colloid labeling technique showed that the amount of adsorbed protein was quite small and decreased with an increase in the MPC moiety.[43] Proteins existing at the plasma-contacting surface after 60-min con-tact with poly(BMA) and poly(MPC-co-BMA) were determined by radioimmunoas-say (Figure 16.9). On every material surface, the major components of plasma proteins, albumin (Alb), fibrinogen (Fib), γ-globulin (IgG), and minor components were observed. Protein adsorption was reduced with an increase in the MPC unit composition. In the case of poly(MPC-co-BMA) with 30 mol% of MPC, every ad-sorbed protein was reduced drastically compared with poly(BMA).[44]

16.5.2 MECHANISM OF PROTEIN ADSORPTION RESISTANCE ON THE PHOSPHOLIPID POLYMERS

The characteristics of the water in the materials or on the surfaces of the materials are important in determining the interactions between proteins and polymeric materials.

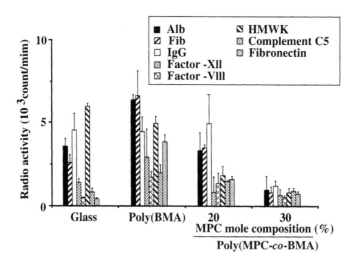

FIGURE 16.9 Amounts of proteins at plasma contact surfaces on MPC polymer and glass. Contact period of plasma was 60 min at 37°C. Factor-XII = coagulation factor XII; Factor-VIII = coagulation factor VIII; HMWK = high molecular weight kininogen.

Particularly, the structure of water surrounding the proteins and the polymer surfaces is considered to influence the protein adsorption.

The equilibrium amounts of bovine serum albumin (BSA) and bovine plasma fibrinogen (BPF) adsorbed on a polymer surface were measured and represented with free water fractions in the hydrated polymers (Figure 16.10).[45-46] The amounts of both proteins adsorbed on poly(HEMA), poly[acrylamide(AAm)-co-BMA] and poly[N-vinylpyrrolidone(VPy)-co-BMA] were larger than those on the MPC polymers. The increase in the MPC mole fraction was effective in reducing the amount of protein adsorption. The theoretical amounts of BSA and BPF adsorbed on the surface in a monolayer state were reported as 0.9 $\mu g/cm^2$ and 1.7 $\mu g/cm^2$, respectively. The amounts of adsorbed proteins on the surfaces of the MPC polymers were less than these theoretical values. This means that the proteins on the surfaces could be detached easily by rinsing. Thus, it is considered that the phosphorylcholine group can reduce protein adsorption effectively.

Lu et al. reported one possible mechanism for understanding protein adsorption on the polymer surface.[47] When a protein adsorbs on a polymer surface, water molecules between the protein and the polymer need to be displaced. Removal of water molecules induces direct contact between the amino acid residues and the polymer surface. A repulsive solvation or hydration interaction, occurs whenever water molecules are associated with surfaces containing hydrophilic groups, and its strength depends on the energy necessary to disrupt the ordered water structure and ultimately dehydrate the surface. When water molecules are associated with hydrophobic surfaces, an attractive solvation interaction (hydrophobic interaction) occurs and its strength depends on the hydrophobicity of the surface or surface groups. The protein adsorbed on the surface loses bound water at its surface-contacting portion. This phenomenon induces a conformational change in the proteins; that is, the hydrophobic

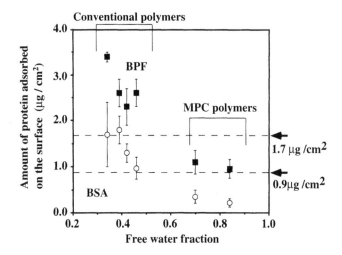

FIGURE 16.10 Relation between free water fraction in the hydrated polymer and amount of protein adsorbed on the surface.

part of the protein is exposed and contacts the polymer surface directly. If the water state at the material surface is similar to that in the aqueous solution, the protein does not need to release the bound water molecules even when the protein molecules contact the surface. This means that no hydrophobic interaction occurs between the proteins and the polymer surface. Moreover, the conformational change during the protein adsorption on or contact with the surface is also suppressed. Andrade and Tsuruta recognized the importance of water structure on biomedical polymers.[48,49] The polymers such as poly(HEMA) that have hydroxyl groups can incorporate water molecules at their surfaces and form network structures of water molecules. The protein adsorption starts with protein trapping by the network structure of water molecules on the surface. The longer the contact of a protein on the surface, the greater the chance that it will interact with the surface, undergo a conformational change, and induce irreversible adsorption. This is an acceptable explanation of the difference in protein adsorption behavior between the MPC polymers and the other amphiphilic polymers including poly(HEMA).

As shown in Table 16.1, most polymeric materials have negative surface charges even if they do not contain any negatively charged groups. The poly(HEMA) hydrated polymer has a negative ζ-potential of -16 mV. On the other hand, when the PET surface was covered with poly(MPC-co-BMA), the ζ-potential was -0.4 mV. This characteristic is important for understanding the surface water structures of these polymers. On PET, poly(BMA), and poly(HEMA), water molecules bind to the surfaces through electrostatic interactions (dipole–dipole interactions). The MPC polymer effectively prevents interactions between the surfaces and water molecules. This also reduces the binding of water at the surfaces of MPC polymers.

16.6 CONCLUSION

When the free water fraction on a polymer surface is kept at a high level, the proteins can contact the surface reversibly without significant conformational change. The free water fraction is an important factor to consider when determining the blood compatibilities of polymeric materials. Thus, a phospholipid polymer having a phosphorylcholine group, such as an MPC polymer, is an effective biomedical material that may be useful in the development of new blood-contacting artificial organs.

REFERENCES

1. Singer, S.J. and Nicolson, G.L., The fluid mosaic model of the structure of cell membranes, *Science*, 175, 720, 1972.
2. Gennis, R.B., Biomembranes: *Molecular Structure and Function*, Springer-Verlag, New York, 1989.
3. Hayward, J.A. and Chapman, D., Biomembrane surface as model for polymer design: the potential for haemocompatibility, *Biomaterials*, 5, 135, 1984.
4. Noishiki, Y., Biochemical response to Dacron vascular prosthesis, *J. Biomed. Mater. Res.*, 10, 795, 1976.

5. Bangham, A.D. and Horne, R.W., Negative staining of phospholipids and their structural modification by surface-active agents as observed in the electron microscope, *J. Mol. Biol.*, 8, 660, 1964.

6. Hall, B. et al., Biomembranes as models for polymer surfaces V. Thrombelastographic studies of polymeric lipids and polyesters, *Biomaterials*, 10, 219, 1989.

7. Kono, K. et al., Platelet adhesion onto polyamide microcapsules coated with lipid bilayer membrane, *Biomaterials*, 10, 455, 1989.

8. Coyle, L.C. et al., Chemisorbed phospholipid monolayer on gold: well-defined and stable phospholipid surface for cell adhesion studies, *Chem. Mater.*, 1, 606, 1989.

9. Kohler, A.S. et al., Platelet adhesion to novel phospholipid materials: modified phosphatidylcholine covalently immobilized to silica, polypropylene, and PTFE materials, *J. Biomed. Mater. Res.*, 32, 237, 1996.

10. Marra, K.G. et al., Cytomimetic biomaterials 1. *in situ* polymerization of phospholipids on an alkylated surface, *Macromolecules*, 30, 6483, 1997.

11. van der Heiden, A.P. et al., A photochemical method for the surface modification of poly(etherurethanes) with phosphorylcholine-containing compounds to improve hemocompatibility, *J. Biomed. Mater. Res.*, 37, 282, 1997.

12. Liu, J-H. et al., Surface modification of polyethylene membrane using phosphorylcholine derivatives and their platelet compatibility, *J. Appl. Polym. Sci.*, 74, 2947, 1999.

13. Ishihara, K. et al., Preparation of phospholipid polymers and their properties as hydrogel membrane, *Polym. J.*, 22, 355, 1990.

14. Ueda, T. et al., Preparation of 2-methacryloyloxyethyl phosphorylcholine copolymers with alkyl methacrylates and their blood compatibility, *Polym. J.*, 24, 1259, 1992.

15. Ishihara, K. et al., Hemocompatibility on graft copolymers composed of poly(2-methacryloyloxyethyl phosphorylcholine) side chain and poly(*n*-butyl methacrylate) backbone, *J. Biomed. Mater. Res.*, 28, 225,1994.

16. Kojima, M. et al., Interaction between phospholipids and biocompatible polymers containing phosphorylcholine moiety, *Biomaterials*, 12, 121, 1991.

17. Ishihara, K. et al., Synthesis of graft copolymers having phospholipid polar group by macromonomer method and their properties in water, *J. Polym. Sci. A Polym. Chem.*, 32, 859, 1994.

18. Oishi, T. et al., Synthesis and polymerization of macromonomer having phospholipid polar group, *Polym. J.*, 32, 378, 2000.

19. Uchida, T. et al., Graft copolymers having hydrophobic backbone and hydrophilic branches XXX. Preparation of polystyrene core nanosphere having a poly(2-methacryloyloxyethyl phosphorylcholine), *J. Polym. Sci. A Polym. Chem.*, 38, 3052, 2000.

20. Iwasaki, Y. et al., Effect of methylene chain length in phospholipid moiety on blood compatibility of phospholipid polymers, *J. Biomater. Sci. Polymer Edn.*, 6, 447, 1994.

21. Ishihara, K. et al., Synthesis of polymers having a phospholipid polar group connected to poly(oxyethylene) chain and their protein adsorption-resistance properties, *J. Polym.Sci. A Polym. Chem.*, 34, 199, 1996.

22. Sugiyama, K. et al., Emulsion copolymerization of 2-(acryloyl)oxyethyl phosphorylcholine with vinyl monomers and protein adsorption at resultant copolymer microspheres, *Macromol. Chem. Phys.*, 196, 1907, 1995.

23. Ruiz, L. et al., Synthesis, structure and surface dynamics of phosphorylcholine functional biomimicking polymers, *Biomaterials*, 19, 987, 1998.

24. Oishi, T. et al., Synthesis and properties of poly(fumaramate) bearing a phosphoryl-choline moiety, Polymer, 38, 3109, 1997.
25. Oishi, T. et al., Synthesis and properties of poly(methacrylate) bearing a phosphoryl-choline analogous group, *Polym. J.*, 30, 17, 1998.
26. Kros, A. et al., Biocompatible polystyrenes containing pendant tetra(ethylene glycol) and phosphorylcholine groups, *J. Polym.Sci. A Polym. Chem.*, 39, 468, 2001.
27. Baumgartner, J.N. et al., Physical property analysis and bacterial adhesion on a series of phosphonated polyurethanes, *Biomaterials*, 18, 831, 1997.
28. Ruiz, L. et al., Phosphorylcholine-containing polyurethanes for the control of protein adsorption and cell attachment via photoimmobilized laminin oligopeptides, *J. Biomater. Sci. Polymer Edn.*, 10, 931, 1999.
29. Iwasaki, Y. et al., Synthesis of novel phospholipid polymers by polycondensation, *Macromol. Rapid Commun.*, 21, 287, 2000.
30. Ueda, T. et al., Adsorption–desorption of proteins on phospholipid polymer surfaces evaluated by dynamic contact angle measurement, *J. Biomed. Mater. Res.*, 29, 381, 1995.
31. Andrade, J.D., Ed., *Surface and Interfacial Aspects of Biomedical Polymers*, Vol. 1, Plenum Press, New York, 1985.
32. Ishihara, K. et al., Improved blood compatibility of segmented polyurethane by poly-meric additives having phospholipid polar group II. Dispersion state of polymeric ad-ditive and protein adsorption on the surface, *J. Biomed. Mater. Res.*, 32, 401, 1996.
33. Ishihara, K. and Iwasaki, Y., Biocompatible elastomers composed of segmented polyurethane and 2-methacryloyloxyethyl phosphorylcholine polymer, *Polym. Adv. Technol.*, 11, 626, 2000.
34. Ishihara, K. et al., Antithrombogenic polymer alloy composed of 2-methacryloy-loxyethyl phosphorylcholine polymer and segmented polyurethane, *J. Biomater. Sci Polymer Edn.*, 11, 1183, 2000.
35. Ishihara, K. et al., Improvement of hemocompatibility on a cellulose dialysis mem-brane with a novel biomedical polymer having a phospholipid polar group, *Artif. Organs*, 18, 559, 1994.
36. Chang, P.C.-T. et al., Heterobifunctional membranes by plasma-induced graft poly-merization as an artificial organ for penetration keratoprosthesis, *J. Biomed. Mater. Res.*, 39, 380, 1996.
37. Iwasaki, Y. et al., The effect of chemical structure of the phospholipid polymer on fi-bronectin adsorption and fibroblast adhesion on the gradient phospholipid surface, *Biomaterials*, 20, 2185, 1999.
38. Ishihara, K. et al., Photoinduced graft polymerization of 2-methacryloyloxyethyl phosphorylcholine on polyethylene membrane surface for obtaining blood cell adhe-sion resistance, *Colloids Surfaces B Biointerfaces*, 18, 325, 2000.
39. Sugiyama, K. and Aoki, H., Surface-modified polymer microspheres obtained by the emulsion copolymerization of 2-methacryloyloxyethyl phosphorylcholine with vari-ous vinyl monomers, *Polym. J.*, 26, 561, 1994.
40. Konno, T. et al., Preparation of blood-compatible nanoparticles bearing phospholipid polar group as a novel drug carrier, *Biomaterials*, 22, 1883, 2001.
41. Brash, J.L. and Horbett, T.A., Eds, *Proteins at Interfaces: Physicochemical and Biochemical Studies*, American Chemical Society, Washington, 1987.
42. Horbett, T.A. and Brash, J.L., Eds., *Proteins at Interfaces: Fundamentals and Applications*, American Chemical Society, Washington, 1995.

43. Ishihara, K. et al., Protein adsorption from human plasma is reduced on phospholipid polymer, *J. Biomed. Mater. Res.*, 25, 1397, 1991.
44. Ishihara, K. et al., Reduced thrombogenicity of polymers having phospholipid polar group, *J. Biomed. Mater. Res.*, 24, 1069, 1990.
45. Ishihara, K. et al., Why do phospholipid polymers reduce protein adsorption? *J. Biomed. Mater. Res.*, 39, 323, 1998.
46. Ishihara, K. et al., Inhibition of cell adhesion on the substrate by coating with 2-methacryloyloxyethyl phosphorylcholine polymers, *J. Biomater. Sci. Polymr. Edn.*, 10, 1047, 1999.
47. Lu, D.R. et al., Calculation of solvation interaction energies for protein adsorption on polymer surface, *J. Biomater. Sci. Polym. Edn.*, 3, 127, 1991.
48. Andrade, J.D. et al., Water as biomaterial, *Trans. Amer. Soc. Artif. Int. Organs*, 19, 1, 1973.
49. Tsuruta, T., Contemporary topics in polymeric materials for biomedical applications, *Adv. Polym. Sci.*, 126, 1, 1996.

17 Supramolecular Approaches for Cellular Modulation

Keiji Fujimoto

CONTENTS

17.1 INTRODUCTION

The surface layer of the cell membrane plays important roles in interactions between the cells and their surroundings, e.g., other cells, soluble biological molecules, and extracelluar matrices (Figure 17.1). Cellular recognition is usually initiated by direct contact with biologically functional molecules at the cell surfaces. The mechanical stress stimulates cell activation in some circumstances. Specific

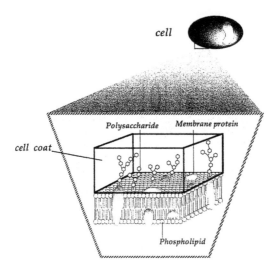

FIGURE 17.1 Hierarchical structures of cell surface. (Reprinted with permission, Copyright 2000, Society for Biomaterials.)

interactions between receptors and ligands are important for cellular recognition. In many cases, multivalent binding (multivalency) can strengthen the ligand–receptor adhesion. In intercellular communication, accessory receptors are often required to stabilize the interaction by increasing the overall strength of the cell–cell adhesion, and co-receptors help activate cells by generating their own intracellular signals. Different combinations of receptors are likely to form complexes that transmit signals across membranes.

In biological systems, dimerization or oligomerization of the receptor-ligand complex is the general control mechanism for generating a cascade of intracellular signals that alter cell behavior. Most biological processes are complex and are not well understood. Greater understanding of cellular functions and machineries will enable us to design and synthesize advanced biological materials and devices. The detailed data of biomedical engineering and materials science have been reduced to a set of interacting theoretical models that describe cellular recognition, signaling, and response. One may wonder whether cellular functions can be controlled or created by combining conventional technologies, and ultimately lead to the design of synthetic materials mimicking biological systems. Multivalent bindings have been used to control receptor occupation and generate biological signaling. Various molecules and chemical scaffolds have been synthesized as nanoscale to microscale supramolecular materials to synthesize antiviral and antibacterial agents, toxin inhibitors, immunorejection shielding, signal transduction controls, and surface modifications for cell delivery. Recently, a variety of techniques have been developed on the basis of further studies on the structures of interacting biological molecules. This chapter will discuss the basic interactions in some biological systems and examples of applications. The reader is referred elsewhere for more detailed discussions on multivalency (polyvalency) in biological systems and principles of design, synthesis, and assay of synthetic multivalent ligands.[1]

17.2 CELLULAR INTERACTIONS AND FUNCTIONS

17.2.1 BIOLOGICAL ASPECTS

Many biological processes follow certain distinct motions. For instance, a binding site on a ligand and a binding site on a receptor stick together in a specific fashion. Multivalent interactions involve the simultaneous attachments of multiple ligands to multiple receptors. Most crucial biological processes such as cell–cell recognition processes and antibody–antigen interactions are mediated by multivalent interactions. Processes such as cell–cell recognition and signal transduction often depend on the formation of multiple receptor–ligand complexes at the cell surfaces. Why does nature require multivalency? The first reason is that multivalency produces strong attachments. The second is that collective properties that emerge from multiple simultaneous interactions are different from those added up from each monovalent interaction. Cells and other biological entities appear to exist in a specific fashion. How do cells create their responses to the external environment in specific ways? Although many biological events are known partially or remain unsolved, we must better understand these biological aspects before we can proceed further with design and synthesis.

17.2.1.1 Cell Adhesion

Cell spreading, adhesion, and migration depend on interactions with extracellular matrices (ECMs).[2] These interactions are mediated by interactions of glycoprotein and proteoglycan receptors on the cell surfaces with proteins existing within the ECMs.[3] Receptor proteins of the selectin family contain lectin-like features and recognize branched oligosaccharide structures in their ligands, namely the sialyl Lewis X and the sialyl Lewis A structures.[4] Members of the immunoglobulin family are also receptors.[5] They bind to other cell surface proteins and are involved in cell–cell interactions. The other adhesion receptor group is the integrin family.[6] The integrins are dimeric proteins, consisting an α and a β subunits assembled noncovalently into an active dimer. The $\beta2$ integrins are involved primarily in cell–cell recognition, whereas the $\beta1$ and $\beta3$ integrins bind to numerous proteins present in ECMs, including collagen, fibronectin, vitronectin, von Willebrand factor, and laminin.

Many of these adhesive proteins share the arginine–glycine–aspartate (RGD) amino acid sequence and bind integrin receptors on the cell surfaces via this tripeptide sequence.[7] There are two models for integrin activation and ligand binding.[8] One is associated with modulation of ligand-binding affinity. Integrin activated by agents such as manganese or monoclonal antibodies acquires an elevated affinity for ligand. Another adhesion is independent of affinity and regulation of integrin diffusion/clustering may be a key step in controlling cell adhesion. Integrin–ligand pairs become clustered in the cell membranes and promote the assembly of actin filaments.

Reorganization of actin filaments into larger stress fibers causes more integrin clustering, thus enhancing matrix binding and organization by integrins in a positive feedback system. Integrins can signal through the cell membranes in both inside–out and outside–in directions.[9]

17.2.1.2 Inflammation

Implantation of biomaterials commonly leads to inflammatory responses. One important aspect of these responses is the adhesion of leucocytes to blood vessel walls. The different receptors of a leukocyte and an endothelial cell are needed for a multistep process of adhesion.[10] The model steps are initial contact, primary adhesion, rolling, activation, secondary adhesion, and transmigration as shown in Figure 17.2.

Following initial contact, leukocytes often roll slowly along the endothelium. The initial adhesion and rolling are mediated by E and P selectins that can bind to the carbohydrate moieties of neutrophil cell surface glycoproteins. Under flow conditions, this weak interaction may enable the rolling which is believed to keep the neutrophil and endothelium cell surfaces at an appropriate distance so that they can be stimulated by substances in the local environment and engage additional binding mechanisms.[11,12] Firm adhesion can follow the rolling step. If neutrophils are not stimulated, the firm adhesion does not take place. The adhesion, which is stronger relative to the binding of E and P selectins to carbohydrate moieties, is mediated by LFA-1 and Mac-1, including the $\beta 2$ integrins which can bind to the endothelial ligand ICAM-1 (intercellular adhesion molecule-1) of the immunoglobulin superfamily. These interactions make important contributions to transmigration. If we consider these events in terms of an interacting distance, the affinity and the precision of cellular recognition strengthen upon reducing the distance between receptors and ligands. Different types of receptor–ligand pairs are in turn selected at certain points of the multistep pathway of the cellular process.

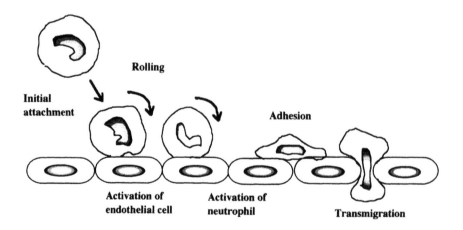

FIGURE 17.2 Schematic diagram of leukocyte extravasation.

17.2.1.3 The Immune Systems of T Cells

Growth factor receptors can be activated by antibodies that cross-link two receptors.[13] Dimerization and oligomerization of the receptor–ligand complex are general mechanisms for the control of many biological processes. In the adaptive immune response, the activation of T lymphocytes is mediated by the interaction of T cell antigen receptors (TCRs) with their ligands, major histocompatibility molecule–peptide complexes (MHC–peptide).[14] Complexes of MHC molecules and bound peptide fragments (the products of viral or bacterial degradation) are displayed on the surfaces of antigen-presenting cells (APCs) and bind to the TCRs, and then a series of signal transduction events are initiated.[15] Class I and class II MHC molecules are the most polymorphic proteins that have genetic variability. Their unique structural features allow the tight binding of peptides differing in length and composition.[16] These early signals may be sufficient to trigger some effector functions such as killer T cell execution of target cells, whereas sustained TCR engagement is essential for more complex functions such as T cell proliferation, and maintaining MHC–peptide strength.

Alteration of an antigenic peptide can have significant effects on the T cell activation.[17] For mature activation, it is believed that T cell receptors require the help of CD4 or CD8 co-receptors and of receptor–ligand pairs, such as LFA–1–ICAM-1, CD2–CD48, and CD28–CD80. CD4 and CD8 bind to polymorphic regions of the MHC molecules as co-receptors, making it possible to increase the strength of the cell–cell adhesion. CD2–CD48 and CD28–CD80 receptor–ligand pairs are thought to function as molecular rulers to keep T cells and APCs at an appropriate distance.

These signaling molecules appear to segregate into distinct areas of the T cell-APC interface, termed the "supramolecular activation cluster."[18] Dynamic pictures of antigen-specific T cell junctions revealed the formation of an "immunological synapse."[19] Grakoui et al. hypothesized that the formation of the immunological synapse provides a mechanism for sustained TCR engagement and signaling as shown in Figure 17.3.

T cell activation was reconstituted by fluorescently labeled MHC–peptide and ICAM-1 molecules in a glass-supported planar bilayer and real-time imaging and quantitative analysis of the formation of a functional immunological synapse were carried out. They identified three stages for TCR engagement during the formation of a stable immunological synapse: junction formation, MHC–peptide transport, and stabilization. After initial contact, T cells stopped migrating and the molecular pattern was formed through the segregation of MHC–peptide complexes into an outer ring and the coalescence of ICAM-1 molecules into a central region. Next, the relocation of the peptide-MHC complexes and the ICAM-1 molecules were relocated into the center and the peripheral ring, respectively, to form the molecular configuration similar to the supramolecular activation cluster. The size and density of the peptide–MHC clusters are directly proportional to the initial density of the peptide–MHC complexes present in the lipid bilayer. Such biologically dynamic pictures leads to novel ideas for supramolecular design and synthesis. To trigger complex biological responses, the immune system may possibly be modulated by organizing or disorganizing the static and dynamic patterns of the supramolecular hierarchies formed at the cell–cell interface.

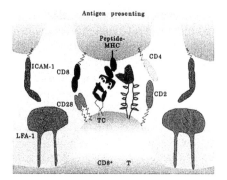

FIGURE 17.3 Formation of immuno-logical synapse between a T cell and an antigen-presenting cell. (Modified and reprinted with permission from *Science,* 1999, 285, 207-208. Copyright 1999, American Association for the Advancement of Science.)

17.2.1.4 Cell Survival and Death

Apoptosis is essential to maintaining cell population balance in tissues and organ de-velopment and is thought to associate with diseases such as cancer and disorders of the self-immune system. Apoptosis is initiated by various external or internal stim-uli. The *Fas* ligand and tumor necrosis factor bind to their receptors and induce apop-tosis. Numerous studies have shown that anchorage-dependent cells must be an-chored to appropriate ECMs to survive. In the absence of any ECM interactions, human endothelial cells rapidly undergo apoptosis.[20] Apoptosis was also induced by disruption of the interactions between normal epithelial cells and ECMs.[21] This phe-nomenon has been termed "anoikis." The $\alpha 5\beta 1$ integrin induced expression of the an-tiapoptotic Bcl-2 protein, thus protecting cells from apoptosis.[22]

Christopher et al. reported that RGD-containing peptides can directly induce apoptosis without any requirement for integrin-mediated cell clustering or signals.[23] RGD peptides were detectable within the cytoplasms of treated cells, indicating that they have to enter cells and are likely to have an intracellular target, the active site of caspase 3. Many researchers utilized RGD peptides to produce adhesive sites on biomaterials. If the RGD motif is selected for the design of a synthetic device, researchers must consider that degraded segments can trigger apoptosis selectively in cancer cells.

17.2.1.5 Infection

The nucleic acids of most viruses are surrounded by protein shells (capsids) that con-tain more than one type of polypeptide chain. In many viruses, lipid bilayer mem-branes containing proteins further enclose the protein capsids. Many of these viruses acquire their envelopes in the process of budding from the plasma membranes. The envelope proteins form heterotrimers that span the lipid bilayer. The glycosylated portions are always on the exterior of the lipid bilayer and are shaped like spikes. The influenza virus attaches to the epithelial cell surface through the binding of multiple trimers of the hemagglutinin (HA) to sialylated oligosaccharides of cell surface glycoproteins and glycolipids.[24] The tips of the external domains of the three subunits of HA contain the three binding sites for sialic acid. This interaction can be inhibited by the sialic acid-based polymeric agents as described below.

Another important feature of HA is that it serves as a trigger for membrane fusion.[25] Bacterial cell walls are made of peptidoglycan which is composed of covalently linked polysaccharide and polypeptide chains. The cell walls of Gram-negative bacteria are coated with thick outer membranes, which consist of lipopolysaccharides, proteins, and phospholipids. In general, bacteria bind directly to a cellular surface or to molecules in the ECMs of preferred tissues. Bacteria that bind sugars and proteins on the surfaces of host cells and in the ECMs are listed elsewhere.[1]

17.3 COLLOIDAL STABILITY AND AGGREGATION

If cells are regarded as simple particles, one can imagine that they diffuse in media, come into contact with each other, and recognize each other in a biological fashion. The net interaction energy of the large particles relative to molecules is proportional to the radius of the particle. The energy level is large at contact and remains appreciable at large separations up to 100 nm or more.[26] If particles experience the same type of interaction, then they will be attracted to each other. However, when the energy barrier is too high to surmount, they will effectively repel each other. Two particles will attract each other only when the energy barrier is negligibly small compared to the kT. If the particles are covered with large molecules such as polymers, attractions will decrease and, in some cases, be almost negligible. As a result, two particles can strongly repel each other and still be well dispersed in a medium (stabilization).

Initial bacterial attraction or repulsion to a material surface can be described in terms of colloidal interactions. Razatos et al. used atomic force microscopy (AFM) to probe the initial interactions of *E. coli* with surfaces coated with poly(ethylene glycol) (PEG)–lysine dendron and Pluronic F127, both of which impede bacterial adhesion.[27] Adsorption of PEG-containing block copolymers at an interface reduced long-range attractive forces between bacteria and the substrate surface while introducing short-range, steric interactions that prevented direct contact between bacteria and the surface.[28]

The adsorption or anchoring of polymer onto a particle surface provides a means of imparting stability.[29] Among synthetic polymers, amphipathic block or graft copolymers have recently emerged as very effective stabilizers. Regarding the concentration profiles of the segments of chains attached terminally to flat plates in a good solvent, Napper et al. described two distinguishable cases of low surface coverage and high surface coverage.[30] The lower limit of surface coverage includes a hemisphere centered at the point of attachment of the terminus of the chain to the surface that has the same Flory radius as a coil in a good solvent. When the average distance between the points of attachment is significantly less than radius of gyration *Rg*, grafted chains overlap and thus expand away from the surface into the bulk.

High surface coverage is of greater practical importance in polymeric stabilization. The cell coat keeps foreign objects and other cells at a distance to prevent undesired contacts and regulate cell recognition. Large glycoproteins like CD43 and CD45 function as steric barriers to the interaction of TCR and MHC described above. When cells come into contact under a large adhesive force derived from affinity, they will deform elastically due to their softness. Thus, contacting cells will not remain spherical and will enable multiple bindings. This phenomenon allows strengthening of cell–cell adhesion.

Multivalent interactions are stronger than corresponding monovalent interactions. This multivalent effect is often explained in terms of a chelate-type binding that begins with the intermolecular association between ligand and receptor followed by intramolecular associations between individual ligand binding sites and individual receptor binding sites. This effect involves cooperativity.[31] A sigmoidal shape found in the O_2 dissociation curve of hemoglobin indicates the system is positively cooperative, based on the Hill equation.

Multivalent interactions are usually interpreted via a model of thermodynamics such as the equilibrium-binding free energy of ligand–receptor pairs cited by Whitesides.[1] Glycoproteins and oligosaccharides reduce the adhesion-free energy, but the physical origin of the enhancement is unknown. In some circumstances, aggregation events make a great contribution to enhancements in binding.[32] Biological and calorimetric analyses of multivalent glycodendrimer ligands for concanavalin A were carried out using ligands containing different kinds of spacers. The performance of ligands was found to be strongly dependent on valency, linker composition, and the protein concentrations used to evaluate them. The apparent enhancements in affinity resulted from entropically driven protein aggregation phenomena that followed the initial intermolecular binding step.

The multivalent effect must be strongly dependent on both the structures and geometries of the receptors and ligands and their arrangements at the interface. Visualization and manipulation of biological systems enhanced our understanding of the mechanisms of monovalent and multivalent binding and unbinding. Transmission electron microscopy (TEM) allows direct visualization of multivalent receptor–ligand complexes.

Colloidal gold particles were employed as labels to monitor receptor position in the presence of a ligand.[33] The unbinding forces between receptor–ligand pairs and domains formed by their pairs were measured by a mesoscopic method.[34] The unbinding force was applied by pulling the vesicle with a point force in the normal direction and using a magnetic bead to measure the binding strengths of focal adhesion sites formed by integrin receptor–RGD ligand pairs. The bond between integrins and RGD ligands can be broken by pulling forces well below 1 pN at force rates of 1 pN/s. This evidence suggests that the strength of either monovalent or multivalent bindings may be lower than expected under certain biological conditions. This study also explains why cells strengthen their tethering forces by receptor clustering and by coupling to the intracellular domains of receptors to actin stress fibers through focal adhesion complexes.

17.4 CHEMICAL APPROACHES TO CELLULAR BEHAVIOR

Binding events are essential to biological processes. Chemists are aware of the importance of these interactions and recently synthesized a variety of biomaterials functioning at the cell surfaces. Approaches ranging from synthesis of small clustered ligands to conjugation with large polymeric aggregates have been used as chemical scaffolds to display ligands with tailored properties applicable to the pharmaceutical and medical fields.

17.4.1 APPROACHES TO HIGHER AFFINITY AND SPECIFICITY

Carbohydrates are essential constituents of biological systems where they handle a multitude of functions in a form presenting on cell surfaces or in a soluble form. Carbohydrate–protein bindings are presumed to mediate cellular responses in a specific manner. However, these bindings are weak and have affinities for different receptors. Some of their dissociation constants (affinities) are in the mM range. In general, carbohydrates are clustered on the cell surfaces whereas complementary receptors contain multiple binding sites. Consequently, we can speculate that multivalency makes the receptor–ligand interaction strong and specific. The effect has been explained in terms of the enthalpy and entropy described above.

Many groups have developed lectin ligands with high affinity through multivalency for various applications, especially in medical fields. Early chemical synthesis involved adding up the binding sites per ligand. Lee et al. synthesized a series of glycopeptides and oligosaccharides with small clusters containing two to three sugar residues to study the ability to inhibit the binding of labeled ligands to mammalian hepatic lectin.[35] The binding affinity of triantennary oligosaccharides increased 1000-fold compared to monoantennary ones. The number of *Gal* residues and the cluster and orientation of *Gal* residues on the ligands were the major determinants of binding affinity.

This study established the affinity enhancements related to multivalency now known as the cluster effect. Recently, Rao et al. reported a trivalent system with an exceptionally high dissociation constant of about 10^{-7} M. It is one of the strongest organic receptor–ligand pairs based on small molecules. Vancomycin and the D-Ala-D-Ala dipeptide found in bacterial cell walls were utilized as receptor and ligand, respectively. Since vancomycin is relatively rigid, there was little loss in conformational entropy on binding.[36]

RGD peptide was also allowed to enhance its cell-adhesive ability by the cluster effect. Danilov et al. reported that the efficiency of adhesion to a substrate coated with bovine RGD-conjugated serum albumin was enhanced upon increasing the valencies of conjugated polymers.[37]

Hirano et al. synthesized a dendritic oligopeptide, $(RGDS)_8K_4K_2KG$, which included eight units of RGD by using lysine residues as linkers to improve the cell attachment activity of the RGD peptide.[38] Attachment of L-929 cells to a fibronectin-coated substrate was inhibited more by adding this clustered RGD than by adding the corresponding monovalent RGD. Horan et al. also immobilized carbohydrates on beads.[39] They screened a library of 1300 di- and trisaccharides immobilized on beads for binding to *Bauhinia purpurea* lectin and found that the protein bound to only one carbohydrate in the library. This high selectivity can be created by multiple binding sites displayed on beads. They synthesized the specific and nonspecific disaccharides with appropriate alkanethiol linkers at the anomeric positions, fabricated self-assembled monolayers presenting different mole fractions of the specific disaccharides, and examined the influence of carbohydrate surface density on carbohydrate-protein interactions.[40] The selectivity of carbohydrate–protein binding depends on the surface densities of carbohydrate ligands. Both the density and the composition of a ligand is important to cellular recognition processes.

17.4.2 NEOGLYCOCONJUGATES

The multivalent forms of ligands have been synthesized to amplify binding by the use of polymers as chemical scaffolds. Chemical conjugation enables macromolecules to possess predetermined properties, such as solubility, molecular weight, ligand density, and capability of biodegradation.[41] Lee et al. synthesized polyacrylamides bearing sialic acid groups on their side chains.[42] Monomers of sialic acid with attached acrylamide moieties were obtained by chemical conjugation of sialic acid with acrylamide and copolymerized with other derivatives of acrylamide. Another approach for the synthesis of neoglycoconjugates has been employed using poly(4-nitrophenyl acrylate) to produce polymeric materials for enzyme-linked immunosorbent assay (ELISA), a dot blot assay, and detection and analysis of lectins.[43]

Mortell et al. synthesized multivalent saccharide derivatives by ring-opening metathesis polymerization (ROMP) to generate different lengths and valencies and display a single saccharide residue per repeat unit.[44] ROMP is a living polymerization process that progresses by rapid initiation followed by slower growth steps; it can generate neoglycopolymers of low polydispersities and various lengths. In an agglutination test of red blood cells by concanavalin A, the inhibitory activity of mannose-substituted derivatives prepared by ROMP exhibited a 2500-fold enhancement relative to monovalent mannoside. Mortell's group also synthesized four kinds of glucose-, mannose-, α-O-glucoside-, and α-O-mannoside-substituted neoglycopolymers by polymerization of bicyclic oxanorbornene derivatives. All four polymers with multivalent ligands showed significant increases in affinity. The enhancement in inhibitory activity observed for the mannose-containing polymer was dramatic. Agglutination was inhibited at a concentration 50,000-fold lower than the corresponding monovalent ligand in assays with concanavalin A.[45] Incorporation of N-hydroxysuccinimide esters into the polymers produced by ROMP was carried out to attach recognition epitopes bearing nucleophilic functional groups.[46] A variety of polyacrylamide-bound selectin ligands, such as β-D-galactose-3-sulfate, Le[a]-trisaccharide, and Le[x]-trisaccharide are available commercially now as carbohydrate probes for laboratory use only (Seikagaku Corporation, Tokyo).

17.4.3 INHIBITION OF INTERACTIONS AMONG BIOLOGICAL ENTITIES

Enhanced affinity and specificity allow the development of highly potent antiviral or antibacterial drugs associated with the receptor–ligand interaction. Inhibitors are required to prevent the attachment of viruses, bacteria, and toxins to the surface of the target cell, which is the initial step in cellular recognition. Inhibition of interactions between external biological entities and the target cells is accomplished by blocking the binding site or by preventing the direct attachment. The ability of small or large molecules to bind specifically to external entities or target cells allows blockage of the binding site, whereas access to target cells is prevented by a steric barrier to this interaction. Some groups succeeded in inhibiting agglutination of erythrocytes by influenza A virus utilizing scaffolds bearing sialic acid groups.[47-49] The enhancement of the affinity and the specificity among interactions was allowed by multiple bindings generated by a multivalent polymeric system. Hemagglutinins (HAs) are known to be fusogenic. Kamitakahara et al. developed a sophisticated method for inhibition of virus based on inhibition of the initial binding and the subsequent membrane fusion mediated by HA.[50] Lysoganglioside GM3 — a molecule that has both sialyl and hydrophobic groups — was conjugated with poly-L-glutamic acid. The polymers became insoluble in aqueous media to form aggregates displaying specific ligands (sialyl groups) on their surfaces. Clustered sialyl groups on the surface of polymeric aggregates attached to hemagglutinin with high affinity through multivalent interactions, and this binding was enhanced by amphiphilic sphingosine. The aggregates were deformed to form a stable complex of polymers with HA through hydrophobic interactions. The hydrophobic region contributed to the enhanced binding and to the conformational change of the HA region. This inhibitor required only picomolar concentrations to inhibit the viral infection.

Synthetic ligands generated by conjugation with polymers are not effective in all cases. The enhancement in affinity is often accomplished by precise controls of the spacing of ligands in terms of the three-dimensional structures of ligand–receptor pairs. Therefore, it is important to find the ideal spacings and orientations for multivalent ligands to interact with the binding sites of targets on cell surfaces. Bacteria such as *Shigella dysenteriae* type 1 and *E. coli* produce toxins that cause serious clinical complications. Synthetic inhibitors of pathogenic Shiga-like bacterial toxins were designed and synthesized on the basis of this concept.[51] Shiga-like toxin 1, (SLT-1), is composed of two kinds of A and B subunits. The B subunit pentamer has a doughnut-shaped structure in complex with the glycolipid Gb3, which serves as a toxin receptor on mammalian cells. This B subunit pentamer allows toxins to present 15 saccharide-binding sites on one face, making it possible to engage the receptors on the cell surface. The crystal structures of the bound ligands in each binding site provided the idea of designing a synthetic inhibitor with a tethered divalent ligand composed of two trisaccharide units. The inhibitor was a molecular assemblage having five tethered arms radiating from a central glucose core; it was named STARFISH. It could bind to two B subunit pentamers so that two toxins were bridged through the multivalent binding. The *in vitro* inhibitory activity of STARFISH was 1 to 10 million times higher than that of the corresponding monovalent ligand.

The structure-based design of ligands was also explored by Fan et al. They selected acylated pentacyclen, 1-β-amidated D-galactose, and the repeat unit of 4,7,10-trioxa-1,13-tridecanediamine as the core, monovalent ligand, and linker, respectively, and synthesized pentavalent ligands with various linkers.[52] These pentavalent galactose ligands were displayed at the tips of the five linkers that project from the core. The affinity was dependent on the lengths of the extended linkers, and the best pentavalent ligand exhibited more than 10^5-fold gain in affinity compared to the corresponding monovalent ligand. They demonstrated that it is important for the dimensions of the ligands to match the distribution of binding sites on the targets.

Manning et al. studied the creation of high affinity selective inhibitors of P selectin which, with L selectin, facilitates leukocyte trafficking to sites of inflammation.[53] The ring-opening metathesis polymerization of norbornene or 7-oxanorbornene conjugated with sulfated saccharides was employed to obtain neoglycopolymers with multiple galactose residues that possess anionic substituents at 3- and/or 6-positions. The inhibitors that had sulfate groups at the 6-positions of the galactose residues were potent and specific to P selectin. In an effort to obtain potent inhibitors of B cell activation associated with allergy, rheumatoid arthritis, and Crohn's disease, a novel multivalent high affinity ligand for a glycoprotein CD22 on the surfaces of B cells has been developed.[54]

17.4.4 MODIFICATION AND REMODELING OF CELL SURFACES

The outermost layer of the cell membrane, the cell coat, plays an important role in interactions between the cell and the external environment, such as cell–cell communication and recognition. It also keeps foreign objects and other cells at a distance to prevent undesired contacts and regulate cell recognition. Signals created at the cell surface and transmitted across the cell membrane through movements and conformational changes of cell surface molecules and their hierarchical organizations make cell responses diverse. Novel techniques in cell–surface engineering are being developed to control cell functions.[55] It can be expected that cell surface modification would allow new responses to external stimuli and living cells modified with these techniques would have biomedical uses.

Shielding of the cell surface can block some cellular recognition processes and is a useful technique to protect cells and tissues against the harmful substances. It may solve problems associated with cellular therapies such as insulin-dependent diabetes mellitus. Furthermore, prevention mechanisms generated by the human immune system would make it possible to use human or animal organs for transplantation. Several types of modifications using inert polymers have been developed to produce shielding layers over the cell surfaces. One example is the adsorption of PEG-containing block copolymers such as Poloxamer 188 onto the surfaces of red blood cells (RBCs) for the purpose of forming a steric barrier. Particles are sterically stabilized by adsorption or attachment of polymer chains onto their surfaces. By utilizing a similar approach, RBC aggregation was inhibited and blood viscosity was reduced *in vitro*.[56] Polymer chains that adhere to cell surfaces must be flexible, amphiphilic, unsusceptible to proteases, and nonimmunogenic. Since PEG chains with appropriate relative molecular masses fulfill these needs, they are widely utilized to protect cells and bodies from undesired influences.

By using water-soluble and nonionic polymers having lipophilic anchor groups at one end, polymer chains were attached to cell surfaces through hydrophobic interaction (Figure 17.4A). Takahashi et al. tried to modify the surfaces of neutrophils with poly(*N,N*-dimethylacrylamide) (M.W. ca.17,000).[57] The extent of cell modification can be evaluated by measuring the amount of active oxygen released from neutrophils. The active oxygen released from modified cells was suppressed when they encountered large structures such as tissue culture dishes and micrometer-sized latex particles. In contrast, modified neutrophils could respond to small molecules such as chemotaxis peptide fMLP and phorbolmyristateacetate (PMA) that can diffuse into the shielding layer. Similar modification to the surfaces of platelets revealed that thrombin-induced agglutination of the modified platelets was inhibited.

Polymer chains can be chemically linked to membrane proteins or saccharides (Figure 17.4B). Yonezawa et al. modified the surfaces of neutrophil-like cells, differentiated from HL-60 cells and platelets using reactive polymer chains.[58] Poly(*N,N*-dimethylacrylamide) chains with amino groups at one end (PDMAA-NH2) were polymerized and allowed to react with cyanuric chloride so as to produce the reactive polymer chain (PDMAA-CC). The average molecular weight was approximately 30,000 g/mol. These reactive chains were conjugated with cells through the reaction of chlorines with hydroxyl and amino groups in the cell surfaces. Neither cytotoxicity nor cell activation was caused by this chemical conjugation.

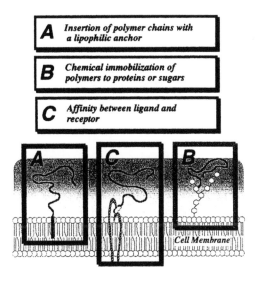

FIGURE 17.4 Approaches to immobilization of polymer chains onto a surface of living cells. (Copyright 2000, Society for Biomaterials. Reprinted with permission.)

Modified neutrophil-like cells produced less active oxygen than unmodified cells or cells treated with PDMAA-NH$_2$ when polystyrene (PS) particles were added to cell suspensions. When the fMLP was added, however, modified cells produced as much active oxygen as unmodified cells did. This indicates that some cellular function is preserved throughout chemical processing.

Modified platelets showed little change in their cytoplasmic free Ca^{2+} concentration and thrombin-induced aggregation was significantly reduced. When calcium ionophore A23187 that can diffuse into the shielding layer was added to the suspension of modified platelets, aggregation could be introduced. Armstrong et al. developed a similar method to coat human red blood cells with PEG chains (M.W. ca. 5000).[59] No apparent adverse effects on RBC morphology or deformability were observed and agglutination by antibodies against blood group antigens was effectively inhibited.

To reduce the immunogenicity and alter cell binding characteristics, rat islets were treated with reactive PEG–isocyanate whose molecular mass was 5000 g/mol in spite of encapsulation of cells.[60] The responses of the treated islets to insulin and glucose were retained even after the chemical treatment. It was concluded that shielding of the cell surface is a novel means of immunoisolation. In all cases, the introduced shielding layer protected the cells against relatively large materials.

Cell modification can be carried out using polymer chains with affinities such as RGD–integrin (Figure 17.4C). Ito et al. prepared nonionic polymer chains carrying cell-adhesive ligands at one end. Neutrophils were treated with a polyacrylamide chain with an RGD end to create cells lacking specific characteristics.[61] No cytotoxicity was observed upon their binding to neutrophils. When the modified cells came into contact with a polystyrene dish, the active oxygen production was reduced to approximately 70% of that of unmodified cells. This shielding effect was dependent upon Ca^{2+} concentration and suppressed by adding soluble RGD peptide. From these findings, it can be expected that the capacity to prevent cells from a direct interaction with large materials could enable the immunological rejection. Immune system rejection is caused by the binding of human anti-*Gal* antibody to carbohydrate epitopes (α-*Gal*) on the cell surface. Thus, carbohydrate polymers conjugated with varying densities of α-*Gal* epitopes were designed and synthesized to inhibit the immune response to transplantation.[62] The synthesized polymer ligands exhibited a 10,000-fold inhibition of binding of anti-*Gal* antibody to mouse laminin glycoproteins and mammalian PK15 cells.

Some researchers tried to install reactive moieties on the cell surface. Valuev et al. developed a method to introduce C=C double bonds into biological compounds containing amino groups for covalent immobilization of microorganisms.[63] The amino groups were allowed to react with acryloyl chloride to produce a cell-bound reactive monomer (cell macromonomer). A variety of membrane-impermeant reagents that cross-link membrane proteins have been synthesized to probe the dynamic interactions among membrane proteins and supramolecular cellular structures and reveal the functions of membrane proteins.[64] A powerful protein engineering technology has been exploited to manipulate the surface protein composition without gene transfer.[65]

One can express any protein of interest as a GPI-anchored derivative by substituting a 3′-mRNA end sequence of natural glycoinositol phospholipid (GPI)-anchored protein for an endogenous 3′-mRNA end sequence. The possibility of using GPI-anchored protein transfer as a cellular engineering tool was also mentioned, e.g., amplification of cell-mediated responses. Recently, Bertozzi et al. elaborated a strategy for engineering the display of chemically defined oligosaccharides on cell surfaces.[66] Decorating cell surfaces with defined carbohydrate epitopes was achieved through sialoside biosynthesis. In the productive pathway, sialic acids were used as vehicles for cell surface functional group display. Displayed ketones and azides could serve as molecular handles for the attachment of biological molecules or small molecular probes to cells.[67,68]

17.4.5 MODULATION OF CELLULAR RESPONSE

Another cell surface engineering technique is signal transduction through cell membrane receptors. The signaling appears to emerge from dynamic motions such as clustering and patterning of distribution of proteins and other molecules in the membrane. Therefore, one may suppose that cellular machinery associated with signal transduction exists. Spencer et al. developed a sophisticated method to control the intracellular oligomerization of specific proteins by using synthetic ligands.[69] Myristylated receptors containing only the domains required for intracellular signaling were expressed as fusion proteins with specific dimerization domains that could be cross-linked by synthetic ligands. The addition of synthetic ligands linked by a covalent tether to initiate dimerization induced signal transmission and specific target gene activation.

Another attempt to achieve signal transduction via dimerization used intracellular antibodies. Tse and Rabbits devised a method by which apoptosis can be triggered by an antibody–antigen interaction using an antibody–caspase 3 fusion protein.[70] Caspase 3 is known to function in apoptosis as an executioner through self-activation caused by dimerization of two caspase 3 molecules.[71] Caspase fused to a single-chain anti-β-galactosidase (β-*Gal*) antibody was expressed inside cells. Two caspase 3 molecules were brought close together by binding four fusion proteins to a β-*Gal*, tetramer at four separate antigenic sites, leading to apoptosis of cells through the self-activation of caspase 3. This technique represents a general approach to induce apoptosis of tumor cells. Kramer et al. synthesized polymer-linked ligands containing two cyclic GMP moieties to activate cyclic nucleotide-gated channels and cGMP-dependent protein kinase. The dimer ligands exhibited enhanced potencies and the optimal chain length for the activation was observed.[72]

Immobilization of signaling molecules on the substrate surface is a unique method for controling cellular functions. Horwitz et al. reported that interleukin-2 immobilized on a polystyrene plate preserved the viability of an interleukin-2-dependent cell line.[73] They presumed that internalization of the receptor was not essential for signal transduction. Ito et al. demonstrated that co-immobilization of insulin and fibronectin was very effective for the acceleration of cell growth.[74] They explained the increased mitogenic effect of immobilized insulin in terms of the inhibition of receptor down-regulation by internalization.[75]

The extracellular matrix separates one tissue space from another and organizes cells in spaces to provide them with environmental signals to direct site-specific regulation.[76] Cell activation is triggered by the clustering of integrin receptors.[77] It has been reported that RGD sequences immobilized on a substrate surface promote adhesion of fibroblasts. This result suggests that the cluster effect of RGD peptides immobilized onto a substrate surface influences cell behavior. The ligand surface concentration is an important determinant for functions such as regulation of cell morphology, growth, differentiation, and motility. The minimal peptide spacing corresponded to 440 nm for spreading and 140 nm for focal contact formation.[78]

Microscale particles presenting RGD ligands at much higher surface concentrations activated platelets to induce aggregation,[79] whereas soluble RGD did not activate them. The RGD-carrying microspheres also induced leukocyte activation while its potency was inhibited by soluble RGD.[80] One can speculate that changes in receptor clustering allows modulation of cellular recognition and control of cellular response. It can be expected that tuning of cellular functions will be provided by dynamic change of the surface concentration. Multivalent ligands can be utilized as artificial "tweezers" to pick up receptors. If a polymer possesses both cell-adhesive and stimuli-sensitive properties, cells bound to stimuli-sensitive polymers are expected to have the ability to control their biological recognitions and responses by the artificial stimuli.[60]

The cell surface modification technique using polymer chains has been employed to control cell recognition and response through the multiple binding of receptor–ligand pairs. Poly(N-isopropylacrylamide) (PNIPAM) was selected as a thermosensitive polymer. Its molecular shape changes from a coil to a globule when temperature increases.[81] Ringsdorf et al. developed model membranes or "molecular accordions" by thermoreversible contraction /expansion of the PNIPAM chain.[82] PNIPAM chains inserted into a liposome membrane via its anchor groups exhibited temperature-dependent conformational changes. This may be the next step toward a more advanced simulation of the natural process, especially the dynamics of the cytoskeleton.

Fujimoto et al. studied activation of cells induced by clustering of receptors using similar thermosensitive polymer chains with cell-adhesive ligands.[60] They synthesized a PNIPAM chain conjugated with RGDS moieties (PNIPAM–nRGDS). The chains were soluble in aqueous media at room temperature and became insoluble upon the shrinking above 32°C. Neutrophils treated with PNIPAM-nRGDS were activated when the temperature was raised to 37°C and the release of active oxygen was controllable by temperature. As a control, the PNIPAM chains that had a single RGD residue at their tips were prepared. When neutrophils were treated with this polymer chain and the temperature was raised to 37°C, no activation was observed. They concluded that this event was caused by the clustering of RGD–integrin complexes based on the temperature-induced shrinking of the polymer chain as shown in Figure 17.5. Moreover, they intended to synthesize stimuli-sensitive copolymers that can bind to any antibody of interest to extend applications of controllable clustering to methods for controlling receptor-mediated biological processes such as immune responses.[83]

Enhanced potency requires clustering the receptor–ligand complexes so that the region of displayed ligands is large enough to cover the receptor–ligand pairs scattered on the cell surface. Microspheres are chemical scaffolds that have large surface areas that allow diverse displays. Kisara et al. developed RGD-carrying particles composed of thermosensitive polymer chains. The obtained particles swelled and shrank reversibly in response to temperature. This reversible change in the surface area led to the variation of the surface concentrations of the ligands. By increasing incubation temperature, neutrophils covered with gel particles were activated to release the active oxygen and thermosensitive polymer chains.[84]

In some circumstances, signaling is mediated through changes in cytoskeletal organization. The dynamic response of the cytoskeleton is thought to be associated with mechanical perturbation although its mechanism is still unclear. Mechanical stresses were applied directly to integrin $\beta1$ on the cell surface with a magnetic twisting device.[85] Spherical ferromagnetic microspheres coated with a synthetic peptide containing the RGD sequence were allowed to bind endothelial cell surfaces and a strong external magnetic field was applied to magnetize the beads. Cytoskeletal stiffness increased in direct proportion to the applied stress. Adherent pulmonary arterial smooth muscle cells exhibited similar stiffness responses. Further developments are emerging from the combination of cell surface chemistry and manipulative

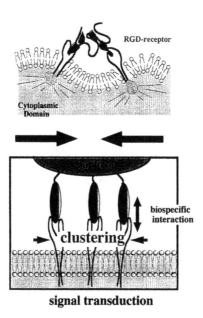

FIGURE 17.5 Control of signal transduction by using ligand-carrying polymeric materials. (Reprinted with permission, Copyright 2000, Society for Biomaterials.)

techniques such as magnetic twisting cytometry. Wider applications to the biotechnological and medical fields are expected.

17.4.6 TISSUE ENGINEERING AND CYTOTHERAPY

A variety of polymeric materials have been utilized to promote or inhibit cell–cell or cell–tissue interactions, isolate transplanted cells from a host immune system, and regulate the secretion and production of cellular products.[86] Cell-adhesive RGD and Tyr–Ile–Gly–Ser–Arg (YIGSR) were conjugated with linear PEG chains at both ends to promote cell aggregation.[87] PEG–peptide conjugates promoted the aggregation of PC12 cells and Neuro-2a cells. This method may enable us to produce three-dimensional cell aggregates with enhanced function and viability, suitable for use in artificial organs or as cell transplants for tissue regeneration.

Four models of polymer conjugates (the dumbbell, double-fork, ladder, and star-dendrimer) were synthesized for development as useful templates to promote cell aggregation. Meier et al. reported that water-soluble polymers carrying small fractions of hydrophobic groups could interconnect different cells to form aggregations.[88] Spheroid-like cell aggregates were observed in hepatocytes when the copolymer of methacrylic acid and methylmethacrylate (Eudragit) was added to the culture medium.[89] The spheroids expressed high liver functions, such as albumin secretion, ammonia removal, and urea synthesis. Synthetic polymers bearing β-galactose residues and poly (vinylbenzyl-β-D-lactonamide) (PVLA) were utilized as polymeric ligands of the asialogylcoprotein receptor (ASGP-R) on hepatocytes.[90] Galactose density is an important factor that determines whether adhering hepatocytes are converted to differentiation or proliferation modes.

Microencapsulation techniques have been employed to prevent destruction of implanted cells by the host's immune system. Okada et al. studied the utilization of microencapsulated living cells as carriers of bioactive drugs. This represents a novel method for effective long-term delivery of bioactive drugs. The technique is designated cytomedical therapy or cytomedicine.[91,92] Modification of the cell surface may allow living cells to function as cytomedicines. Kanai et al. carried out modifications with bifunctional PEO chains to make the cell surfaces suitable for shielding and delivery (Figure 17.6).[93] By adding excess of polymers bearing RGD peptides at both ends to the cell suspension, RGD-displayed cells were produced. Cell aggregation took place when RGD-displayed cells were mixed with unmodified cells. The size of aggregates was dependent on Ca^{2+} concentration in a buffered solution. Moreover, aggregates were not observed when cells were pretreated with soluble RGDS before modification. This indicates that cell aggregation was caused by the specific interaction between RGD moieties displayed on modified cells and integrins on unmodified cells.

N-Succinimidyl-3(2-pyridyl dithio)propinate (SPDP) was used to obtain heterofunctional PEO chains. Cells modified with this polymer displayed disulfide bonds on their surfaces. Modified cells adhered to the thiol group-bearing dish surface to form multilayers or aggregates of cells at 25°C and monolayers at 4°C, whereas they did not adhere to the hydroxyl group-bearing surface. Unmodified cells did not adhere to either surface. This indicates that cell adhesion was caused

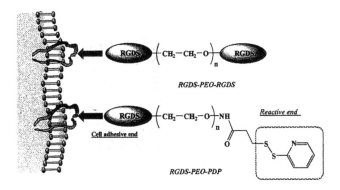

FIGURE 17.6 Cell-surface modification with bifunctional polymers.

by the thiol–disulfide exchange reaction. Adhering cells could be detached from the surface by the addition of reducing agents. This method may be useful for the recovery of adhered cells and regenerated tissues and for cell delivery. Cell surfaces were modified using unsymmetrically substituted PEO chains carrying hydrophobic cholesteryl groups at one end and hydrophilic biotin groups at the other end. Cells presenting biotin residues could be reversibly aggregated through the biotin–streptavidin interaction.[94]

Nanoscale particles are commonly prepared by interchain aggregation or chemical cross-linking of polymer chains. Since they are capable of incorporating a drug through physical or chemical entrapment, they have been applied to the delivery of drugs for cancer therapy. Fujimoto et al. reported a novel drug delivery system involving apoptosis induction by a "smart" polymer vehicle possessing thermosensitivity and bioaffinity.[95] This nanometer-sized vehicle possesses targeting ability and a cavity for incorporation of the drugs (Figure 17.7).

To achieve specific targeting through the immobilization of various ligands, reactive and thermosensitive polymer chains (M.W. 130,000) were prepared by copolymerization of N-isopropylacrylamide with N-methacryloyloxysuccinimide. RGD peptides were chemically linked to the copolymer chains to render the site specificity for the generic cell targeting to the copolymer chain. Aggregates of RGD-conjugated copolymers were formed around 31°C and kept monodisperse in size at temperatures from 33 to 44°C. Their diameter was 133 nm at 37°C. The polymeric nanospheres incorporating an apoptotic inducer, dol-p, were added to a human promonocytic leukemia U937 cell suspension at 37°C. By lowering temperature to 25°C, cells underwent apoptosis in the presence of Ca^{2+}. Copolymer vehicles probably were concentrated on cell surfaces through the binding of RGD and integrin and the release of lipid inducers was caused by the disruption of vehicles in response to temperature. This technique allows cells to induce apoptosis in response to stimuli such as temperature, and enables us to program cell death without genetically engineered procedures. Engineered cells may be used for gene therapy and cytomedical therapy. Death-programmed cells may serve as tools to control tissue regeneration.

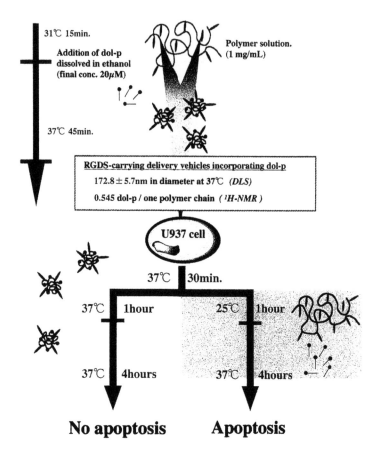

FIGURE 17.7 Control of cell death by nanoscale particle. (Reproduced with permission from *Biomacromolecules* 2000, 1, 515-518. Copyright 2000, American Chemical Society.)

17.4.7 DENDRIMERS AS NOVEL CHEMICAL SCAFFOLDS

Dendrimers are three-dimensional architectures fabricated from branching polymers attached to a center core. Their advantages include precise nanometer size, high functionality, and regular structural features. The functional groups displayed at their outermost surfaces can be utilized for the conjugation of desirable ligands. They are suited for multvalent interactions due to the densely packed end-groups on their surfaces. A number of reports have discussed multivalent effects with dendrimers incorporating recognition elements such as amino acids or carbohydrates.[96]

Poly(amidoamine) dendrimers (PAMAMs) synthesized by the divergent growth procedure are used commercially as building blocks for mutilayered assemblages.[97] Carbohydrate-protein binding interactions can be greatly amplified using the cluster or multivalent effect.[98] Aoi et al synthesized a novel globular "sugar ball" dendrimer with a fully sugar-substituted surface (Figure 17.8).[99] They synthesized lactose and maltose derivative persubstituted dendrimers by the reactions of amine-terminated PAMAM dendrimers with excess amount of O-β-D-galactopyaranosyl-(1→4)-D-glucono-1,5-lactone and O-α-D-glucopyaranosyl-(1→4)-D-glucono-1,5-lactone, respectively. The recognition ability of sugar balls was investigated by the assay using peanut agglutinin (PNA) and concanavalin A (ConA).

They found selective recognition between lectin and the terminal carbohydrate residues of the sugar balls. Binding between ConA and maltose derivative persubstituted dendrimers was broken by the addition of 1200-fold molar excess of D-glucose. This is attributable to cooperative binding to dendrimer surface units. In the convergent approach to dendrimer synthesis, the use of dendrimers for targeted delivery has been studied. Kono et al. designed and synthesized dendrimers containing folate residues as models for drug carriers with tumor cell specificity.[100] Guest molecules can be physically entrapped in the internal cavities of dendrimers when they are utilized for drug delivery systems. Utilization of the dendritic framework as a ligand for lanthanide metals allows their entrapment at the center of built-up dendrimers, and carbohydrates are displayed on their surfaces as cellular recognition sites.[101]

Conjugation with multiple sialic acid (SA) residues may provide the ability to inhibit virus adhesion and block infection of mammalian cells.[102] The potency of the inhibitors increased to approximately that of a polyacrylamide conjugated with SA residues to its backbone. Because dendritic polymers have low cytotoxicity relative to the conjugated acrylamide, dendrimers with SA residues may be a new therapeutic modality for viruses that employ SA as their target receptors.

Reuter et al. synthesized a variety of SA-conjugated dendritic polymers and screened them for the ability to prevent adhesion of several strains of virus based on

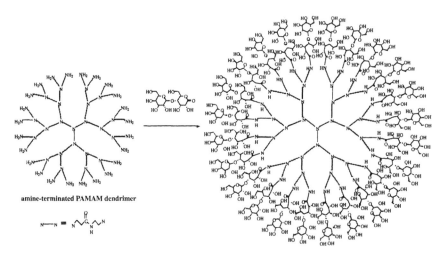

FIGURE 17.8 Sugar-ball dendrimer. (Reproduced with permission from *Macromolecules* 1995, 28, 5391-5393. Copyright 1995, American Chemical Society.)

molecular architectures including linear polymer, comb-branched polymer, dendri-graft polymer, spheroidal dendrimer, and linear-dendron copolymers.[103] While spheroidal dendrimer architecture might be expected to have limited ability to interact with a virus due to its rigid size and shape, its activity was 32- to 256-fold more effective than monomeric SA. The most effective inhibitors were the comb-branched and den-drigraft architectures. The studies confirmed that these conjugates can prevent viral infections in mammalian cells.

Fulton and Stoddart developed a synthetic strategy for β-cyclodextrin (CD)-based carbohydrate cluster compounds.[104] Carbohydrate residues were attached to different parts of a β-CD core by the photoaddition of thiols to allyl ethers in an anti-Markovnikov fashion.

Flexible and biocompatible polyamide chains with defined numbers of repeat units were prepared by automated solid-phase synthesis.[105] The obtained polyamide chains could replace polypeptides and PEG as linkers since protecting groups are not needed for the synthesis process. Tetrameric molecules were fabricated to display phage-derived binding peptides at each tip. The assembled polyamide molecules can bind simultaneously to complementary structures in a multivalent fashion and their flexible linkers would allow control of spacing of ligands for the enhanced affinities and activities.

17.5 CONCLUSIONS

Most molecular mechanisms by which individual cells recognize and respond to bi-ological entities and the forces generated by the external environment are still un-known. However, marvelous clues have been found in the studies described in this review. Some characteristics required for molecular and supramolecular designs have been defined, and various techniques to synthesize materials that can interact with bi-ological entities in specific ways have been developed. Crystal structures of proteins and other biological molecules have been reported. Many synthetic receptors have been fabricated via combinatorial chemistry and other techniques to produce the syn-thetic tools with binding properties rivaling those of their natural counterparts. Peptides that bind to a range of semiconductor surfaces with high specificity have been prepared by the use of combinatorial phage-displayed libraries.[106] These ap-proaches are new and different from chemical ones. It can be expected that diverse and attractive materials will be produced by such cross-fertilization. Our task now is to design and synthesize materials to meet practical needs. Studies in this field will hopefully lead to successful practical applications.

ACKNOWLEDGMENTS

Our work was supported by a grant in aid for scientific research from the Ministry of Education, Science, Sports, and Culture of Japan.

REFERENCES

1. Mammen, M., Choi, S.-K., and Whitesides, G.M., Polyvalent interactions in biological systems: implications for design and use of multivalent ligands and inhibitors, *Angew. Chem. Int. Ed.*, 37, 2754, 1998.
2. Huttenlocher, A., Sandborg, R.R., and Horwitz, A.F., Adhesion in cell migration, *Curr. Opin. Cell Biol.* 7, 697, 1995.
3. Albelda, S.T. and Buck, C.A. Integrins and other cell adhesion molecules, *FASEB J.,* 4, 2868, 1990.
4. Varki, A., Selectin ligands, *Proc. Natl. Acad. Sci. U.S.A.*, 91, 7390, 1994.
5. Hunkapiller, T. and Hood, L., Diversity of the immunoglobulin gene superfamily, *Adv. Immunol.* 44, 1, 1989.
6. Ruoslahti, E., Integrins, *J. Clin. Invest.* 87, 1, 1991.
7. Ruoslahti, E. and Pierschbacher, M.D. New perspectives in cell adhesion: RGD and integrins, *Science*, 238, 491, 1987.
8. Bazoni, G. and Hemler, M.E., Are changes in integrin affinity and conformation overemphasized? *Trends Biochem. Sci.,* 23, 30, 1998.
9. Giancotti, F.G. and Ruoslahti, E., Integrin signaling, *Science*, 285, 1028, 1999.
10. Smith, C.W., Endothelial adhesion molecules and their role in inflammation, *Can. J. Physiol. Pharmacol.,* 71, 76, 1993.
11. Goldman, A.J., Coox, R.G., and Brenner, H., Slow viscous motion of a sphere parallel to a plane wall, *Chem. Eng. Sci.*, 22, 637, 1967.
12. Atherton, A. and Born, G.V.R., Relationship between the velocity of rolling granulocytes and that of the blood flow in venules, *J. Physiol.*, 233, 157, 1973.
13. Ullrich, A. and Schlessinger, J., Signal transduction by receptors with tyrosine kinase activity, *Cell*, 61, 203, 1990.
14. Unanue, E.R., Antigen-presenting function of the macrophage, *Annu. Rev. Immunol.,* 2, 395, 1984.
15. Marrack, P. and Kappler, J., The antigen-specific, major histocompatibility complex-restricted receptor on T cells, *Adv. Immunol.*, 38,1, 1986.
16. Madden, D.R., The three-dimensional structure of peptide-MHC complexes, *Annu. Rev. of Immunol.,* 13, 587,1995.
17. Allen, P.M. et al., Identification of the T-cell and Ia contact residues of a T-cell antigenic epitope. *Nature*, 327, 713, 1987.
18. Monks, C.R.F., Three-dimensional segregation of supramolecular activation clusters in T cells, *Nature*, 395, 82, 1998.
19. Grakoui, A. et al., The immunological synapse: a molecular machine controlling T cell activation, *Science*, 285, 221, 1999.
20. Meredith, J.E., Fazeli, B., and Schwartz, M.A., The extracellular matrix as a cell survival factor, *Mol. Biol. Cell,* 4, 953, 1993.
21. Frisch, S.M. and Francis, H., Disruption of epithelial cell-matrix interactions induces apoptosis, *J. Cell Biol.*, 124, 619, 1994.
22. Zhang, Z.K. et al., The $\alpha5\beta1$ integrin supports survival of cells on fibronectin and upregulates BCL-2 expression, *Proc. Natl. Acad. Sci. U.S.A.,* 92, 6161, 1995.
23. Christopher, D. et al., RGD peptides induce apoptosis by direct caspase-3 activation, *Nature*, 397, 534, 1999.
24. Paulson, J.C., Interactions of animal viruses with cell surface receptors, in *Receptors*, Conn, P.M., Ed., Academic Press, Orlando, FL, 1985, vol. 2, 131.

25. Doms, R.W., Influenza virus hemagglutinin and membrane fusion, in *Membrane Fusion*, Wilschut, J. and Hoekstra, D., Eds., Marcel Dekker, New York, 1991, chap. 15.

26. Israelachvili, J.N., *Intermolecular and Surface Forces*, Academic Press, London, 1987, chap.10.

27. Razatos, A. et al., Molecular determinants of bacterial adhesion monitored by atomic force microscopy, *Proc. Natl. Acad. Sci. U.S.A.*, 95, 11059, 1998.

28. Razatos, A. et al., Force measurements between bacteria and poly(ethylene glycol)-coated surfaces, *Langmuir*, 16, 9155, 2000.

29. Russel, W.R., Saville, D.A., and Schowalter, W.R., *Colloidal Dispersion*, Cambridge University Press, New York, 1989, chap.6.

30. Napper, D.H., *Polymeric Stabilization of Colloidal Dispersions*, Academic Press, London, 1983, chap.4.

31. Connors, K.A., *Binding Constants*, John Wiley & Sons, Toronto, 1987, p. 78.

32. Corbell, J.B., Lundquist, J.J., and Toone, E.J., A comparison of biological and calorimetric analyses of multivalent glycodendrimer ligands for concanavalin A, *Tetrahedron Asymmetry*, 11, 95, 2000.

33. Gestwicki, J.E., Strong, L.E., and Kiessling, L.L., Visualization of single multivalent receptor–ligand complexes by transmission electron microscopy, *Angew. Chem. Int. Ed.*, 39, 4567, 2000.

34. Guttenberg, Z. et al., Measuring ligand-receptor unbinding forces with magnetic beads: molecular leverage, *Langmuir*, 16, 8984, 2000.

35. Lee, Y.C. et al., Binding of synthetic oligosaccharides to the hepatic Gal/GalNAc lectin, *J. Biol. Chem.*, 258, 199, 1983.

36. Rao, J. et al., A trivalent system from vancomycin-D-Ala-D-Ala with higher affinity than avidin-biotin, *Science*, 280, 708, 1998.

37. Danilov, Y.N. and Juliano, R.L., (Arg-Gly-Asp)n-albumin conjugates as a model substratum for integrin-mediated cell adhesion, *Exp. Cell. Res.*, 182, 186, 1989.

38. Hirano, Y. et al., Synthesis and evaluation of cell-attachment activity of RGDS-related molecules, in *Proceedings of The Second Far-Eastern Symposium on Biomedical Materials*, Zhang, X. and Ikada, Y., Eds., Koubunshi Kankokai, Kyoto, 1995, p. 147.

39. Liang, R. et al., Parallel synthesis and screening of a solid phase carbohydrate library, *Science*, 274, 1520, 1996.; Liang, R. et al., Polyvalent binding to carbohydrates immobilized on an insoluble resin, *Proc. Natl. Acad. Sci. U.S.A.*, 94, 10554, 1997.

40. Horan, N. et al., Nonstatistical binding of a protein to clustered carbohydrates, *Proc. Natl. Acad. Sci. U.S.A.*, 96, 11782, 1999.

41. Bovin, N.V., Synthesis of polymeric neoglycoconjugates based on N-substituted polyacrylamides, *Glycoconjugate J.*, 10, 142, 1993.

42. Lees, W.J. et al., Polyacrylamides bearing pendant alpha-sialoside groups strongly inhibit agglutination of erythrocytes by influenza A virus: multivalency and steric stabilization of particulate biological systems, *J. Med. Chem.*, 37, 3419, 1994.

43. Bovin, N.V. and Gabius, H.-J., Polymer-immobilized carbohydrate ligands: versatile chemical tools for biochemistry and medical sciences, *Chem. Soc. Rev.*, 1995, p. 413.

44. Mortell, K.H., Weatherman, R.V., and Kiessling, L.L., Recognition specificity of neoglycopolymers prepared by ring-opening metathesis polymerization, *J. Am. Chem. Soc.*, 118, 2297, 1996.

45. Kanai, M., Mortell, K.H., and Kiessling, L.L., Varying the size of multivalent ligands: the dependence of concanavalin A binding on neoglycopolymer length, *J. Am. Chem. Soc.*, 119, 9931, 1997.

46. Strong, L.E. and Kiessling, L.L., A general synthetic route to defined, biologically active multivalent arrays, *J. Am. Chem. Soc.,* 121, 6193, 1999.

47. Matrosovich, M.N. et al., Synthetic polymeric sialoside inhibitors of influenza virus receptor-binding activity, *FEBS Lett.,* 272, 209, 1990.

48. Spaltenstein, A. and Whitesides, G.M., Polyacrylamides bearing pendant alpha-sialoside groups strongly inhibit agglutination of erythrocytes by infuenza virus, *J. Am. Chem. Soc.,* 113, 686, 1991.

49. Gamian, A. et al., Inhibition of influenza A virus hemagglutinin and induction of interferon by synthetic sialylated glycoconjugates, *Can. J. Microbiol.,* 37, 233, 1991.

50. Kamitakahara, H. et al., A lysoganglioside/poly-L-glutamic acid conjugate as a picomolar inhibitor of influenza hemagglutinin, *Angew. Chem. Int. Ed.,* 37, 1524, 1998.

51. Kitov, P.I. et al., Shiga-like toxins are neutralized by tailored multivalent carbohydrate ligands, *Nature,* 403, 669, 2000.

52. Fan, E. et al., High-affinity pentavalent ligands of *Escherichia coli* heat-labile enterotoxin by modular structure-based design, *J. Am. Chem. Soc.,* 122, 2663, 2000.

53. Manning, D.D. et al., Synthesis of sulfated neoglycopolymers: selective P-selectin inhibitors, *J. Am. Chem. Soc.,* 119, 3161, 1997.

54. Sliedregt, L.A.J.M. et al., Design and synthesis of a multivalent homing device for targeting to murine CD22, *Bioorg. Med. Chem.,* 9, 85, 2001.

55. Fujimoto, K., Modification and functionalization of cell surface by polymer chains, paper presented at *6th World Biomaterials Congress,* Hawaii, May 15, 2000.

56. Carter, C. et al., Hemorheological effects of a nonionic copolymer surfactant (P188), *Clin. Hemorheol.,* 12, 109, 1992.

57. Takahashi, T., Fujimoto, K., and Kawaguchi, H., Surface modification of cell with a nonionic polymer and assessment of the hybrid function, *Polymer Preprints Jpn.,* 47, 572, 1996.

58. Fujimoto, K., Yonezawa, T., and Kawaguchi, H., Cell surface modification by reactive polymer chains and control of cell recognition and response, in *Proceedings of The Fourth Asian Symposium on Biomedical Materials,* Zhang, X. and Ikada, Y., Eds., Kobunshi Kankokai, Kyoto, 1999, p. 106.

59. Armstrong, J.K., Meiselman, H.J., and Fisher, T.C., Covalent binding of PEG to the surface of red blood cells inhibits aggregation and reduces low shear blood viscosity, *Am. J. Hematol.,* 56, 26, 1997.

60. Panza, J.L. et al., Treatment of rat pancreatic islets with reactive PEG, *Biomaterials,* 21, 1155, 2000.

61. Fujimoto, K., Ito, K., and Kawaguchi, H., Modification and functionalization of cell surface by polymer chains with cell-adhesive ligands, *Abstr. Pap. Am. Chem. Soc.,* 216, 318, 1998.

62. Wang, J.-Q. et al., Enhanced inhibition of human anti-Gal antibody binding to mammalian cells by synthetic α-Gal epitope polymer, *J. Am. Chem. Soc.,* 121, 8174, 1999.

63. Valuev, L.I., Chupov, V.V., and Plate, N.A., Covalent immobilization of microorganisms in polymeric hydrogels, *J. Biomater. Sci., Polym. Edn.,* 5, 37, 1993.

64. Staros, J.V., Membrane-impermeant cross-linking agents: probes of the structure and dynamics of membrane proteins, *Acc. of Chem. Res.,* 21, 435, 1988.

65. Medof, M.E., Nagarajan, S., and Tykocinski, M.L., Cell-surface engineering with GPI-anchored proteins, *FASEB J.,* 10, 574, 1996.

66. Mahal, L.K., Yarema, K.Y., and Bertozzi, C.R., Engineering chemical reactivity on cell surfaces through oligosaccharide biosynthesis, *Science,* 276, 1125, 1997.

67. Yarema, K.J. et al., Metabolic delivery of ketone groups to sialic acid residues, *J. Biol. Chem.*, 273, 31168, 1998.
68. Saxon, E. and Bertozzi, C. R., Cell surface engineering by a modified Staudinger reaction, *Science*, 287, 2007, 2000.
69. Spencer, D.M. et al., Controlling signal transduction with synthetic ligands, *Science*, 262, 1019, 1993.
70. Tse, E. and Rabbitts, T.H., Intracellular antibody-caspase-mediated cell killing: an approach for application in cancer therapy, *Proc. Natl. Acad. Sci. U.S.A.*, 97, 12266, 2000.
71. MacCorkle, R.A., Freeman, K.W., and Spencer, D.M., Synthetic activation of caspase: artificial death switchers, *Proc. Natl Acad. Sci. U.S.A.*, 95, 3655, 1998.
72. Kramer, R.H. and Karpen, J.W., Spanning binding sites on allosteric proteins with polymeric-linked ligand dimers, *Nature*, 395, 710, 1998.
73. Horwitz, J.I. et al., Immobilized IL-2 preserves the viability of an IL-2 dependent cell line, *Mol. Immunol.*, 30, 1041, 1993.
74. Ito, Y. et al., Cell growth on immobilized cell growth factor 6. Enhancement of fibroblast cell growth by immobilized insulin and/or fibronectin, *J. Biomed. Mater. Res.*, 27, 901, 1993.
75. Ito, Y. et al., Protein-free cell culture on an artificial substrate with covalently immobilized insulin, *Proc. Natl. Acad. Sci. U.S.A.*, 93, 3598, 1996.
76. Hubbell, J.A., Matrix effects, in *Principles of Tissue Engineering*, Lanza, R.P. et al., Eds., Academic Press, San Diego, 2000, chap. 20.
77. Kornberg, L.J., Signal transduction by integrins: increased protein tyrosine phosphorylation caused by clustering of β1 integrins, *Proc. Natl. Acad. Sci. U.S.A.*, 88, 8392, 1991.
78. Massia, S.P. and Hubbell, J.A., An RGD spacing of 440 nm is sufficient for integrin αvβ3-mediated fibroblast spreading and 140 nm for focal contact and stress fiber formation, *J. Cell. Biol.*, 114, 1089, 1991.
79. Kasuya, Y. et al., Preparation of peptide-carrying microspheres with bioactivity on platelets, *J. Biomater. Sci. Polym. Edn.*, 4, 369, 1993.
80. Kasuya, Y. et al., Activation of human neutrophils by Arg-Gly-Asp-Ser immobilized on microspheres, *J. Biomed. Mater. Res.*, 28, 397, 1994.
81. Schild, H.G., Poly(N-isopropylacrylamide): experiment, theory and application, *Prog. Polymer Sci.*, 17, 163, 1992.
82. Ringsdorf, H., Venzmer, J., and Winnik, F.M., Interaction of hydrophobically modified poly-N-isopropylacrylamides with model membranes — or playing a molecular accordion, *Angew. Chem. Int. Ed.*, 30, 315, 1991.
83. Tsushima, Y., Preparation of the polymer chains for controlling cell functions through the clusterization of receptors, M.S. thesis, Keio University, Yokohama, 2000.
84. Kawaguchi, H. et al., Versatility of thermosensitive particles, *Macrom. Symp.*, 151, 591, 2000.
85. Wang, N., Butler, J.P., and Ingber, D.E., Mechanotransduction across the cell surface and through the cytoskeleton, *Science*, 260, 1124, 1993.
86. Baldwin, S.P. and Saltzman, W.M., Polymers for tissue engineering, *TRIP*, 4, 177, 1996.
87. Dai, W., Belt, J., and Saltzman, W.M., Cell-binding peptides conjugated to poly(ethylene glycol) promote neutral cell aggregation, *Biotechnology*, 12, 797, 1994.
88. Meier, W.M., Hotz, J., and Gunter-Ausborn, S., Vesicle and cell networks: interconnecting cells by synthetic polymers, *Langmuir*, 12, 5028, 1996.

89. Yamada, K. et al., Efficient induction of hepatocyte spheroids in a suspension culture using a water-soluble synthetic polymer as an artificial matrix, *J. Biochem.*, 123, 1017, 1998.

90. Tobe, S. et al., Tissue reconstruction in primary cultured rat hepatocytes on asialoglycoprotein model polymer, *Artif. Organs*, 16, 526, 1992.

91. Okada, N. et al., Medical application of microencapsulating hybridoma cells in agarose microbeads: cytomedicine. Therapeutic effect on IgG1 plasmacytosis and mesangio-proliferative glomerulonephritis in the interleukin 6 transgenic mouse, *J. Controlled Release*, 44, 195, 1997.

92. Okada, N. et al., Cytomedical therapy for IgG1 plasmacytosis in human interleukin-6 transgenic mice using hybridoma cells microencapsulated in alginate-poly(L)lysine-alginate membrane, *Biochim. Biophys. Acta*, 1360, 53, 1997.

93. Kanai, K. and Fujimoto, K., Cell-surface modification by polymer chains carrying ligands to produce the sites of signal recognition, *Polymer Preprints, Jpn.*, 49, 3904, 2000.

94. Meier, W., Reversible cell aggregation induced by specific ligand-receptor coupling, *Langmuir*, 16, 1457, 2000.

95. Fujimoto, K. et al., Control of cell death by the smart polymeric vehicle, *Biomacromolecules*, 1, 515, 2000.

96. Jayaraman, N., Nepogodiev, S.A., and Stoddart, J.F., Synthetic carbohydrate-containing dendrimers, *Chem. Eur. J.*, 3, 1193, 1997

97. Tomalia, D.A. et al., A new class of polymers: starburst-dendritic macromolecules, *Polymer J.*, 17, 117, 1985.

98. Zanini, D. and Roy, R., Synthesis of new thiosialodendrimers and their binding properties to the sialic acid specific lectin from *Limax flavus*, *J. Am. Chem. Soc.*, 119, 2088, 1997.

99. Aoi, K., Itoh, K., and Okada, M., Globular carbohydrate macromolecule "sugar balls" 1. Synthesis of novel sugar-persubstituted poly(amido amine) dendrimers, *Macromolecules*, 28, 5391, 1995.

100. Kono, K., Liu, M., and Frechet, J.M.J., Design of dendritic macromolecules containing folate or methotrexate residues, *Bioconjugate Chem.*, 10, 1115, 1999.

101. Takahashi, M. et al., Utilization of dendritic framework as a multivalent ligand: a functionalized gadolium(III) carrier with glycoside cluster periphery, *Tetrahedron Lett.*, 41, 8485, 2000.

102. Roy, R. et al., Solid-phase synthesis of dendritic sialiside inhibitors of influenza A virus haemagglutinin, *J. Chem. Soc., Chem. Commun.*, 1869, 1993.

103. Reuter, R. et al., Inhibition of viral adhesion and infection by sialic-acid-conjugated dendritic polymers, *Bioconjugate Chem.*, 10, 271, 1999.

104. Fulton, D.A. and Stoddart, J.F., An efficient synthesis of cyclodextrin-based carbohydrate cluster compounds, *Organic Lett.*, 2, 1113, 2000.

105. Rose, K. and Vizzavona, J., Stepwise solid-phase synthesis of polyamides as linkers, *J. Am. Chem. Soc.*, 121, 7034, 1999.

106. Whaley, S.R. et al., Selection of peptides with semiconductor binding specificity for directed nanocrystal assembly, *Nature*, 405, 665, 2000.

SECTION III

Future Aspects of
Supramolecular Architectures

18 Supramolecular Architectures toward Biological Applications

Nobuo Kimizuka

CONTENTS

0-8493-0965-4/02/$0.00+$1.50
© 2002 by CRC Press LLC

18.1 SUPRAMOLECULAR CHEMISTRY IN THE MESOSCOPIC DIMENSION

18.1.1 HIERARCHY OF SUPERMOLECULES IN BIOLOGICAL AND SYNTHETIC SYSTEMS

Biological supramolecular assemblies, as exemplified by nucleic acid multiplexes, multimeric proteins, nucleic acid–protein complexes and viruses provide a variety of soluble superstructures in the mesoscopic range (ca. 10 to 1000 nm in scale).[1] They spontaneously self-assemble in aqueous media by ingeniously employing multiple noncovalent interactions such as electrostatic interactions, hydrogen bonding, dipole–dipole interactions, and hydrophobic association. Figure 18.1 illustrates the hierarchy of molecular assemblies in biological and synthetic systems. Amino acids are arranged into peptides and proteins that fold into nanostructures. These units may further assemble into mesoscopic structures, such as the tobacco mosaic virus, actin fibers, or microtubules.[2]

Nature offers a wide spectrum of mesoscopic self-assemblies with exquisite architectural controls. The information for forming many of the supramolecular complexes is contained in their subunits. There are several advantages to using smaller subunits for building larger structures. First, building a large structure from one or a few repeating smaller subunits reduces the amount of genetic information required. Second, since the subunits associate through multiple bonds of relatively small energy, assembly and disassembly can be readily controlled. This allows dynamic and reversible transformations between molecular components and mesoscopic scale entities — one of the outstanding features of mesoscopic supramolecular systems.

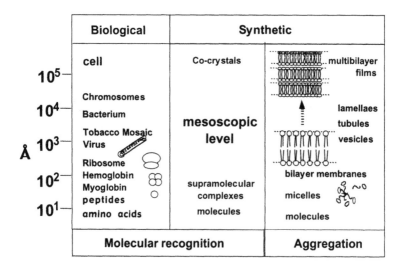

FIGURE 18.1 Hierarchy of molecular assemblies in biological and synthetic systems.

The development, characterization, and exploitation of synthetic materials based on the assembly of molecular components are active fields of research. One example of artificial mesoscopic molecular assemblies is the synthetic bilayer membrane, first reported by Kunitake and Okahata in 1977.[3] It launched the concept of chemical self-assembly discussed in subsequent works.[4] Mesoscopic morphologies such as tubes, tapes, disks, lamellae, and even chiral helices are available from a large variety of synthetic amphiphiles (Figure 18.1), and these aggregate structures and assembling properties are controlled by tuning chemical structures of the unit amphiphiles.[4] While the chemistry of self-organization influenced the biomimetic chemistry that evolved into supramolecular chemistry,[4,5] one can point out that the mesoscopic superstructures formed from conventional bilayer membranes are based on molecular aggregation. The element of molecular recognition has been less eminent in mesoscopic bilayer assemblies, in contrast to biological, mesoscopic supramolecular assemblies.[4]

Construction of mesoscopic supramolecular systems directed by molecular recognition is a new trend in supramolecular chemistry. This chapter focuses on our ability to design such mesoscopic entities and their structural characteristics. It also discusses supramolecular materials for biological applications from a chemical perspective, along with the elements essential for progress in this field.

18.1.2 HYDROGEN BOND-DIRECTED SUPERMOLECULES IN ORGANIC MEDIA

Hydrogen bonding interactions play a pivotal role in biological molecular recognition processes,[2] and multiple hydrogen bonds between complementary molecular components have been popularly used to drive the formation of dimers and oligomeric aggregates in organic media.[6-15] Complementary hydrogen bond pairs are also formed in bulk materials such as organic gels,[16] liquid crystals,[17-20] and molecular co-crystals.[21-27] The combination of melamine and cyanuric acid (or barbituric acid) has been used to create a variety of supramolecular motifs such as linear tapes, crinkled tapes, and circular structures.[26] These architectures are in principle controlled by steric interactions among the bulky substituents introduced in the molecular components. This steric control approach enables us to preorganize hydrogen bond donor and acceptor groups in desired configurations, thus reducing the entropic disadvantages in the assembling process. Unfortunately, however, introduction of such bulky groups inevitably prevented assembly growth into mesoscopic dimensions.[26] The mesoscopic dimension of conventional supramolecular chemistry is still unexplored.

In order to design soluble, mesoscopic-scale supramolecular assemblies, we have developed a new concept — imparting amphiphilicity to the complementary hydrogen bond pairs.[28-34] 1,8:4,5-Naphthalenebis(dicarboxyimide) (**1**, Scheme 1), which is hardly soluble in common organic solvents except for DMSO, was complexed with dialkylated melamines (**2**, Scheme 1).[32] Upon formation of the complementary hydrogen bond pairs, **1** became soluble in common organic solvents. UV-vis spectrum in methylcyclohexane showed significant broadening of naphthalenediimide

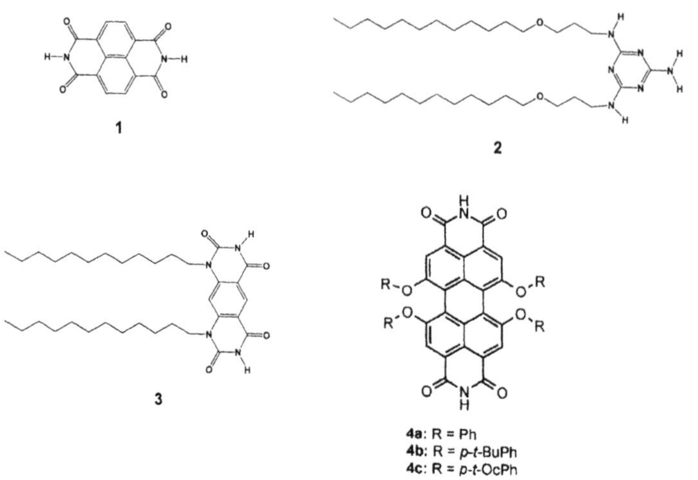

1

2

3

4a: R = Ph
4b: R = p-t-BuPh
4c: R = p-t-OcPh

SCHEME 1

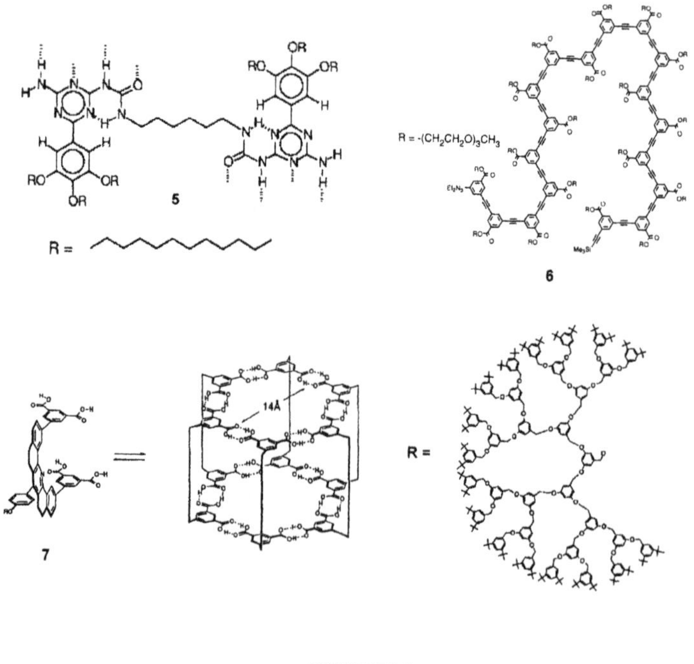

R = -(CH₂CH₂O)₃CH₃

5

6

R =

7

14Å

SCHEME 1a

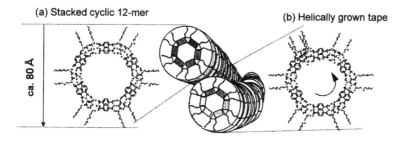

FIGURE 18.2 Solvophobically organized mesoscopic supramolecular assemblies formed from Subunits 1 and 2.[32]

absorption band due to the stacking of naphthalene chromophores. Electron microscopy revealed flexible, mesoscopic fibrous structures with widths of ca. 10 nm. These observations are compatible with either the stacked cyclic structure (a) or the helically grown structure (b) shown in Figure 18.2. Formation of these structures has been further supported by AFM observations.[35]

Amphiphilic design of the supermolecules directed the packing and folding of the complementary subunits in which solvophilic moieties (alkyl chains) are oriented toward the solvents while solvophobic moieties (stacked aromatic hydrogen bond networks) are hidden inside the assembly. The amphiphilic superstructure provides solubility in organic media and determines the folding patterns of hydrogen bond networks in solution.[32]

The formation of mesoscopic supramolecular assemblies has been extended to the combinations of Janus molecules (**3**, Scheme 1) with dialkylated melamines,[33] perylenebisimide (**4**, Scheme 1) with dialkylated melamines,[36] and self-aggregates of ureidotriazine derivatives (**5**, Scheme 1a).[37-38] The solvophobicity-driven folding is also highlighted in the single oligomers of phenylene ethynylene (**6**, Scheme 1a) reported by Moore et. al.[39-40] and the foldamers of Iverson et. al.[41] An alternative approach to constructing mesoscopic supramolecular structures in organic media has been developed by Zimmerman et. al.[14,42] Starting with large dendric subunits (**7**, Scheme 1a), they constructed nanosized, self-assembling dendrimers.

18.1.3 MESOSCOPIC SUPRAMOLECULAR SYSTEMS IN WATER

18.1.3.1 Molecular Recognition by Hydrogen Bonding in Aqueous Environments

In contrast to biological systems, formation of hydrogen bond-directed assemblies has been mostly carried out in nonaqueous media, due to the highly deteriorating action of water molecules against hydrogen bonding. Generally, enthalpic gain by the formation of hydrogen bonds in water is cancelled by the enthalpy required to break hydrogen bonds between these molecules and water.[43-44] Therefore, hydrogen bonding in aqueous media requires integration of other noncovalent interactions such as hydrophobic interactions or aromatic stacking to compensate for the entropic disadvantage.

A hydrophobic microenvironment is a prerequisite for proteins that bind their hydrated substrates by hydrogen bonding. For example, when lectins capture their sugar substrates, water molecules are excluded from the sugar binding sites.[45] In synthetic systems, hydrogen bond recognition of cyclic dipeptides by an amide microcycle guest required hydrophobic interaction together with amide–amide-hydrogen bonds.[46]

Aoyama et al., reported that phosphate anions bind oligosaccharide-derivatized calix[4]resorcarenes (**8** Scheme 2) via hydrogen bonding (binding constant K = 3 × 10^3 M^{-1}).[47] This value is comparable with those reported for the hydrogen-bonded saccharide–phosphonate complexes in organic media.[48] Formation of complementary hydrogen bonds in water also takes advantage of the hydrophobic microenvironments provided by aromatic surfaces[49-51] or by the interiors of aqueous micelles.[52-54] Meijer et al. reported hydrogen bond-directed self-association of bis-ureidotriazine derivatives in water; hydrophobic interactions also played a pivotal role in the assembling process.[37] Recent studies showed that the formation of complementary hydrogen bonding at the air-water interface is greatly facilitated compared to bonding observed at the surfaces of aqueous micelles or bilayers (see Chapter 15).[55-65] For example, binding constants (*K*) obtained for the combination of alkyl guanidium and phosphates are ca. 10^2 to 10^4 M^{-1} at the micellar and bilayer surfaces, while those at the air-water interfaces are on the order of 10^6 to 10^7 M^{-1}. Physical properties of water molecules at the interface are different from properties of those in bulk. These studies clearly demonstrate the importance of interfacial phenomena in supramolecular chemistry.

18.1.3.2   SUPRAMOLECULAR MEMBRANES: RECONSTITUTION OF AMPHIPHILIC SUPERMOLECULES IN WATER

We previously reported that the preformed, amphiphilic hydrogen bond pairs of quaternary ammonium-derivatized cyanuric acids (hydrophilic subunits **9** and **10**) and alkylated melamines (hydrophobic subunits **2** and **11**) were maintained in aqueous dispersions (supramolecular membranes).[28-31] The hydrogen bond networks in the

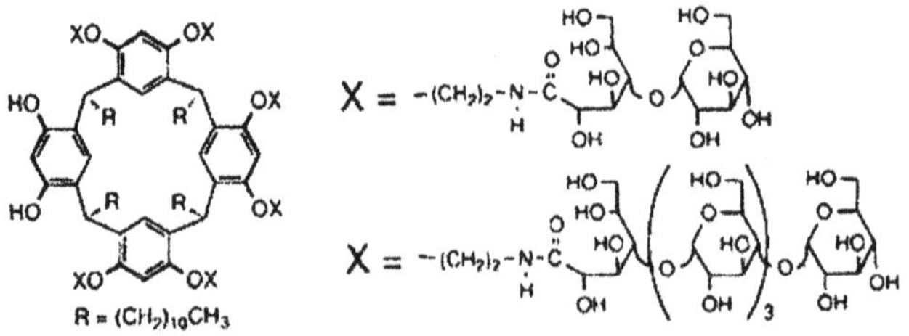

8

SCHEME 2

supramolecular membranes are stabilized in water by molecular stacking, similarly to the stacking of nucleic acid base pairs in DNA. Complementary hydrogen bond networks are *in situ*-reconstituted in water, and undergo hierarchical self-assembly into mesoscopic supramolecular membranes.[34]

When chiral hydrophobic melamine subunit (**11**) and an ammonium-derivatized cyanuric acid subunit (**10**) were mixed in water, helical superstructures (thickness 14 to 28 nm; width 30 to 50 nm; pitches 180 to 430 nm) were observed (Figure 18.3). These helical structures were stably dispersed in water and were distinct from those

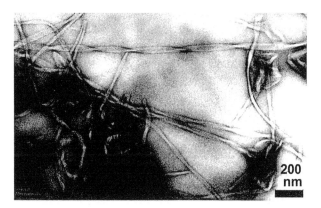

SCHEME 3

FIGURE 18.3 Transmission electron micrograph of helical superstructures self-assembled from **10** and **11** in water.[34]

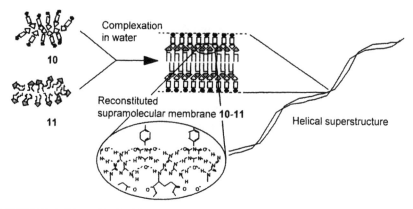

FIGURE 18.4 Hierarchical self-assembly in water. Amphiphilic networks of complementary hydrogen bonds are spontaneously reconstituted in water and further assembled into helical superstructures.[34]

observed for the individual subunits. Several lines of evidence show that these nanohelices are comprised of supramolecular membranes hierarchically self-assembled from the *in situ* formed, amphiphilic complementary hydrogen bond networks (Figure 18.4). The complexation of complementary subunits is stoichiometric, and spectral titration experiments indicated that **10** binds to **11** with an association constant of 1.13×10^5 M^{-1}. This is a significantly larger value than those reported for hydrogen bonding in aqueous media (binding of hexylthymine to acetylpentyladenine in SDS micelle; K = 48 M^{-1})[54] or at the air–water interface (barbituric acid to a surface monolayer of dialkylated melamine,[60] 2530 M^{-1}; 2,4,6-triaminopyrimidine to a cyanurate lipid monolayer,[65] 3500 M^{-1}). Amphiphilic supramolecular design is crucial to achieve such efficient complementary hydrogen bonding in water.

Water plays an essential role in directing the hydrogen bonding and hierarchical molecular organization. Bulk water directs the supramolecular organization in which more hydrophobic melamine subunits are organized in the interior of the assembly, and the ammonium-containing counterparts constitute the outer surface of the assembly (Figure 18.4). This amphiphilic supramolecular organization satisfies the solubility and maintenance requirements of complementary hydrogen bond networks in water. These hydrogen bonds are effectively shielded from the bulk water by their packing in the bilayer. The hydrophobically driven supramolecular organization is reminiscent of the biological self-assemblies and protein folding.

18.1.4 METAL ION-DIRECTED SUPRAMOLECULAR ASSEMBLIES

18.1.4.1 Supramolecular Chemistry of Discrete Transition Metal Complexes

A variety of molecular architectures have been prepared by metal coordination. The simplest approach is the template syntheses of macrocycles that utilizes the ability of metal ions to organize reactive sites.[66,67] Elegant developments in metal ion templating include the synthesis of catenanes and knots by Sauvage et al.[68] and double-helical metal complexes (helicates) by Lehn et al.[69] Studies on the formation of tetranuclear macrocyclic complexes by Fujita et al.[70-71] attracted widespread interest.[72] Paneling of organic ligands by metal complexation has been extended to produce nanobowls and nanoboxes (Figure 18.5).[73,74] Fujita's smart approach enables molecules to self-assemble into finite nano-sized objects with well-defined shapes.

These supramolecular architectures consist of discrete metal complexes,[68-74] and therefore the focus has been on shape and shape-related functions such as host–guest characteristics. The control of magnetism and electronic states in the solid metal complexes represents another important issue in inorganic chemistry.[75] It is natural to predict that the supramolecular complexes in the next generation will integrate these two features and display electronic states that are turned on and off by self-assembly. In the next section, our approach toward this goal is introduced.

18.1.4.2 Mesoscopic or Nanometal Complexes

Molecular wires are indispensable elements of future molecular-scale electronic devices, and their fabrication is one of the central issues in nanochemistry. Conventional research focused on the synthesis of π-conjugated oligomers and polymers.[76] They suffer from limitations on the types of elements that can be incorporated into the wires. We recently developed a new strategy to manipulate mesoscopic metal complexes by supramolecular packaging of one-dimensional inorganic complexes $[M(en)_2][M'Cl_2(en)_2]$ (M, M' = Pt, Pd, and Ni; en = 1,2,-diaminoethane).[77-80]

A family of halogen-bridged one-dimensional M^{II}/M^{IV} mixed valence complexes $[M(en)_2][M'X_2(en)_2]Y_4$ (X = Cl, Br, I, Y, counterions such as ClO_4) has been attracting considerable interest due to their unique physicochemical properties such as intense intervalence charge transfer (CT) absorption, semiconductivity, and large third-order nonlinear optical susceptibilities.[81] Their 1-D electronic structure is composed of d_{z^2} orbital of the metals and p_z orbital of the bridging halogens, where the z axis is parallel to the chain (Figure 18.6a). However, these one-dimensional complexes are not considered as candidates for molecular wires because they exist only in three-dimensional solids. They are not soluble in organic media. When dispersed in water, their one-dimensional structures are disrupted and dissociate into constituent molecular complexes.

We prepared ternary inorganic/organic polyion complexes $[Pt(en)_2][PtCl_2(en)_2]($**12** and **13**$)_4$, which displayed yellow (**12**) or indigo color (**13**) depending on the amphiphilic chemical structure.[77,79] These colors are typical of the intervalence charge transfer (CT) of halogen-bridged Pt^{II}/Pt^{IV} complexes, and they are dispersed in organic media with the basic amphiphilic supramolecular structure shown in Figure 18.6b. Thus, supramolecular packaging of the one-dimensional complex provides solubility to the solvophobic Pt-chains. It is noteworthy that the structures of lipids exert remarkable influence on the CT band, and thus the electronic structures of one-dimensional complexes are tunable (supramolecular band gap engineering).

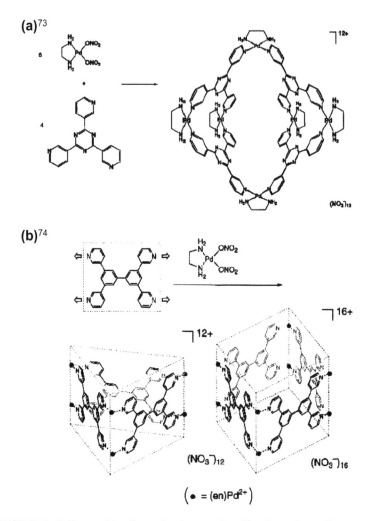

FIGURE 18.5 Self-assembly of coordination nanobowl[73] and nanoboxes.[74]

One of the most significant features of these mesoscopic metal assemblies is thermochromism. When an indigo-colored chloroform solution of [Pt(en)$_2$][PtCl$_2$(en)$_2$](**13**)$_4$ was heated, its CT absorption intensity disappeared completely at 60°C. Upon cooling, the indigo color reappeared reversibly. The observed thermochromism indicates that the one-dimensional complex underwent dissociation into component complexes at elevated temperatures (Figure 18.6c) and re-assembled upon cooling.[79,80] Electron microscopy revealed fibrous nanostructures with minimum widths of 18 nm and lengths of 700 to 1700 nm. Because the widths of these nanostructures are larger than the bimolecular lengths of the amphiphile, they must consist of bundles of amphiphilic supramolecular polyion complexes.

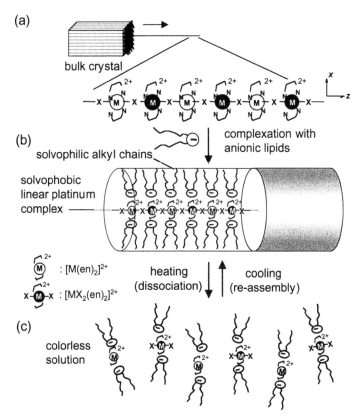

FIGURE 18.6 (a) Pseudo-1D halogen-bridged complex $[M(en)_2][MX_2(en)_2]$. (b) A soluble supramolecular wire consisting of $[M(en)_2]$, $[MX_2(en)_2]$, and anionic amphiphiles in organic media. (c) Molecularly dissociated complexes of $[M(en)_2](lipid)_2$ and $[MX_2(en)_2](lipid)_2$ formed at elevated temperatures.[80]

The self-assembling characteristics are reminiscent of biological supramolecular assemblies. The packaging of low-dimensional inorganic solids aids the creation of novel polymer molecules. This strategy should open new dimensions in mesoscopic supramolecular assemblies and molecular wire research.[80]

18.2 TOWARD BIOLOGICAL APPLICATIONS: SUPRAMOLECULAR BIOARCHITECTURES

Assemblies incorporating biomolecules and their components are particularly attractive as supramolecular biomaterials. While biomolecules possess nanosized structures, supramolecular architectures of biological interest inevitably have mesoscopic

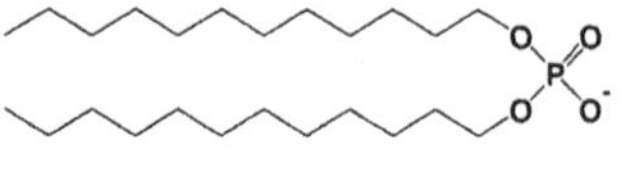

12

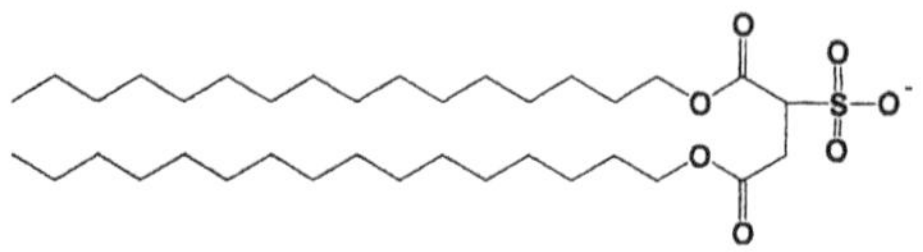

13

SCHEME 4

dimensions. In this section, molecular recognition of proteins and examples of meso-scopic supramolecular assemblies that contain proteins are introduced as new trends in supramolecular chemistry. In addition, their possible roles in biological applications will be discussed.

18.2.1 MOLECULAR RECOGNITION OF PROTEIN SURFACES

With the Human Genome Project approaching closure, researchers are turning to the task of converting the DNA sequence into practical application. Proteomics is one of the next directions and the study of protein–protein interactions in the cellular protein cascade is a key issue. The interactions are known to play a critical role in signal transduction and apoptosis. Recognition of proteins by synthetic molecules will provide insights into how proteins interact. However, it is not easy for small molecules to effectively recognize proteins.

Strategies for recognition of peptide secondary structures and protein surfaces were recently reviewed by Hamilton et al.[83] Inspired by the immune system, they introduced a calix[4]arene scaffold with pendant cyclic peptide units as a mimetic of antibody Fab fragments (Figure 18.7).[84] The arrangement of several peptide loops mimics the hypervariable antibody loops of the complementary determining regions. The synthetic receptor containing cyclic peptide sequences 3-amb–Gly–Asp–Gly–Asp (3amb = 3-aminomethylbenzoic acid) complexed with cytochrome c with K_a values in the 10^5 to 10^7 M^{-1} range. This preorganization of cyclic peptide allows targeting of fairly large protein surface areas (>6 nm^2), with possible control by the amino acid sequences and structures of the central scaffolds. Attainment of specific orientations in the binding groups seems to be crucial. This approach may become important in the areas of separations, biosensors, and biomedical materials.

An alternative approach to manipulating nanostructured surfaces that are complementary to proteins is molecular imprinting. There are a number of excellent reviews on molecular imprinting,[85,86] but attempts to imprint proteins have met with only limited success.[87,88] A smart technique was developed by Ratner et al.,[89] in which proteins on mica surfaces were first coated with disaccharide molecules, and polymeric films formed on them by plasma deposition (Figure 18.8). The disaccharides

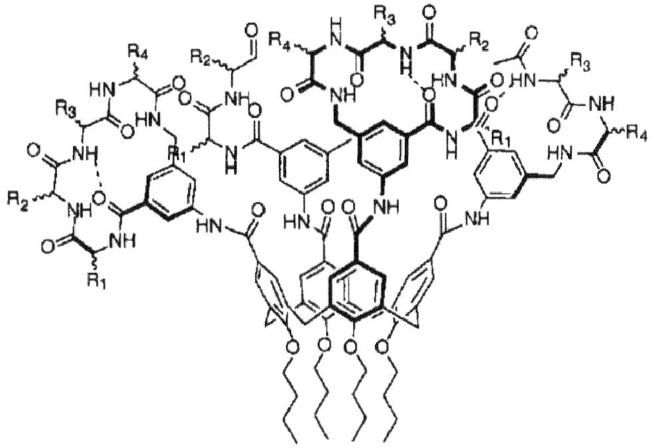

FIGURE 18.7 Hamilton's synthetic protein receptor.[84]

became covalently attached to the polymer films, and provided polysaccharide-like cavities that exhibited highly selective recognition for a variety of template proteins, including albumin, immunoglobulin G, lysozyme, ribonuclease, and streptavidin. The observed protein recognition can be ascribed to the specificity conferred by shape selectivity and hydrogen bonding.

Inorganic gels also provide imprinted surfaces. Kunitake et al. have shown that ultrathin films of TiO_2 gel can be prepared by the surface sol–gel technique.[90] Films produced in the presence of carbobenzyloxy L-amino acids showed selective binding to the original template molecules.[91] This technique has not been extended to protein recognition yet, possibly due to the unavoidable use of organic $Ti(O^nBu)_4$ solutions in the layer-by-layer absorption steps that might lead to protein denaturation. This issue may be circumvented by the use of aqueous phase synthesis of metal oxides, whose combination with layer-by-layer absorption has shown to afford alternate multilayers of Cyt c and TiO_2 gels.[92]

18.2.2 PROTEIN–PROTEIN INTERACTIONS

Protein–protein interactions play key roles in many physiological and pathological processes, particularly those involving cell signaling. After a hormone binds at the cell surface, the messenger molecule cyclic AMP (cAMP) is generated inside the cell and the subsequent actions inside the cell are mediated by cAMP-dependent protein kinase (PKA). PKA is a tetrameric protein composed of two monomeric catalytic subunits that phosphorylate serine residues on the proteins (C) and a dimeric regulatory subunit (R) that prevents the enzyme from working when cAMP is scarce (Figure 18.9).[93] The R subunit includes a homodimerization domain, two tandem cAMP-binding domains, and an autoinhibitory domain that blocks the kinase activity of the C subunit when cAMP is not bound. The holoenzymatic regulation of PKA by cAMP provides an effective strategy for supramolecular control of protein functions.

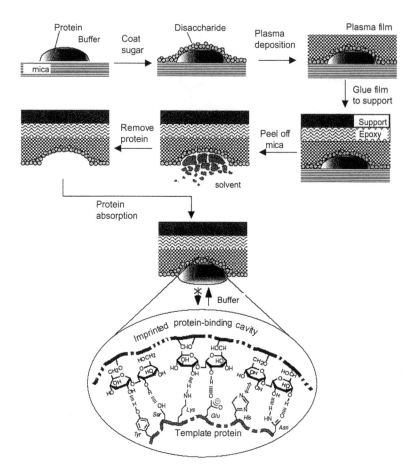

FIGURE 18.8 Ratner's protein imprinting.[89]

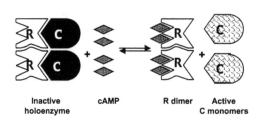

FIGURE 18.9 Regulation of protein kinase A by cyclic AMP.[93]

Designing small cofactor molecules capable of controlling protein–protein interactions is also important to manipulate super-protein structures and control their functions. 2,3-Diphosphoglycerate (2,3-DPG) binds human hemoglobin at a specific site that involves a cluster of eight positively charged amino acid residues (Val–NA1, His–NA2, Lys–EF6, and His–H21 of each β–chain) located on the dyad axis of the hemoglobin tetramer. It acts as a major modulating factor for human adult hemoglobin *in vivo*.[94] However, modulation of protein functions by such a gluing molecular subunit is not generally applicable to the control of multimeric proteins. Schultz et. al. introduced mutations into human growth hormone (hGH) and its cellular receptor that create a gap at the interface between the two proteins.[95] This resulted in reducing binding affinity by a factor of 10^6.

Combinatorial screening of indole compounds indicated that 5-chloro-2-trichloromethylimidazole is capable of filling the gap and restoring the affinity of the mutant hormone for its receptor. This approach may be generally extended to allow other protein–protein and protein–nucleic acid interactions to be switched on and off by the addition or depletion of exogenous small molecules. Manipulation of protein–protein interactions *in vivo* has also employed dimeric ligands as chemical inducers of dimerization (CIDs). The majority of CIDs described to date are dimers of FK506.[96-98] A recently synthesized heterodimeric CID that dimerizes a DNA-binding protein chimera and a transcription activation protein chimera effectively reconstituted a transcriptional activator and stimulated transcription of DNA.[99]

18.2.3 SUPERPROTEIN ASSEMBLIES

Another supramolecular approach in developing protein nanoassemblies is to utilize the superprotein architectures omnipresent in nature. As described in section 18.1.1, supramolecular structures are formed by the noncovalent assembly of many preformed subunits.[1,2] Examples of such protein aggregates include linear chains of sickle cell hemoglobin fibers, formed by polymerization of deoxyhemoglobin S that induce gelation and alter intraerythrocytic rheology.[100] Annelid hemoglobins form giant hexagonal bilayer structures that consist of two superimposed hexagons of pentagonally shaped substructures and a central cavity (height ca. 20 nm; diameter ca. 30 nm).[101]

Supramolecular functionalization of protein assemblies has been achieved by incorporating photofunctional groups in the protein subunits. Actin, a key protein of muscle cells, is induced to polymerize *in vitro* by millimolar concentrations of divalent cations and/or physiological ionic strength.[102,103] By the labeling of actin at cysteine 373 with an energy donor (5-iodoacetamidofluorescein, D) or an energy acceptor (tetramethylrhodamine iodoacetamide, A), the assembly and disassembly of actin filaments were detected by using photoinduced energy transfer (Figure 18.10).[104] Upon polymerization of D- and A-labeled actins, energy transfer from the attached fluorescein to the rhodamine chromophores occurred between the actin subunits.

When unlabeled actin filaments were added to these donor–acceptor labeled filaments, interchange of actin subunits diluted the D- and A- labeled actins in the filaments. This resulted in separation of donor-acceptor distance in the filaments, leading to loss of energy transfer characteristics. Energy transfer in chromophore-labeled

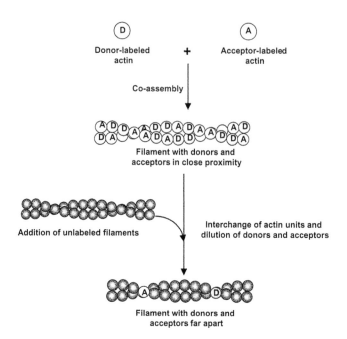

FIGURE 18.10 Copolymerization of donor- and acceptor-tagged G-actins into actin filaments and succeeding interchanges of actin subunits.[104]

actins is a classic example. Recent advances in single-molecule observation and manipulation[105] allows us to elucidate the dynamic mechanisms of such protein assembling phenomena. Semisynthetic self-assembling proteins provide basic information on protein–protein dynamic interactions and act as powerful biological tools for the design of nanoprotein devices.

18.2.4 MESOSCOPIC PROTEIN ASSEMBLIES HYBRIDIZED WITH NANOMATERIALS

Potentially interesting materials properties may be produced from mesoscopic architectures including biomolecules and nanomaterials such as metal nanoparticles, carbon nanotubes, and organic molecular assemblies. The diversity of components and processes requires cross-disciplinary research in the fields of chemistry, biochemistry, physics, and the engineering disciplines.

Alivisatos et al. demonstrated the use of DNA as a rigid template to direct the spatial dispositions of nanoclusters.[106] DNA does not fulfill a biological role in this situation; it directs the cluster to the desired site via sequence-specific hydrogen-bonding interactions. Mirkin et al. have shown that nanoparticles with several single strands of DNA attached can be used to create reversible arrays of nanoparticles, thus providing a quick testing method for specific sequences.[107-109] The DNA cluster example highlights the potential of biomolecules in constructing novel organic–inorganic composites.

A fluorescent biological detection system involved covalently coupling the transfer protein with highly luminescent CdSe–ZnS semiconductor quantum dots (QDs, Figure 18.11).[110] The properties of QDs result from quantum-size confinement that occurs when metal and semiconductor particles are smaller than their exciton Bohr radii (about 1 to 5 nm).[111] QDs have the potential to overcome the problems of fluorescent labeling such as lower chemical stability, ease of photo-breaching and limited spectral variety. Transferrin–QD bioconjugates were transported into cultured HeLa cells by receptor-mediated endocytosis. The attached transfer molecules are active and are recognized by the receptors of the cell surface.[110] QDs are apparently biocompatible with living cells.

Supramolecular strategy can be also employed to prepare protein–QD bioconjugates. Protein-modified QD dispersions were obtained by electrostatic attractions between negatively charged QDs and positively charged leucine zipper domains in genetically engineered recombinant proteins.[112] This supramolecular approach may be limited to QDs with charged surfaces, but its utility in conjugate formation may have a variety of biological applications. Surface modification of gold nanoparticles has been well studied, and the formation of giant, chiral nanometer-scale metal structures was suggested for glutathione-based gold cluster compounds.[113] Bioderived inorganic materials may become powerful tools of bionanotechnology.

Since their discovery in 1991, carbon nanotubes have attracted considerable interest due to their outstanding mechanical and electronic properties, particularly for the development of new nanotechnologies. The selective opening at the ends of nanotubes by oxidants[114] has promoted extensive experiments on the filling of the inner hollow cavity. Studies on capillarity and wetting of carbon nanotubes have shown that the surface tension is sufficiently high to allow wetting by water.[115] However, biological application of carbon nanotubes is still in its infancy. An example of biological application is provided by the immobilization of Zn-Cd methallothionein in side nanotubes.[116]

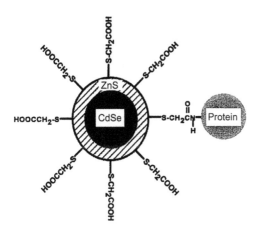

FIGURE 18.11 ZnS-capped CdSe QD covalently coupled to a protein.[110]

Streptavidin is adsorbed on multiwalled nanotubes (MWNTs), presumably via hydrophobic interactions between the nanotubes and the hydrophobic domains of the proteins (Figure 18.12a).[117] DNA molecules are also adsorbed on MWNTs via non-specific interactions.[118] Dai et al. developed a smart approach to noncovalently functionalize the side walls of single-walled carbon nanotubes (SWNTs) and subsequent immobilization of proteins (Figure 18.12b).[119] In the first step, noncovalent functionalization involves adsorption of 1-pyrenebutanoic acid succinimidyl ester onto the surfaces of SWNTs. The highly aromatic pyrenyl group strongly interacts with the side walls of SWNTs which are highly resistant to desorption in aqueous solutions. The second step is nucleophilic substitution of N-hydroxysuccinimide by an amine group on the proteins. This approach resulted in immobilization of ferritin and streptavidin onto the noncovalently functionalized SWNTs. This approach will be applicable to many biological molecules, and may promote the development of new biosensors and bioelectronic nanomaterials that take advantage of their biological properties. It is expected that other organic nanomaterials such as π-conjugated molecular wires,[120] organic nanotubes,[121] inorganic nanowires[122] supramolecular membranes[31,34] and oganic–inorganic nanowires[78-79] that can serve as nanotemplates will enrich this area of chemistry.

18.2.5 Mesoscopic Assembly of Proteins on Molecular Assemblies

Most bacteria possess supramolecular-layered cell-wall structures outside their cytoplasmic membranes. Commonly observed surface structures are crystalline arrays of proteinaceous subunits termed surface layers (S layers).[123] They are planar assemblies of identical protein or glycoprotein subunits that can be aligned in lattices with oblique (p1, p2), square (p4), or hexagonal (p3, p6) symmetry with center-to-center spacings of the morphological units of approximately 2.5 to 30 nm (Figure 18.13).[124] The surface layer subunits can recrystallize on liposomes.[125] Such liposomes coated

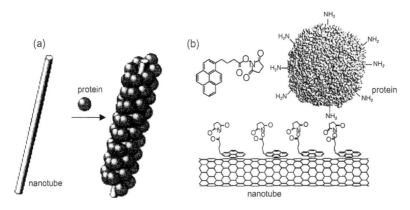

FIGURE 18.12 (a) Helical crystallization of proteins on the outer surface of a carbon nanotube.[117] (b) Adsorption of 1-pylenebutanoic acid succinimidyl ester onto the side wall of SWNT.[119]

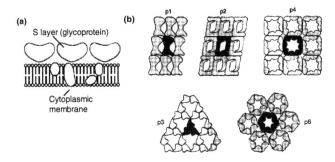

FIGURE 18.13 (a) Prokaryotic cell envelopes containing crystalline bacterial cell surface layers (S layers). (b) Protein organization in S layers.[124]

with S layers are similar to biomimetic structures such as virus envelopes. The mechanical and thermal stability of S layer-coated liposomes may have broad application in drug delivery and gene therapy. In addition, the intrinsic property of S layer proteins to form extended crystalline arrays on solid supports provides unique opportunities for organization of functional materials.[126]

Polymerization of actin by charged liposomes is another example of protein assemblies formed on bilayer membranes. When positively charged liposomes prepared from phosphatidyl choline and 1 to 20% stearylamine are mixed with G-actin, they are polymerized at the bilayer surfaces even at low salt concentrations.[127] Wong et. al describe spontaneous polymerization of actins. The self-assembling actin rods sandwich a cationic lipid bilayer and form trilayered membranes that curl up into tubes (Figure 18.14).[128] These protein-bilayer conjugates may find possible uses as drug carriers.

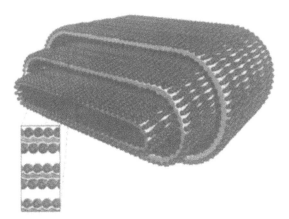

FIGURE 18.14 Polymerized actin rods self-organized at the surfaces of cationic lipid bilayers.[128]

Chemical modification has been used to regulate protein functions,[129-136] and introduce signal-responsible groups such as photofunctional groups[129,132,133] and affinity ligands[134] into proteins. Site-directed modification of proteins requires a uniquely reactive residue on the protein surface, and such covalent modifications generally lower their activity. On the other hand, supramolecular regulation is ubiquitously employed in biological systems. For example, protein kinase C (PKC), a key enzyme in the intracellular signal transduction system, is activated at the plasma membrane surface by intracellular messengers of diacylglycerol, anionic phosphatidylserine, and Ca^{2+}.[137] PKC then activates a protein kinase cascade that leads to the phosphorylation of a DNA-bound gene regulatory protein.[2,138]

Such messenger-induced activation of dormant enzymes preorganized at bilayer surfaces ensures their rapid response to an extracellular signal molecule, and provides a supramolecular basis for designing artificial protein-regulation systems. We have reported construction of supramolecular holoenzymes by the use of bilayer membrane as a regulatory co-factor.[139] Cleavage of λ-DNA by a restriction enzyme, HindIII is suppressed when it is electrostatically bound to glutamate-based, phosphate bilayer membrane **14** at 37°C. The membrane-bound HindIII is not irreversibly denatured, since its cleavage activity is restored by heating the aqueous mixture to 45 to 55°C, or by the addition of Ca^{2+}. The intact phosphate bilayer surfaces provided by amphilphile **14** in the gel state serve as regulatory co-factors, and HindIII is preorganized at these bilayer surfaces in a dormant form (Figure 18.15). An increase in temperature (i) or the addition of Ca^{2+} (ii) liberates active HindIII from the bilayer surfaces, thus switching on the hydrolysis of DNA. Liberation of HindIII is also achieved by photochemical release of Ca^{2+} ions from Nitr-5/Ca^{2+} (iii). HindIII is irreversibly denatured upon binding to bilayer **12** or SDS micelles.

The Ca^{2+} ion is a ubiquitous intracellular messenger, and the use of suitably designed phosphate bilayers converts the restriction enzyme to a supramolecular holoenzyme that requires Ca^{2+} for activation. The present system provides a novel means to thermally regulate enzymatic activities. Bilayer membranes have been involved also in the activation of enzymes such as β-hydroxybutyrate dehydrogenase[140] and DNA A protein[141] and the functional conversion of lipase[142] and heme proteins.[143,144] This simple approach applicable to the control of biological functions exerted by proteins, enzymes, and functional peptides.

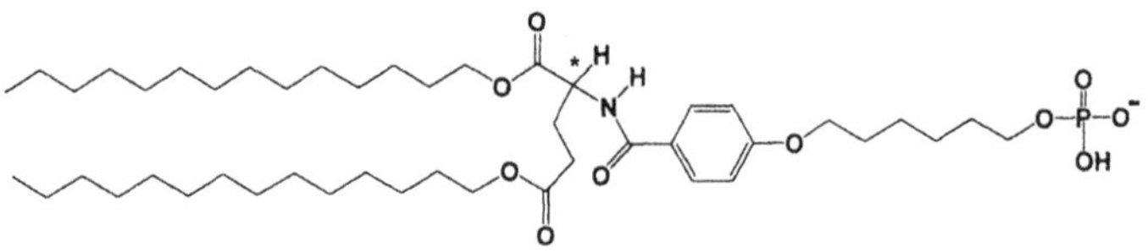

14

SCHEME 5

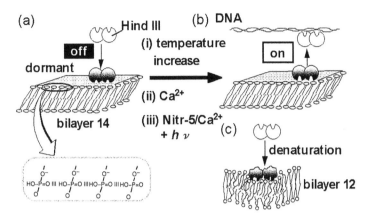

FIGURE 18.15 Supramolecular holoenzymatic system.[139] (a) Hind III becomes dormant upon binding to bilayer **14** (off-state). (b) Triggered release of Hind III from the bilayer surface (on-state). (c) Hind III is irreversibly denatured upon binding to dialkyl phosphate bilayer **12**.

18.3 PROSPECTS: TOWARD SUPRAMOLECULAR FACTORIES

The fields of supramolecular chemistry and molecular self-assembly have undergone explosive growth during the last two decades. Mesoscopic supramolecular assemblies seem to provide new ways to design and control biomolecular functions. The approaches described in this chaper represent the incredible diversity of mesoscopic biomaterials. The ability to control spatial arrangements of these supramolecular systems and to position them as desired remains an important area for future research. The use of techniques such as soft lithography-mediated submicrometer patterning[144] and topographical micropatterning[146] may help fabricate supramolecular factories for biological applications. The mastery of lab-on-a-chip technology will lead to supramolecular factories in which the functions of each supramolecular system are spatiotemporally integrated. Our growing ability to design and synthesize biomolecules with desired functions suggests continuous advances during the decades ahead.

REFERENCES

1. Klug, A., *Angew. Chem. Int. Ed. Engl.* 22, 565, 1983.
2. Alberts, B. et al., *Molecular Biology of the Cell*, 3rd ed., Garland Publishing, New York, 1994.
3. Kunitake, T. and Okahata, Y., *J. Am. Chem. Soc.* 99, 3860, 1977.
4. Kunitake, T., *Angew. Chem. Int. Ed. Engl.* 31, 709, 1992.
5. Fuhrhop, J.-H. and Köning, J., *Membranes and Molecular Assemblies: The Synkinetic Approach*, Royal Society of Chemistry, Cambridge, 1994.

6. Rebek, J., Jr., *Angew. Chem. Int. Ed. Engl.* 29, 245, 1990.
7. Lehn, J.-M., *Angew. Chem. Int. Ed. Engl.*, 29, 1304, 1990.
8. Whitesides, G.M., Mathias, J.P., and Seto, C.T. *Science*, 254, 1312, 1991.
9. Lawrence, D.S., Jiang, T., and Levett, M. *Chem. Rev.,* 95, 2229, 1995.
10. Prins. L.J., Reinhoudt, D.N., and Timmerman, P., *Angew. Chem. Int. Ed. Engl.*, 40, 2383, 2001.
11. Zimmerman, S.C. and Duerr, B.F., *J. Org. Chem.*, 57, 2215, 1992.
12. Mathias, J.P. et al., *J. Am. Chem. Soc.*, 116, 1725, 1994.
13. Yang, J. et al., *Tetrahedron Lett.*, 22, 3665, 1994..
14. Zimmerman, S.C. et al., *Science*, 271, 1095, 1996.
15. Drain, C.M. et al., *J. Chem. Soc. Chem. Commun.*, 337, 1996.
16. Hanabusa, K. et al., *J. Chem. Soc. Chem. Commun.*, 1382, 1993.
17. Mariani, P. et al., *J. Am. Chem. Soc.*, 111, 6369, 1989.
18. Lehn, J.-M., *Makromol. Symp.*, 69, 1, 1993.
19. Kotera, M., Lehn, J.-M., and Vigneron, J.-P., *J. Chem. Soc. Chem. Commun.*, 197, 1994.
20. Suárez, M. et al., *J. Am. Chem. Soc.*, 120, 9526, 1998.
21. Voet, D., *J. Am. Chem. Soc.,* 94, 8213, 1972.
22. Shimizu, N. and Nishigaki, S., *Acta Cryst.*, B38, 2309, 1982.
23. Etter, M.C., *Acc. Chem. Res.*, 23, 120, 1990.
24. Lehn, J.-M. et al., *J. Chem. Soc. Chem. Commun.*, 479, 1990.
25. G-Tellado, F. et al., *J. Am. Chem. Soc.*, 113, 9265, 1991.
26. MacDonald, J. C. and Whitesides, G. M., *Chem. Rev.,* 94, 2383, 1994.
27. Holman, K. T. et al., *J. Am. Chem. Soc.*, 123, 4421, 2000.
28. Kimizuka, N., Kawasaki, T., and Kunitake. T. J., *Am. Chem. Soc.,* 115, 4387, 1993.
29. Kimizuka, N., Kawasaki, T., and Kunitake. T., *Chem. Lett.,* 33, 1994.
30. Kimizuka, N., Kawasaki, T., and Kunitake. T., *Chem.Lett.*, 1399, 1994.
31. Kimizuka, N. et al., *J. Am. Chem. Soc.*, 120, 4094, 1998.
32. Kimizuka, N. et al., *J. Am. Chem. Soc.*, 117, 6360, 1995.
33. Kimizuka, N. et al., *J. Chem. Soc. Chem. Commnun.*, 2103, 1995.
34. Kawasaki, T. et al., *J. Am. Chem. Soc.*, 2001, 123, 6792.
35. Kuramori, M. et al., *Rept. Prog. Polym. Phys. Jpn.*, 39, 401, 1996.
36. Würthner, F., Thalacker, C., and Sautter, A., *Adv. Mater.*, 11, 754, 1999.
37. Hirshberg. J.H.K.K. et al., *Nature*, 407, 167, 2000.
38. Schenning, A. P. H. et al., *J. Am. Chem. Soc.*, 123, 409, 2001.
39. Nelson, J. C. et al., *Science*, 277, 1793, 1997.
40. Lahiri, S., Thompson, J.L., and Moore, J.S., *J. Am. Chem. Soc.*, 122, 11315, 2000.
41. Lokey, R.S. and Iverson, B.L., *Nature*, 375, 303, 1995.
42. Thiyagarajan, P. et al., *J. Mater. Chem.*, 7, 1221, 1997.
43. Doig, A.J. and Williams, D.H., *J. Am. Chem. Soc.*, 114, 338, 1992.
44. Searle, M.S., Williams, D.H., and Gerhard, U., *J. Am. Chem. Soc.*, 114, 10697, 1992.
45. Swaminathan, C.P., Surolia, N., and Surolia, A., *J. Am. Chem. Soc.*, 120, 5153, 1998.
46. Allot, C. et al., *J. Chem. Soc. Chem. Commun.*, 2449, 1998.
47. Hayashida, O. et al., *J. Am. Chem. Soc.,* 121, 11597, 1999.
48. Das, G. and Hamilton, A.D., *J. Am. Chem. Soc.*, 116, 11139, 1994.
49. Constant, J.F. et al., *Tetrahedron Lett.*, 28, 1777, 1987.
50. Rotello, V. M. et al., *J. Am. Chem. Soc.*, 115, 797, 1993.
51. Kato, Y., Conn, M., and Rebek, J., Jr., *Proc. Natl. Acad. Sci. U.S.A.*, 92, 1208, 1995.
52. Nowick, J.S. and Chen, J.S., *J. Am. Chem. Soc.*, 114, 1107, 1992.

53. Nowick, J.S., Chen, J.S., and Noronha, G., *J. Am. Chem. Soc.*, 115, 7636, 1993.
54. Nowick, J.S., Cao, T., and Noronha, G., *J. Am. Chem. Soc.*, 116, 3285, 1994.
55. Kurihara, K. et al., *J. Am. Chem. Soc.*, 113, 5077, 1991.
56. Ikeura, Y., Kurihara, K., and Kunitake, T., *J. Am. Chem. Soc.*, 113, 7343, 1991.
57. Sasaki, D.Y., Kurihara, K., and Kunitake, T., *J. Am. Chem. Soc.*, 114, 10994, 1992.
58. Taguchi, K., Ariga, K., and Kunitake, T., *Chem. Lett.*, 701, 1995.
59. Cha, X., Ariga, K., and Kunitake, T., *J. Am. Chem. Soc.*, 118, 9545, 1996.
60. Koyano, H. et al., *Chem. Eur. J.*, 3, 1077, 1997.
61. Kitano, H. and Ringsdorf, H., *Bull. Chem. Soc. Jpn.*, 58, 2826, 1985.
62. Ahlers, M. et al., *Colloid Polym. Sci.*, 268, 132, 1990.
63. Ahuja, R., et al., *Angew. Chem. Int. Ed. Engl.*, 32, 1033, 1993.
64. Bohanon, T.M. et al., *Angew. Chem. Int. Ed. Engl.*, 34, 58, 1995.
65. Onda, M. et al., *J. Am. Chem. Soc.*, 118, 8524, 1996.
66. Curtis, N.F., *J. Chem. Soc.*, 4409, 1960.
67. Tompson, M.C. and Busch, D.H., *J. Am. Chem. Soc.*, 86, 213, 1964.
68. Chambron, J.-C., Buchecker, C.D., and Sauvage, J.P., in *Comprehensive Supramolecular Chemistry*, Vol. 9, Atwood, J.A. et al., Eds., Elsevier Science, New York, 1996, Chap. 2.
69. Lehn. J.-M., *Angew. Chem. Int. Ed. Engl.*, 29, 1304. 1990.
70. Fujita, M., Yazaki, J., and Ogura, K., *J. Am. Chem. Soc.*, 112, 5645, 1990.
71. Fujita, M., *Acc. Chem. Res.*, 32, 53, 1999.
72. Leininger, S., Olenyuk, B., and Stang, P., *J. Chem. Rev.*, 100, 853, 2000.
73. Yu, S.-Y. et al., *J. Am. Chem. Soc.*, 122, 2665, 2000.
74. Yamanoi, Y. et al., *J. Am. Chem. Soc.*, 123, 980, 2001.
75. Gatteschi, D., *Adv. Mater.*, 6, 635, 1994.
76. Huang. S. and Tour, J. M., *J. Org. Chem.*, 64, 8898, 1999.
77. Kimizuka, N., Oda, N., and Kunitake,T., *Chem. Lett.*, 695, 1998.
78. Kimizuka, N., Lee, S.H., and Kunitake,T., *Angew. Chem. Int. Ed. Engl.*, 39, 389, 2000.
79. Kimizuka, N., Oda, N., and Kunitake, T., *Inorg. Chem.*, 12, 2684, 2000.
80. Kimizuka, N., *Adv. Mater.*, 12, 1461, 2000.
81. Okamoto, H. and Yamashita, M., *Bull. Chem. Soc. Jpn.*, 71, 2023, 1988.
82. Wada, Y. et al., *J. Phys. Soc. Jpn.*, 54, 3143, 1985.
83. Peczuh, M.W. and Hamilton, A.D., *Chem. Rev.*, 100, 2479, 2000.
84. Hamuro, Y. et al., *Angew. Chem. Int. Ed. Engl.*, 36, 2680, 1997.
85. Shea, K.J., *Trends Polym. Sci.*, 2, 166, 1994.
86. Wulff, G., *Angew. Chem. Int. Ed. Engl.*, 34, 1812, 1995.
87. Kempe, M., Glad, M., and Mosbach, K., *J. Mol. Recogn.* 8, 35, 1995.
88. Venton, D.L. and Gudipati, E., *Biochim. Biophys. Acta*, 1250, 117, 1995.
89. Shi, H. et al., *Nature*, 398, 593, 1999.
90. Ichinose, I., Senzu, H., and Kunitake, T., *Chem. Lett.*, 831, 1996.
91. Lee, S.W., Ichinose, I., and Kunitake, T., *Chem. Lett.*, 1193, 1998.
92. Kimizuka, N., Tanaka, M., and Kunitake, T., *Chem. Lett.*, 1333, 1999.
93. Lowell, B.B., *Nature*, 382, 585, 1996.
94. Marta, M. et al., *Biochemistry*, 37, 14024, 1998.
95. Guo, Z., Zhou, D., and Schultz, P.G., *Science*, 288, 2042, 2000.
96. Spencer, D. et al., *Science*, 262, 1019, 1993.
97. Belshaw, P. et al., *Proc. Natl. Acad. Sci. U.S.A.*, 93, 4604, 1996.
98. Diver, S. and Schreiber, S., *J. Am. Chem. Soc.*, 119, 5106, 1997.
99. Lin, H. et al., *J. Am. Chem. Soc.*, 122, 4247, 2000.

100. Briehl, R.W., Mann, E.S., and Josephs, R.J., *Mol. Biol.*, 211, 693. 1990.
101. Lamy. J.N. et al., *Chem. Rev.*, 96, 3113, 1996.
102. Frieden, C., *Proc. Natl. Acad. Sci. U.S.A.*, 80, 6513, 1983.
103. Lal, A., Brenner, S., and Korn, E.D., *J. Biol. Chem.*, 259, 13061, 1984.
104. Taylor, D.L. et al., *J. Cell Biol.*, 89, 362, 1981.
105. Mehta, A. et al., *Science*, 283, 1689, 1999.
106. Alivisatos, A.P. et al., *Nature*, 382, 609, 1996.
107. Mirkin, C.A. et al., J. *Nature*, 382, 607, 1996.
108. Mitchell, G.P., Mirkin, C.A., and Letsinger, R.L., *J. Am Chem. Soc.*, 121, 8122, 1999.
109. Mirkin, C.A., *Inorg. Chem.*, 39, 2258, 2000.
110. Chan W.C. and Shuming, W.N., *Science*, 281, 2016, 1998.
111. Alivisatos, A.P., *Science*, 271, 933, 1996.
112. Mattoussi, H. et al., *J. Am. Chem. Soc.*, 122, 12142, 2000.
113. Schaaff, T.G. and Whetten, R.L., *J. Phys. Chem. B.*, 104, 2630, 2000.
114. Tsang, S. C. et al., *Nature*, 372, 159, 1994.
115. Dujardin, E. et al., *Science*, 265, 1850, 1994.
116. Tsang, S. C. et al., *J. Chem. Soc., Chem. Commun.*, 1803, 1995.
117. Balavoine, F. et al., *Angew. Chem. Int. Ed. Engl.*, 38, 1912, 1999.
118. Guo, Z., Sadler, P.J., and Tsang, S.C., *Adv. Mater.*, 10, 701, 1998.
119. Chen, R. J. et al., *J. Am. Chem. Soc.*, 123, 3838, 2001.
120. Tsuda, A. and Osuka, A., *Science*, 293, 79, 2001.
121. Hartgerink, J. D. et al., *Chem. Eur. J.*, 4, 1367, 1998.
122. Tremel, W., *Angew. Chem. Int. Ed. Engl.*, 38, 2175, 1999.
123. Beveridge, T., *J. Curr. Opin. Struct. Biol.*, 4, 204, 1994.
124. Sleytr. U.B. et al., *Angew. Chem. Int. Ed. Engl.*, 38, 1034, 1999.
125. Küpcü, S., Sára, M., and Sleytr. U.B., *Biochim. Biophys. Acta*, 1235, 263. 1995.
126. Shenton, W. et al., Nature, 389, 585, 1997.
127. Laliberte, A. and Gicquaud, C., *J. Cell. Biol.*, 106, 1221, 1988.
128. Wong, G. C. et al., *Science*, 288, 2035, 2000.
129. Martinek, K. and Berezin, I.V., *Photochem. Photobiol.*, 29, 637, 1979.
130. Aizawa, M., Namba, K., and Suzuki, S., *Arch. Biochem. Biophys.*, 182, 305, 1977.
131. Mendel, D., Ellman, J. A., and Schultz, P.G., *J. Am. Chem. Soc.*, 113, 2758, 1991.
132. Willner, I., *Acc. Chem. Res.*, 30, 347,1997.
133. Hamachi, I. et al., *Chem. Lett.*, 537, 1998.
134. Hamachi, I. et al., *Chem. Eur. J.*, 3, 1025, 1997.
135. Westmark, P. R. et al., *J. Am. Chem. Soc.*, 115, 3416, 1993.
136. Hohsaka, T., Kawashima, K., and Sisido, M., *J. Am. Chem. Soc.*, 116, 413, 1994.
137. Mosior, M. and McLaughlin, S., *Biophys. J.*, 60, 149, 1991.
138. Nishizuka, Y. *Nature*, 308, 693, 1984.
139. Kimizuka, N., Baba, A., and Kunitake, T., *J. Am. Chem. Soc.*, 123, 1764. 2001.
140. Jain, M. K. and Zakim, D., *Biochim. Biophys. Acta*, 906, 33, 1987.
141. Sekimizu, K. and Kornberg, A., *J. Biol. Chem.*, 263, 7131, 1988.
142. Okuda, H. and Fujii, S. *J. Biochem.*, 64, 377, 1968.
143. Hamachi, I., Fujita, A., and Kunitake, T., *J. Am. Chem. Soc.*, 116, 8811, 1994.
144. Hamachi, I., Fujita, A., and Kunitake, T., *J. Am. Chem. Soc.*, 119, 9096, 1997.
145. Black, A. J. et al., *J. Am. Chem. Soc.* 121, 8356, 1999.
146. Takayama, S. et al., *Adv. Mater.*, 13, 570, 2001.

Index

C

Milton Keynes UK
Ingram Content Group UK Ltd.
UKHW031125141024
449569UK00006B/430